An
American
Physical
Therapy
Association
Monograph

Pediatric Orthopedics

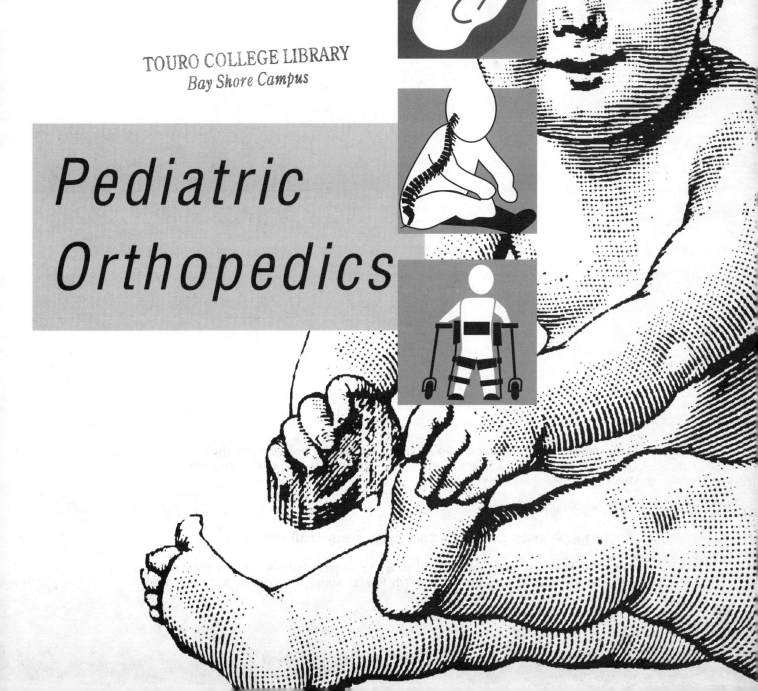

Bay Shore

This monograph is a compilation of articles originally published in the December 1991 and January 1992 issues of *Physical Therapy*. It is printed on recycled/recyclable paper using soy-based inks.

ISBN # 0-912452-80-3

For more information about this and other APTA publications, contact the American Physical Therapy Association, 1111 North Fairfax Street, Alexandria, VA 22314-1488. [Publication No. P-83]

3/14/00

Table of Contents

Editor's Note

The Special Series

As the world begins its celebration of Christmas, we present the first part of a special two-part series on pediatric orthopedics. The confluence stirs images that I had hoped to use in this Editor's Note. Reading through the variety of articles published in this issue and those that will appear in January, I cannot help but marvel at the remarkable growth of the field. Where once pediatric orthopedics was little more than splinting of deformities caused by wholly preventable birth defects or malnourishment syndromes, it is now touched by the wonders of modern medicine, and we physical therapists play a vital role in guaranteeing our young patients the best possible outcome. Thanks to the superb efforts of our guest editors, Dr Susan Harris and Dr Loretta Knutson, and Deputy Editor Dr Gary Soderberg, who coordinated the special series, that role has been documented and hopefully will be facilitated through this presentation.

We have come a long way from the image that I thought I would be using to start this Editor's Note, that of Tiny Tim who beseeched his father to take cheer because perhaps when others saw him on Christmas Day they would find it pleasant to remember ". . . [He] who made lame beggars walk and blind men see." I had planned to begin this note with one of Dickens's remarkably descriptive passages, one that would describe Tiny Tim in detail, but upon re-reading Dickens I found that there is no such passage. Tiny Tim, who has charmed generations in various incarnations of *A Christmas Carol*, is sparsely described. But all Dickens tells us is, "Alas for Tiny Tim, he bore a little crutch, and had his limbs supported from an iron frame!" And pages later, Dickens mentions that Tiny Tim reaches for his father with a withered hand.

I wondered why Dickens, for whom no paragraph was too long and no detail too minute for elaboration, gave us so little about Tim when he spent nearly half a page describing the chains that bound Jacob Marley and more than that telling us every particular about the Ghost of Christmas Present. I also wondered where the finely detailed image of Tim in my mind's eye had come from, because it was certainly not painted by the author of the original book.

The image of Tiny Tim, like so many elements in our minds, has come from an amalgamation of experiences; the sources have long since dissociated themselves from the content they leave behind. It was Dickens's genius that told him to paint Tiny Tim with faint brush work so that the small child would come more alive through the detail each of us brings to his creation. How unlike our task with this journal! We bring forth information for the reader to fully digest, and often we hope it will change the way our readers practice. We also hope that readers always remember the source of their information and do not function from fixed ideas created from unidentifiable elements in an amalgam. In the case of this special series, we ask for therapists to consider what is in their minds and to consider new approaches to the pediatric orthopedic patient.

In fiction, the good author creates images and often challenges the reader to complete the details. The author chooses when to be vague, when to be specific, and when to guide the reader along the path of imagination. We cannot do that in this journal because it would deter us from our mission to contribute to and document the "evolution and expansion of the scientific and professional body of knowledge in physical therapy." In this season of holidays, as we present this special series, I have some envy for those whose mission is less constraining as they speak to the human condition.

Perhaps I can greatly alter the meaning and shift the emphasis of part of Dickens's last paragraph in *A Christmas Carol* to alleviate my envy. Reflecting upon the change that took place in Scrooge after his sojourns with the spirits, Dickens wrote that Scrooge knew how to keep Christmas because the one-time miser now had all the knowledge he needed. Let us take the message more globally, beyond knowing how to keep the Christmas holiday. Let it "truly be said of us, and of all us!" that we possess the knowledge and spirit to do in our personal and professional lives what needs to be done and that we are indeed worthy of the blessings that should be all of ours in this special season and throughout the year. Because that is a message that we, all of us—scientists, poets, painters, clinicians, and even Tiny Tim—may agree upon.

Jules M Rothstein, PhD, PT
Editor

Guest Contributors

The following individuals have contributed articles to the two-part special series on pediatric orthopedics. The December 1991 issue is devoted entirely to this topic; the other articles in this series are presented in this issue of the Journal.

Robert W Armstrong, MD, PhD, FRCPC
Coordinator of Research and Medical Director of the Neuromotor Program, Sunny Hill Hospital for Children, 3644 Slocan St, Vancouver, British Columbia, Canada V5M 3E8, and Assistant Professor, Department of Pediatrics, and Associate Member, School of Rehabilitation Medicine, University of British Columbia, T325-2211, Wesbrook Mall, Vancouver, British Columbia, Canada V6T 2B5.

Michelina C Cassella, PT
Associate Director, Department of Physical Therapy and Occupational Therapy Services, Children's Hospital, 300 Longwood Ave, Boston, MA 02115, Physical Therapy Consultant to the Spinal Program, Children's Hospital, and Lecturer on Orthopaedic Surgery, Harvard Medical School, 25 Shattuck St, Boston, MA 02115.

Dennis E Clark, CPO
Prosthetist/Orthotist and Owner of Clark Prosthetics in Waterloo, Coralville, and Dubuque, Iowa.

Beverly D Cusick, PT
Clinical Specialist, Lucille Packard Children's Hospital at Stanford, 725 Welch Rd, Palo Alto, CA 94304, Teacher, Consultant, and Private Practitioner.

Peter A DeLuca, MD
Co-Director, Gait Analysis Laboratory, Director, Cerebral Palsy Service, and Director, Hip and Foot Service, Newington Children's Hospital, 181 E Cedar St, Newington, CT 06111; Assistant Professor, Department of Orthopaedic Surgery, School of Medicine, University of Connecticut Health Center, 10 Talcott Notch Rd, Farmington, CT 06032; and Assistant Clinical Professor, Department of Orthopaedic Surgery and Rehabilitation, Yale New Haven Hospital, 333 Cedar St, New Haven, CT 06510.

Joan E Edelstein, PT
Associate Professor of Clinical Physical Therapy, Columbia University, 630 W 168th St, New York, NY 10032.

John B Emans, MD
Associate in Orthopaedic Surgery, Department of Orthopaedics, and Clinical Director, Myelodysplasia Clinic, Children's Hospital, 300 Longwood Ave, Boston, MA 02115, and Assistant Clinical Professor, Department of Orthopedic Surgery, Harvard University, Cambridge, MA 02138.

Debbie Field, OT
Occupational Therapist, Positioning Assessment Unit, Sunny Hill Hospital for Children, 3644 Slocan St, Vancouver, British Columbia, Canada V5M 3E8.

Susan E Fife, PT
Research Therapist, Therapy Department, Sunny Hill Hospital for Children, 3644 Slocan St, Vancouver, British Columbia, Canada V5M 3E8.

Janice L Gregson, PT
Physical Therapist, Positioning Assessment Unit, Sunny Hill Hospital for Children, 3644 Slocan St, Vancouver, British Columbia, Canada V5M 3E8.

John E Hall, MD
Orthopaedic Surgeon-in-Chief, Department of Orthopaedics, Children's Hospital, 300 Longwood Ave, Boston, MA 02115, and Professor of Orthopaedic Surgery, Harvard Medical School, 25 Shattuck St, Boston, MA 02115.

Susan R Harris, PhD, PT, FAPTA
Associate Professor, School of Rehabilitation Medicine, University of British Columbia, T325-2211, Wesbrook Mall, Vancouver, British Columbia, Canada V6T 2B5.

Susan E Harryman, PT
Director of Physical Therapy, Kennedy Institute for Handicapped Children, 707 N Broadway, Baltimore, MD 21205, and Instructor, Department of Pediatrics, Johns Hopkins School of Medicine, Baltimore, MD 21218.

Loretta M Knutson, PhD, PT, PCS
Lecturer, Physical Therapy Graduate Program, and Senior Physical Therapist, Division of Developmental Disabilities, The University of Iowa, 2600 Steindler Bldg, Iowa City, IA 52242.

David E Krebs, PhD, PT
Associate Professor, Graduate Program in Physical Therapy, MGH Institute of Health Professions, 15 River St, Boston, MA 02018-3402.

Beverley D Lundgren, PT
Instructor, School of Rehabilitation Medicine, University of British Columbia, T325-2211, Wesbrook Mall, Vancouver, British Columbia, Canada V6T 2B5, and Private Practice, Vancouver, British Columbia, Canada.

Address all correspondence to first author of article unless otherwise indicated by specific footnote in article.

Guest Reviewers

Robert Rosenthal, MD
Associate in Orthopedic Surgery and Assistant Clinical
Professor of Orthopedic Surgery, Department of Orthopedics,
Children's Hospital, 454 Brookline Ave, Boston, MA 02215.

Shirley A Scull, PT
Director, Department of Physical Therapy, Children's Seashore
House, 3405 Civic Center Blvd, Philadelphia, PA 19104, and
Adjunct Assistant Professor, Philadelphia College of Pharmacy
and Sciences, 43rd St & Kingsessing Mall, Philadelphia, PA
19104.

Donald G Shurr, PT, CPO
Eastern District Manager, American Prosthetics Inc, 2203
Muscatine Ave, Iowa City, IA 52245.

David Sutherland, MD
Medical Director, Motion Analysis Laboratory, Children's
Hospital and Health Center, 8001 Frost St, San Diego, CA
92123, and Professor Emeritus, Department of Orthopedics and
Rehabilitation, University of California at San Diego, La Jolla, CA
92092.

Marilynn P Wyatt, PT
Research Physical Therapist, Motion Analysis Laboratory,
Children's Hospital and Health Center, 8001 Frost St, San
Diego, CA 92123.

Foreword: Pediatric Orthopedics in Physical Therapy

Harris SR, Knutson LM. Foreword: pediatric orthopedics in physical therapy. Phys Ther. 1991;71:877.]

Susan R Harris
Loretta M Knutson

Management of the child with an orthopedic impairment should be of interest not only to pediatric therapists but to all physical therapists who deal with clients with any type of musculoskeletal disorder. An understanding of normal musculoskeletal development, as provided in the first article of this two-part special series, is critical to the conscientious management of any individual with disease or abnormality of muscles, bones, or joints. Because it is impossible within this special series to provide a comprehensive review of the entire field of pediatric orthopedics, we have chosen to focus on some of the more common orthopedic concerns of children with developmental disabilities, limb deficiencies, juvenile rheumatoid arthritis, and idiopathic scoliosis.

Landmark federal legislation implemented during the past two decades has greatly expanded the role of physical therapists in both assessment and management of infants, children, and adolescents with orthopedic and neurologic disabilities. Both Public Law 94-142 and Public Law 99-457 identify physical therapists as primary team members in providing services to infants, preschoolers, and school-aged children with handicapping conditions. Despite an increase in the number of physical therapists employed in early intervention centers and public school systems, the extent of the service needs and demands cannot be met without assistance from physical therapists in private practice and hospital settings. Thus, it is incumbent on *all* physical therapists to expand their knowledge base concerning the care and management of children with orthopedic and other disabilities.

The articles in this special series encompass a wide range of topics related to the assessment and management of children with a variety of orthopedic impairments. This issue begins with a review of musculoskeletal development and is followed by articles that discuss the topics of joint mobilization, contemporary physical therapy management of scoliosis and juvenile rheumatoid arthritis, prosthetic management of children with limb deficiencies, physical therapy management of myelodysplasia, and the use of lower-extremity orthoses for children with cerebral palsy and myelomeningocele. The final two articles in this issue review current approaches to gait analysis and the assessment of postural control during adapted seating.

The remaining articles in this series will appear in the January issue of the Journal and will include articles on assessment of lower-extremity torsional alignment, the role of weight bearing and standing for children with developmental disabilities, preoperative and postoperative physical therapy for the child with cerebral palsy who is undergoing orthopedic surgery, and physical therapy management prior to and following the Ilizarov limb-lengthening procedure.

As co-editors of this special series, we would like to thank the authors of these papers for their patience, persistence, and superb contributions to updating our knowledge of pediatric orthopedics. We would also like to thank the manuscript reviewers, who included both regular reviewers and guest reviewers. We are pleased to note that both the authors and the reviewers for these invited manuscripts represent a wide range of health professionals, including physical therapists, occupational therapists, orthopedists, pediatricians, orthotists, prosthetists, and kinesiologists, thus providing a truly interdisciplinary focus to this special series on the care and management of the pediatric orthopedic client.

SR Harris, PhD, PT, FAPTA, is Associate Professor, School of Rehabilitation Medicine, University of British Columbia, T325-2211, Wesbrook Mall, Vancouver, British Columbia, Canada V6T 2B5.

LM Knutson, PhD, PT, PCS, is Lecturer, Physical Therapy Graduate Program, and Senior Physical Therapist, Division of Developmental Disabilities, The University of Iowa, 2600 Steindler Bldg, Iowa City, IA 52242.

Musculoskeletal Development: A Review

The early development of the limbs, the skeletal and muscular systems, and the joints and early changes in joint mobility are reviewed. The musculoskeletal system is vulnerable to failures of specific morphogenetic processes in the embryonic period. Congenital anomalies and postural deformities also may arise in the fetal period. Awareness of prenatal and postnatal events and their timing will assist health care workers in management of pediatric clients. [Walker JM. Musculoskeletal development: a review. Phys Ther. 1991;71:878–889.]

Joan M Walker

Key Words: *Infant; Joints; Musculoskeletal system; Orthopedics, general; Pediatrics, development.*

Increasing survival rates of prematurely born infants and the frequency of pediatric orthopedic problems necessitate a sound understanding of prenatal and postnatal development of the musculoskeletal system. In this article, I will review early development of the limbs, the skeletal and muscular systems, and the joints, as well as early changes in joint mobility.

The stages, timing, and major events of prenatal development are well described in the literature and are outlined in Table 1. To precisely establish the sequence and timing of developmental events, the embryonic period is divided into 23 stages, which are based on external and internal morphological criteria elicited from studies on staged embryos at the Carnegie Institute.[1,2] These stages will be referred to when reviewing the development of the musculoskeletal system. Development, encompassing differentiation, maturation, and growth, occurs at disparate rates throughout the body. Development in the premature infant is significantly different than that in a full-term infant.

During the embryonic period (2–8 weeks), major development of all systems occurs. This period is distinguished by a series of spatially controlled cellular events primarily dependent on the sequential switching on and off of specific gene activities that define the enzyme activity of a cell and hence its ultimate biological nature. From the initial stage, characterized by a homogeneous structure and variable potential for all cells, development proceeds toward a stage in which differentiation prescribes a precise biological role for each cell. Through cytodifferentiation, a process of change in the morphology or chemistry of embryonal cells that renders them more specialized than their antecedents, the predestination becomes visible in the heterogeneous structure of cells. Other important cellular activities of the embryonic period are pattern formation; cell-to-cell and cell- and tissue-contact interactions; morphogenetic movements, defined as the coordinated and directed migrations of individual cells or masses of cells; and mass cell necrosis.[3] All are important in the modeling process.

The fetal period, commencing at the beginning of the eighth week, is characterized by continued, but less spectacular, differentiation and growth. Increasing complexity of structure and function is noted, with a marked increase in fetal weight in the third trimester secondary to development of adipose tissue. These processes continue to varying degrees in the different systems in the postnatal period. Normal dynamics of cell growth give an orderly increase in size in three phases: initial hyperplasia (increase in cell number), hyperplasia with hypertrophy, and hypertrophy alone.

Critical periods in development of limbs and the central nervous system are shown in Figure 1.[4] Major morphological abnormalities occur only during the embryonic period, although minor morphological abnormalities of the limbs can occur in the early fetal period.[4,5] Distinction must be made between *malformation*, which indicates a primary problem in morphogenesis of a tissue; *disruption*, or a breakdown of a previously normal tissue; and *deformation*, or anomalies that represent normal response of a tissue to unusual mechanical force.[5,6] Disruption and deformation can arise at any time during the fetal period,

JM Walker, PhD, PT, is Professor and Director, School of Physiotherapy, Dalhousie University, 5869 University Ave, Halifax, Nova Scotia, Canada B3H 3J5.

Table 1. *Stages, Timing, and Events in Prenatal Development*

Name	Timing (wk)	Event	Trimester (wk)
Zygote	0–2	implantation	1 (0–12)
Embryo	2–8	major development, all systems	1 (0–12)
Fetus	8–38/42	maturation, increased complexity	2 (12–24)
		viability	3 (24–38/40)

with deformation more frequent in the third trimester when the fetus is subjected to greater constraint.

Limb Development

Most of the tissues differentiating in the newly formed limb bud arise from mesenchymal cells.[7,8] Neural elements invade the limb at a later stage. Mesenchymal cells destined to become myoblasts appear to be a distinct population, are derived from somites, and have a different lineage than other limb-bud cells. The ectodermal covering of the limb bud plays an important role and will form the skin. The lower limb bud lags behind that of the upper limb, appearing about the 28th day, 2 days later than that of the upper limb. The sequence of limb-bud development between 26 and 42 days is shown in Figure 2. (Most of our knowledge of limb-bud development evolves from studies in avian models.)

Under the influence of the underlying mesenchymal cells, the apical ectodermal ridge (AER) forms as a thickened specialization of ectoderm. By 33 days, mesenchymal cells commence differentiation into cartilage. Structures are laid down in a proximodistal sequence; thus, the humerus and femur appear before the digits. How the AER exerts its influence on spatial organization of the developing limb is not clearly established. Experiments in which portions of the AER in avians were removed, however, demonstrate the important role of the AER.[7] Experiments with a chick embryo model have shown that removing the AER at an early stage results in loss of distal parts; removal of a small portion results in loss of one to two digits.[7] Influence of the AER is no longer thought to be a simple cell-to-cell interaction. The subadjacent mesenchymal cells may produce an AER-maintenance factor, with the AER playing a more "permissive" than "instructive" role during pattern formulation on the proximodistal axis. The AER may have mitogenic properties that mediate its ability to stimulate limb-bud outgrowth. More is known of pattern formulation in the proximodistal and anteroposterior axes than in the ventrodorsal axis in which the dorsal ectoderm appears in avians to have more dominant effect.[9] Regions in which cell death will occur, such as between the digits, have thinner ectoderm. Cell death is a programmed and ontogenic mechanism, which, if poorly timed, reduced, or excessive, can lead to abnormal limb development.

Figure 3A demonstrates the basically parallel arrangement of the longitudinal axes of the limb buds. The preaxial borders, bearing the thumb and the great toe, face cranially, whereas the postaxial borders face caudally. By the end of the embryonic period, the upper limbs have altered such that the preaxial border has become medial rather than cranial; this position corresponds to pronation (Fig. 3B).[2] Postnatally, the limb can be rotated so that the palm of the hand faces forward because of the greater mobility of the upper limb.

At stage 23, the preaxial border of the lower limb, as indicated by the great toe, is still directed cranially with the soles directed medially, the so-called "praying feet." Translational movements, during the fetal and early postnatal periods, move the preaxial border medially so that the sole of the foot can be applied to the ground. These translational movements should not be referred to as "medial rotation," with the implication of mature

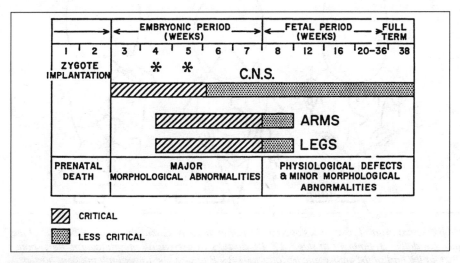

Figure 1. *Critical periods in development of limbs and the central nervous system (CNS). (Asterisks indicate limb-bud appearance.) (Modified with permission from Moore KL. The Developing Human. 4th ed. Philadelphia, Pa: WB Saunders Co; 1988.)*

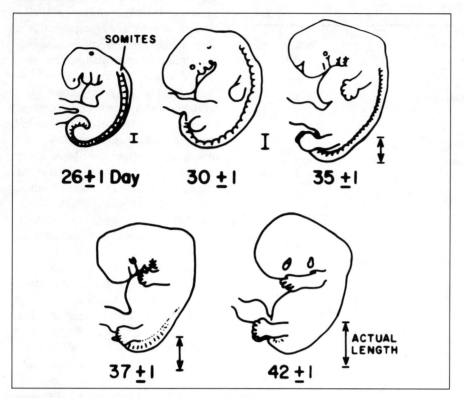

Figure 2. *Limb-bud development in a series of human embryos from 26 to 42 days. Note that the upper limb bud appears below the lower limb bud, and at 42 days digits are visible but are not separated. Actual length of embryos shown by vertical arrows. (Modified with permission from O'Rahilly R, Gardner E. The embryology of moveable joints. In: Sokoloff L, ed. The Joints and Synovial Fluid. New York, NY: Academic Press Inc; 1978;1:29-103.[8])*

movement produced by muscle action. These alterations are completed after differentiation of the muscle mass, innervation of the muscles, and definition of the joint cavities have occurred. They are secondary to complex changes in all of the limb components, especially the skeletal and articular components.[2] According to Tickle and Wolpert, "The mechanisms involved are not understood but the pattern of growth may be a factor."[7(p556)] Blechschmidt and Gasser[10] related growth changes in the limb anlagen in part to the restraining function of vessels and nerves, which exhibit a slower growth rate than other limb tissues. Limb pattern formation may involve interplay between mesenchymal and vascular cells. Caplan[11] theorized that "the presence of particular vascular elements may, indeed, be 'positional information.'"

From the earliest stage, blood vessels invade the limb as it grows, except where cartilage differentiates. Neural crest cells invade the limb bud at about the same time as the nerves (about the 33rd day, when the hand bud is visible) and give rise to sensory nerves and skin-pigment cells. All other limb structures develop *in situ*.

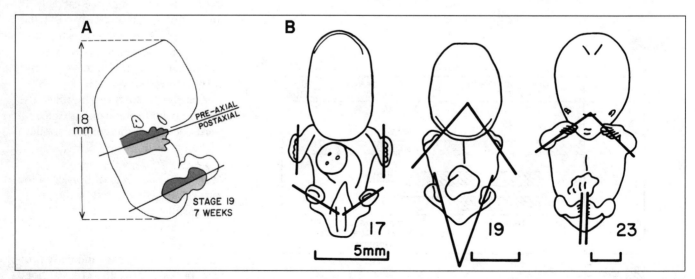

Figure 3. *Development of limb axes: (A) Limb orientation and axes in a stage-19, 7-week embryo. Note that the preaxial borders of the limbs face cranially and the postaxial borders face caudally. (B) Embryos at stages 17, 19, and 23, at decreasing magnification. Bars show the transverse axes of the hands and feet. Note that, at the end of the embryonic period (stage 23, 8 weeks), the upper-limb preaxial border has changed from cranial to medial, but the lower-limb preaxial border is still cranially directed. (Reprinted with permission from O'Rahilly R, Gardner E. The embryology of moveable joints. In: Sokoloff L, ed. The Joints and Synovial Fluid. New York, NY: Academic Press Inc; 1978;1:29-103.[8])*

Skeletal Development

During the first month of fetal life, the matrix of the future skeleton is laid down. In the second month, bone formation commences. Except for the clavicle, mandible, and bones of the skull vault in which bone mineral is deposited directly in mesenchyme (membranous bone, endosteal or periosteal ossification), collagen is laid down to form the template on which bone mineral is deposited (endochondral ossification). Formation of matrix must precede deposition of bone mineral until growth ceases. Because the availability of oxygen in the cellular microenvironment is a factor in ossification, conditions that affect the oxygen supply may influence differentiation of precursor cells. Osteogenesis requires a good oxygen supply, whereas chondrogenesis occurs in the presence of a poor oxygen supply.[12]

Embryonic bone has an irregular arrangement of collagen fibers, is highly mineralized, and has a high number of osteocytes. Gradually, lamellar bone, which is less mineralized and has fewer and smaller osteocytes, covers the connective tissue vascular spaces seen in embryonic bone. Fetal bone, in comparison with mature bone, has a very compact cortex; little remodeling occurs during prenatal life.[11] The accumulation of calcium in bone parallels the increase in fetal weight. Thus, premature birth deprives the skeleton of an important component of calcium and phosphorus. Hormones (ie, somatotrophic hormone, sulphation factor, thyroxine, sex hormones, cortisol) and vitamins appear to play a larger role in development postnatally.[12] Anomalies of calcium metabolism, such as hypocalcemia or hypercalcemia in either the mother (osteomalacia, hypothyroidism or hyperthyroidism) or in the fetus, influence mineralization of the skeleton. For example, maternal osteomalacia causes rickets in the infant.[12] Human breast milk provides more calcium and inorganic phosphorus, which is vital to mineralization, than does cow's milk.

The infant exhibits a much higher rate of remodeling than does the adult, estimated at 50% per annum and 5% per annum, respectively. During the first 2 years, marked remodeling of the cortex of the long bones occurs, resorption increases, and secondary osteons are formed. It is thought that all primary bone has been remodeled by the age of 2 years.[11] Mechanical forces appear to have a negligible role during prenatal development of the skeleton, except for architectural details such as tendon attachments, but are important postnatally. Decreases in pressure parallel to the growth axis in long bones (as in weightlessness) favor growth in length, whereas increases inhibit and may even stop epiphyseal growth.[12,13] Carter et al,[13] using finite-element computer analysis, hypothesized that mechanical stress influences all features of skeletal morphogenesis, from development of primary ossification sites to the existence and thickness of articular cartilage.

The timing of ossification is clearly detailed in anatomical texts.[14-16] Whereas in long bones ossification begins in the periphery (perichondrial) and proceeds distally (enchondral), the vertebral bodies ossify from the center outward (endochondral). Each vertebra is the result of fusion of the caudal half of one somite and the cranial half of the adjacent somite. Both the notochord and the spinal cord appear to play a role in chondrogenesis of the vertebrae.[8,17,18] Ossification from three primary centers commences in the lower thoracic bodies about the eighth week, then proceeds in both cranial and caudal directions. Ossification of the arches commences in the upper cervical vertebra and proceeds caudally.[12] Union of ossified portions occurs postnatally; arches unite in the midline, starting in year 1 with the lumbar region. Fusion of the arches with the vertebral bodies starts in the third year in the cervical region and in the sixth year in the lumbar region.[19]

Skull sutures in the young child have relatively smooth edges, but progressively acquire the mature features of jagged, interlocking, and overlapping edges. Fusion follows a staggered schedule. Between years 1 and 2, the maxillary-premaxillary sutures normally fuse; the temporal sutures fuse between age 2 and 4 years. Closure of other sutures does not occur until adulthood (25–30 years of age); however, sutures bounding the temporal bone close about 5 years later and may only "be partially united even in the aged skull."[20]

Muscle Development

Primary myotubes (multinucleated muscle cells) appear at about the 5th week of human gestation. Early muscle fibers begin to appear in about the 11th week. Few myotubes remain after the 20th week when most muscle fibers are packed with myofibrils, have peripheral nuclei, and are similar to those of adult muscle.[21] "Fibroblastlike" cells associated with fetal muscle fibers are thought to remain as satellite cells, which are presumed to play a role in postnatal growth and regeneration following injury.[22] Whereas initial myogenesis can occur normally in the absence of a nerve supply, innervation (about 20–24 weeks) is shown to enhance muscle development and differentiation.

That functional demands influence muscle development is clearly demonstrated by the observation that diaphragmatic fibers are twice the size of intercostal and limb muscle fibers at birth, a reflection of the primacy of respiration in the neonate.[22] Clear distinction between the two main histochemical fiber types cannot be made until the 18th to 20th prenatal week. Immature fibers all show physiological characteristics of slow-twitch fibers.[22] Type I (slow-twitch, oxidative) fibers predominate in earlier development. Type II (fast-twitch, glycolytic) fibers increase after the 26th week, and fiber types are about equal at term.[23] Given the extent of malnutrition in parts of the world, it is worthy of note that protein-calorie malnutrition in the rat is shown to lead to failure of normal postnatal growth of muscle fibers and is only partially reversible by normal diet.[24]

In the full-term infant, skeletal muscle contains less than 20% of the adult number of cells and accounts for about 25% of the weight of the average baby. Up to the 25th prenatal week, skeletal muscle shows a hyperplastic phase, with cells increasing in number but with little increase in size. After that time, cell size increases more rapidly and cell number more slowly.[22] Although some investigators hypothesize that fiber number continues to increase into the 5th decade, others believe the full fiber number is attained soon after birth.[22] Once differentiation is complete, subsequent growth occurs through hypertrophy of existing fibers. Histological and biochemical analyses confirm that there is a 14-fold increase in sarcolemma nuclei throughout muscle growth, slightly smaller in girls than boys.[25] Widdowson stated that "in no respect has skeletal muscle reached its mature chemical composition at the time of a full-term birth."[26(p338)]

Muscle Neural Elements

Primitive nerve branches ramify among muscle fibers by the 10th week. Myoneural junctions form in the 11th week, and early motor endplate formation has been observed by electron microscopy at 10 weeks. In the early stages, several motor axons innervate a single muscle fiber; eventually, however, only one axon will remain. In the rat, this changeover is related to "increase in speed of contractions and myosin light chain patterns of muscle fibres which occurs in early postnatal life."[27(p25)] By the 14th week, the muscle spindle has all the essential components; myelination of spindle fibers occurs after the second trimester. Golgi tendon organs (GTOs) commence innervation in the 12th week. Subsequently, the GTO structure becomes encapsulated, and myelination of its fibers occurs from 16 weeks.[22]

Tissue-Tissue Attachments

Figure 4 demonstrates the differences between the myotendinous junction of human paravertebral muscle at term, in the adolescent, and in the adult. The neonatal myotendinous junction is less closely packed and interdigitated; the myofibrils at the end of the muscle cells vary in thickness and are less developed.[28]

The question of how soft tissues, such as muscles, maintain their appropriate attachments during long bone growth has long interested investigators. It is theorized that compensatory movement of soft structures must accompany the growth of long bones to ensure that muscles attached to the metaphysis are not "left behind" as length of the bones increases. Hurov[29] studied the attachment of several soft tissue structures about the medial side of the rabbit knee. His findings contradicted earlier theory that the periosteum/perichondrium directly slides along the tibial diaphysis. He demonstrated that collagen-fiber bundles link the periosteum to the subadjacent bone. Ligamentous and muscular structures attach only to the periosteum at birth. At 60 days, however, only the popliteus was attached solely to the periosteum. With aging, the attachment of ligaments to the fibrous periosteum penetrates the fibrocartilage, which is gradually replaced by chondroid and lamellar bone and subsequently remodeled into compact lamellar bone.[29] These changes produce the strong ligament-bone attachment of maturity. Further research is needed to elucidate the roles of long bone growth and periosteal expansion in maintaining the relative positions of soft tissues during growth.

Joint Development

Embryonic Period

Most of the tissues differentiating in the newly forming limb rise from mesenchymal cells. These cells give rise to the various articular tissues, with the exception of neural elements and blood vessels.[8,9] As the skeletal template begins to chondrify, joint formation commences. A region of flattened, undifferentiated cells forms between the two areas that are differentiating into cartilage. Experiments suggest that joint cells are prespecified and that the joint area is a specialized region.[30] The initial joint formation does not appear to be dependent on mechanical pressure that is generated by growth of the skeletal elements. At least in avians, however, movement is important. Paralysis may cause failure of joint cavitation (breakdown of interzonal mesenchyme to form precursor joint cavity).[31–33] Early limb movements by human embryos (about 54 days) may contribute to joint cavitation.

Figure 5 displays a diagrammatic representation of the events in synovial joint formation. Cellular activities in the homogeneous interzone between the skeletal elements transform the initially flattened area into a three-layered interzone that consists of two chondrogenous layers, which are continuous at the periphery of the future joint with the perichondrium, and a middle loose layer, which later forms the joint cavity (Fig. 5C). Synovial mesenchyme will give rise to the synovial membrane, the fibrous capsule, and such intra-articular structures as menisci, tendons, and ligaments. Vascularization of these structures then follows.

The next event is the formation of the joint cavity, which begins at about the same time as other joint tissues differentiate. The precise nature of cavitation is not well established. It is thought, however, to begin centrally. Cavities appear in the middle layer; these cavities coalesce and form a single cavity. Many bursae and synovial sheaths are formed and start cavitation by the end of the embryonic period.[8]

The differentiation of the limb joints, from the early template to structures similar to those in the adult, occurs over a relatively short period of time and in the human occurs between 4½ to 7 weeks. The limbs are most susceptible to the action of teratogens during this embryonic period. Individual variability in the general sequence of the joint morphogenetic events described does occur. Some joints show considerable delay between differentiation and cavitation. The joints of the hand and foot may not develop a three-layered interzone

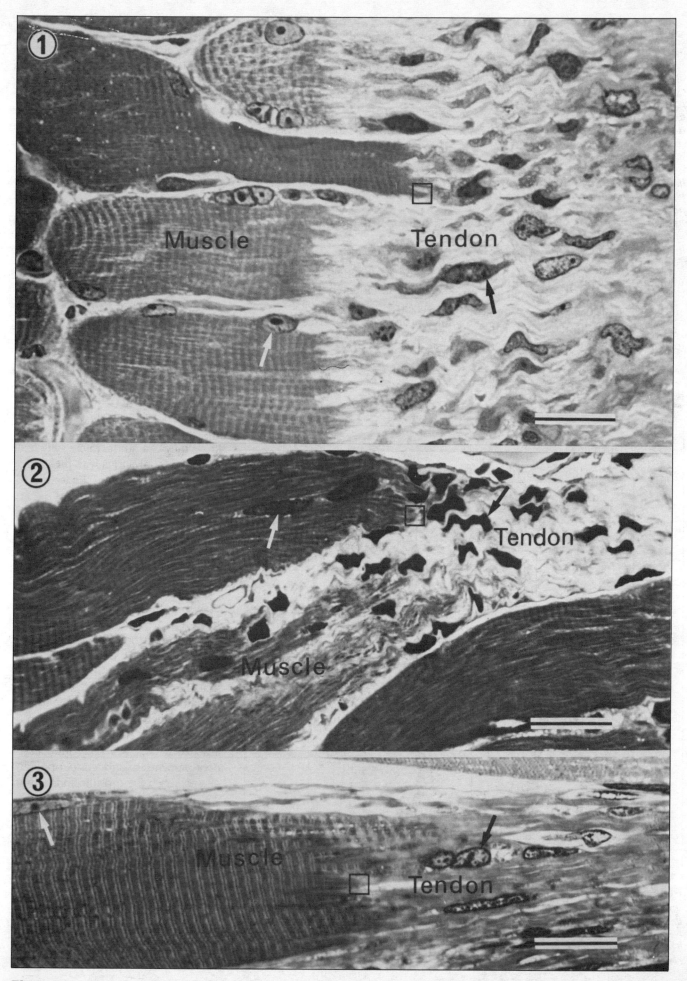

Figure 4.

Figure 4. *Figure is on preceding page. Light microscopic views of human multifidus showing muscle-tendon junction development: neonatal (1), adolescent (2), and adult (3). These sections are parallel to the longitudinal axis of the tendon. Nuclei of muscle fibers (white arrows), tendon fibroblasts (black arrows), terminal extensions of ends of muscle fibers inserting into tendon (squares) are indicated. (×1,050, bars=20 μ.) Note the greater interdigitation of the muscle fibers with the tendon fibers in the adult. (Reprinted with permission from Ovalle WK. The human muscle-tendon junction. Anat Embryol [Berl]. 1987;186:281-294.[28])*

until early in the fetal period.[8] The sacroiliac joint starts cavitation in the 10th week, but does not complete the process until the 7th month.[34,35] For most joints, however, cavitation is

complete in the early fetal period. Other differences in developmental sequence are that the acromioclavicular joint does not show the usual homogeneous then three-layered interzone, the temporomandibular joint develops where a continuous blastema never existed, and the sternochondral joints show cartilaginous continuity in the early stages with subsequent cavitation uncertain.[8]

The sequence of events in joint formation thus may vary slightly within specific human joints. Figure 6 gives the timing for the main events of knee joint development. A number of investigators[36–43] have provided detailed analyses of the development of individual joints. Ligaments tend to appear between stages 19 and 21, os-

sification commences in stages 21 to 23, and cavitation usually commences in the larger joints by stage 23 (end of the seventh week). The role of the developing vessels (and their location) and of the limb flexures (denoted by skin creases) in joint development is not known.

Fetal Period

Developmental changes in the fetal period consist of an increase in the size and maturation of formed structures; an increase in the amount of collagen, resulting in clearer definition of fibrous tissues such as ligaments; and extension of the joint cavity.[8] Even in early development, ligaments are thought to act as restraining structures.[10] There is increased vascularization of epiphyseal cartilages from the third month, with the appearance, and then increase in number, of synovial villi. More bursae appear, and, in joints such as the knee, they extend the joint cavity by their communications with the cavity. Fat cells appear around the fourth to fifth months, marking the sites of future fat pads. Some elastic fibers appear in the fibrous capsule late in the fetal period when tendons and ligaments become increasingly avascular.[8]

Nerve fibers begin to enter the joint tissues in the fetal period, but specialized structures such as Ruffini and Pacini endings only occur late in the fetal period. Dee[44] observed that Hilton's law (ie, nerves, in which branches supply muscles moving a joint, give an articular contribution) is substantially true for all joints. Each joint has a dual nerve supply: Specific articular nerves, which are independent branches of adjacent peripheral nerves, reach the capsule, and nonspecific secondary articular branches arise from related muscle nerves.[44]

Role of Movement

The nature of cavitation and its dependence on movement for its initiation has been shown in avians but not in humans.[7,8] Although the role of movement for initiation and maintenance of cavitation is not clearly dem-

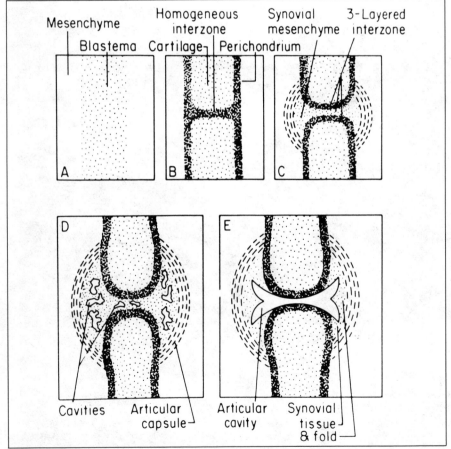

Figure 5. *Sequential events of joint development in the embryological period: (A) initial formation of skeleton in mesenchyme; (B) chondrification of future skeleton and three-layered interzone at future joint site; (C) early development of joint tissues; (D, E) early formation of joint cavity. (Modified with permission from O'Rahilly R, Gardner E. The embryology of moveable joints. In: Sokoloff L, ed. The Joints and Synovial Fluid. New York, NY: Academic Press Inc; 1978;1:29-103.[8])*

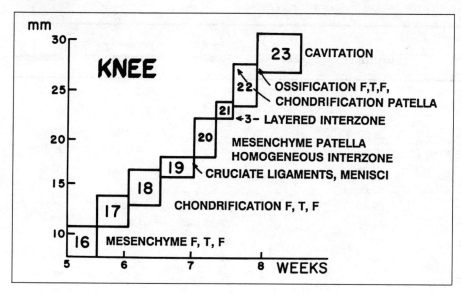

Figure 6. *Main events of knee joint development. (F, T, F=femur, tibia, fibula.) (Modified with permission from O'Rahilly R, Gardner E. The embryology of moveable joints. In: Sokoloff L, ed. The Joints and Synovial Fluid. New York, NY: Academic Press Inc; 1978;1:29-103.[8])*

onstrated for human joints, movement is very important in maintaining and in molding the articular form of human joints once the form is established.[7,8,31] This process continues in the postnatal period.

Movement, as a modeling force, may be more critical to joints such as the hip joint, characterized as a shallow concave socket for a spherical partner. When the hip joint is first formed, the acetabulum is a deep cavity that almost completely surrounds the femoral head.[38,45] As the fetus ages, the depth of the socket increases at a significantly slower rate than does the transverse diameter of the femoral head and the socket. Although acetabular and femoral head diameters increase more than fourfold from 12 weeks to term, depth increases less than threefold.[46,47] The net effect of these differential rates of growth is a change in the shape of the socket.[47] The hip joint at birth is the most unstable joint in the body.

In the immediate postnatal period, depth again increases in relation to diameter, creating a mature and secure ball-and-socket joint.[48] It is theorized that the shallowness of the socket at birth facilitates the passage

of the fetus through the vaginal canal. Initially, the femoral head forms as a spherical structure. Because of restrictions imposed on fetal movement, such as tightness of the uterine wall (Appendix),[5] the femoral head becomes increasingly less round.[49] Postnatally, the cartilaginous femoral head again assumes a more spherical shape, presumably in response to the increased range of motion (ROM). The growth potential of the hip joint decreases steadily after birth. Significant acetabular growth may not occur after 18 months, and probably not after 3 years of age.[50,51] Thus, early diagnosis and management of congenital hip dysplasia is important.

The reported relationship between sleeping position and hip dysplasia suggests that the postnatal sleeping posture can influence acetabular development. When a preferred side-lying posture was demonstrated, hip dysplasia occurred in the upper hip of 19 of 41 children.[52] Presumably, the adducted and medially rotated position of the upper hip reduced the stimulus for growth in the acetabular cup. These changes demonstrate that movement plays an important role in modeling the joint surfaces in the early postnatal period and during in-

fancy. The shallowness of the hip joint at term also means, however, that the neonatal hip joint is vulnerable and may subluxate or dislocate through forceful extension,[53] or simply because of the greater available mobility ex utero. Care should be exerted when moving the hip of premature babies and neonates toward extension, and extension should never be forced. It also is suggested that infants should not be consistently positioned on one side, but alternated between sides.

Skeletal Angles, Axes, and Curves

Stability of the mature hip joint is enhanced by the inclination of the acetabular socket and by the neck shaft and torsion angles of the proximal femur. The neck-shaft (anteversion or inclination) angle is apparently formed very early in the fetal period and changes little with age.[47] Mean birth values have been shown to differ little from the established adult values of 125 degrees.[47,54,55] Torsion (deinclination), the angle that the proximal femur makes with the distal femoral condyles, however, shows marked change during the fetal and postnatal periods.[47] Initially, this angle is negative or retroverted. Although torsion values at birth are about 35 degrees, they decrease to the adult value of about 11 degrees. This decrease is more marked in infancy, but continues gradually to puberty.[50,56–58]

The femoral-tibial axis is minimally greater in the neonate than in the adult (180° versus 171°) and changes spontaneously from the initial varus (bowing) to a valgus position (knock-knee) at about age 2 to 3 years. After age 6 years, the valgus position almost completely straightens out in most children.[59] Variability in values reported is related to selection of anatomic axis. There is a valgus angle of between 4.2 and 5.8 degrees in the mature limb.[60] Persistence of physiologic infantile tibial varus or exaggeration of the subsequent valgus change requires observation and possibly clinical intervention. Substantially greater change is reported for tibial

Table 2. *Reported Mean Values (in Degrees) for Hip Motion in Neonates and Infants[a]*

Authors	Sample	N	Extension[b]	Flexion	Medial Rotation	Lateral Rotation	Abduction
Waugh et al[66]	neonate	40	46 (9)				
			22–68				
Drews et al[72]	0–6 d	54	28 (6)		80 (9)	114 (10)	69 (9)
Haas et al[68]	0–3 d	237–400	28 (8)		62 (13)	89 (14)	76 (12)
			10–75		35–100	45–110	50–90
Hoffer[67]	0–3 d	20	50–80		40–80	−30–0	
	12 mo	11	20–40		40–80	0–50	
	15 mo	11	10–25		40–80	40–70	
Phelps et al[70]	9 m	25	10[c]		41[c]	56[c]	59
	12 mo	25	9		44	58	54
	18 mo	18	4		45	52	59
	24 mo	18	3		52	47	60
Coon et al[69]	6 wk	44	19		24	48	
	3 mo	44	7		26	45	
	6 mo	40	7		21	46	
Watanabe et al[71]	birth	62	25	120	21	77	48
	4 wk	62	12	138	24	66	51
	4–8 mo	54	4	136	39	66	55
	8–12 mo	45	−3	138	38	79	60
	1 y	64	−15	141	49	74	66
	2 y	57	−21	143	59	58	63

[a]Standard deviations shown in parentheses.

[b]Negative values indicate real extension; positive values indicate physiological "flexion contracture."

[c]Significant differences between groups.

torsion, which is zero at birth and changes by puberty to a lateral tibial torsion value of 23 degrees.[61]

Differing cultural practices of baby carrying can influence changes in angles and axes and contribute to conditions such as bowleg and knock-knee. African mothers tend to carry their infants over one hip. Inuit and Chinese mothers carry their infants in a deep coat hood or sling on their backs. In contrast, mothers in several American Indian tribes (eg, Cree-Ojibwa, Navajo) carry their infants on a straight board with a leather harness, which positions the infants' limbs close to the standing position. This position has been considered detrimental to hip joint development because of association between cradling and congenital hip dysplasia (CHD).[53,62] Congenital hip dysplasia is almost unknown among the Inuit and Chinese and has a low incidence in Africans compared with Caucasians. Populations that cradle their infants have the highest reported incidences of CHD; however, other factors such as inbreeding may play a greater role in causation.

Fetal position also has been demonstrated to be an important contributor to the initial limb alignment and joint mobility of the neonate.[5,6,63] Fetal positions, particularly if abnormal (not vertex), or a size disparity between the fetus and the mother subject the growing fetus to unusual forces over a number of weeks and can result in unusual facies and limb postures and restrictions of neonatal joint mobility. Such presentations as face-brow (1 in 500 births) and transverse lie (1 in 300–600 births) maintain the cervical spine in hyperextension and are associated with abnormal facies.[5] The effect on the developing cervical spine and its musculature is unknown. Breech posture and presentation has an established correlation with congenital postural deformities (nonstructural, such as torticollis and hip dysplasia) and severe limitation of hip extension and knee flexion; genu recurvatum is often present.[5,6] Posture of the feet is especially affected by intrauterine space limitations. It has been shown that distraught infants can be more easily settled in their fetal position, or "position of comfort."[5(p41)] Therapists might recreate this position to detect potential developmental problems, such as

Table 3. *Mean Values (in Degrees) for Motions[a] That Decreased or Increased by ≥15 Degrees Between Birth and 2 Years of Age[71]*

Age	N	ShLR[b]	Elbow Extension[c]	Knee Extension[c]	Ankle Dorsiflexion	Ankle Plantar Flexion
Birth	62	134	14	16	54	43
2–4 wk	57	126	6	12	53	58
4–8 mo	54	120	0	4	51	60
8–12 mo	45	124	−1	1	50	60
1 y	64	116	−3	−4	45	62
2 y	57	118	−5	−7	41	62

[a]Passive range of motion.

[b]Shoulder lateral rotation.

[c]Negative values indicate real extension motion.

weak deep cervical flexors in a transverse-lying infant.

Dunn[6] has described a "wind-swept" posture in which both limbs are twisted in the same direction, as well as a "locked" posture in which the femoral rotational element is opposite to that of the tibia. Such fetal postures can produce rotational malalignments such as medial rotation of the tibia associated with lateral femoral torsion (retroversion).[58] Especially in the premature infant, where medical attention often focuses on viability, the therapist should be attentive to the presence of deformities attributable to the fetal position.

Although many writers relate the development of cervical and lumbar curves to postnatal events such as head lifting, crawling, and upright stance, a forward cervical curvature has been observed in young fetuses. Bagnall et al,[64] in a study of fetuses between the ages of 8 and 23 weeks, found that 83% showed a secondary cervical curvature. It appears, therefore, that the forward convexity of the cervical curve may only be accentuated after birth. The early appearance of the secondary cervical curvature is thought to be related to the early ossification of the occipital bone, an event associated with neck extensor muscle activity in the gasp reflex that is present from 6½ weeks of prenatal age.[65] Another factor in development of the secondary lumbar curve may be the relative tightness of the iliopsoas muscle.

Joint Mobility

At birth, the full-term neonate exhibits physiological limitation of hip and knee extension and ankle plantar flexion.[66–68] In contrast, the premature infant may show no limitation and hypermobility of most joints. The term "physiological limitation of motion" should not be confused with flexion contractures in mature joints. It is secondary to restriction of motion generally (ie, in utero), especially in the third trimester. Birth brings release from constraint and freedom of movement. Motion into extension evolves without need for intervention.

Tables 2 through 4 give reported values for joint ROM in neonates and infants.[67–72] Differences in ROM values relate to variability in testing techniques, reporting of active versus passive ROM, measurement precision, and observer variability in end-range detection. Changes in joint mobility with age are paralleled by age-related changes in locomotor abilities. All investigators reported hip extension limitation at birth, which may still be present, though reduced, at 2 years of age. Except for Hoffer,[67] who reported ranges rather than mean values, the investigators demonstrated a clear trend for hip lateral rotation to exceed medial rotation in neonates and infants; both motions have similar values by 2 years of age.

Both the restriction of motion and the hypermobility seen in the neonate are criteria used in gestational assessment, such as the popliteal angle and the scarf and square-window signs.[73,74] Persistence of these characteristic motions may indicate pathology, such as arthrogryposis multiplex congenita and cutis laxa (cutaneous laxity).[5,74]

Table 4. *Ranges of Mean Values for Passive Range of Motion (PROM) Reported for Japanese Infants from Birth to 2 Years of Age[71,a]*

Joint Motion	PROM (°)
Shoulder	
Flexion	172–180
Extension	79–89
Abduction	177–187
Medial rotation	72–90
Elbow	
Flexion	148–158
Pronation	90–96
Supination	81–93
Wrist	
Extension	82–89
Flexion	88–96
Knee	
Flexion	148–159

[a]Age groups: birth, 2–4 wk, 4–8 mo, 8–12 mo, 1 y, 2 y; all groups with n≥45.

Appendix. *Constraint Factors That May Result in an Unusual Fetal Position*

Primigravida
Tight uterus
Malformed uterus
Oligohydramnios
Fetal/maternal size disparity
Multiple fetuses
Malformed fetus
Unusual placental site

Derivation of estrogen intrinsically and extrinsically from the mother may account for the reported greater mobility of female infants compared with male infants. This at-birth difference is generally short-lived. No significant differences between sides of the body have been demonstrated, except where an abnormal fetal posture existed. As reported differences in ROM lie chiefly between neonates and children, or individuals under and over 18 years of age,[75] average adult values are probably achieved by late childhood and well before completion of growth.

Conclusion

Major development of the musculoskeletal system occurs in the embryonic period. In the fetal period, development continues with increase in size and complexity of structure and function. The musculoskeletal system is vulnerable to failures of specific morphogenetic processes, resulting in limb fusions and ameli in the embryonic period. Congenital anomalies, however, may arise during the fetal period and are especially characterized by growth retardation. Late fetopathies, or congenital postural deformities, are probably produced by mechanical factors in utero, such as fetal position, amount of amniotic fluid, and tightness of the uterine wall. These deformities are essentially nonstructural and often resolve spontaneously. Awareness of prenatal and postnatal events and their timing will assist the therapist in management of pediatric patients.

References

1 O'Rahilly R. *Developmental Stages in Human Embryos, Including a Survey of the Carnegie Collection, Part A: Embryos of the First Three Weeks (Stages 1 to 9)*. Washington, DC: Carnegie Institution of Washington, 1973.

2 O'Rahilly R, Gardner E. The timing and sequence of events in the development of the limbs in the human embryo. *Anat Embryol (Berl)*. 1975;148:1–23.

3 Bolande RP. Developmental pathology. *Am J Pathol*. 1979;94:627–683.

4 Moore KL. *The Developing Human*. 2nd ed. Philadelphia, Pa: WB Saunders Co; 1977:136.

5 Smith DW. *Recognizable Patterns of Human Deformation: Major Problems in Clinical Pediatrics*. Philadelphia, Pa: WB Saunders Co; 1981: vol 21.

6 Dunn PM. Congenital postural deformities. *Br Med Bull*. 1976;32:71–76.

7 Tickle C, Wolpert L. Limb development. In: Davis JA, Dobbing J, eds. *Scientific Foundations of Paediatrics*. Baltimore, Md: University Park Press; 1981:544–564.

8 O'Rahilly R, Gardner E. The embryology of moveable joints. In: Sokoloff L, ed. *The Joints and Synovial Fluid*. New York, NY: Academic Press Inc; 1978;1:29–103.

9 Krey AK, Dayton DH, Goetinck PF. NICHD Research workshop: normal and abnormal development of the limb. *Teratology*. 1984;29:315–323.

10 Blechschmidt E, Gasser RF. *Biokinetics and Biodynamics of Human Differentiation: Principles and Applications*. Springfield, Ill: Charles C Thomas, Publisher; 1978:156–175.

11 Caplan AI. The vasculature and limb development. *Cell Differ*. 1985;16:1–11.

12 Royer P. Growth and development of bony tissues. In: Davis JA, Dobbing J, eds. *Scientific Foundations of Paediatrics*. Baltimore, Md: University Park Press; 1981:565–589.

13 Carter DR, Orr TE, Fyhrie DP, Schurman DJ. Influences of mechanical stress on prenatal and postnatal skeletal development. *Clin Orthop*. 1987;219:237–250.

14 Gardner E, Gray DJ, O'Rahilly R. *Anatomy: A Regional Study of Human Structure*. 5th ed. Philadelphia, Pa: WB Saunders Co; 1986.

15 Warwick R, Williams PL. *Gray's Anatomy*. 35th ed. Norwich, England: Longman Group Ltd; 1973:200–385.

16 Lowrey GH. *Growth and Development of Children*. 7th ed. Chicago, Ill: Year Book Medical Publishers Inc; 1978:286–293.

17 Sensenig EC. The early development of the human vertebral column. *Contrib Embryol Carnegie Inst*. 1949;33:23–41.

18 Kunitomo F. The development and reduction of the tail and of the caudal end of the spinal cord. *Contrib Embryol*. 1918;8:161–198.

19 Gusnard DA, Naidich TP, Yousefzadeh DK, Haughton VM. Ultrasonic anatomy of the normal neonatal and infant spine: correlation with cryomicrotome sections and CT. *Neuroradiology*. 1986;28:493–511.

20 Enlow DH. Normal craniofacial growth. In: Cohen MM Jr, ed. *Craniosynotosis: Diagnosis, Evaluation, and Management*. New York, NY: Raven Press; 1986:155.

21 Minguetti G, Mair WGP. The developing human muscle: ultrastructural differences between myoblasts and fibroblasts. *Rev Bras de Pesquisas Med e Biol*. 1980;13:1–8.

22 Mastaglia FL. Growth and development of skeletal muscle. In: Davis JA, Dobbing J, eds. *Scientific Foundations of Paediatrics*. Baltimore, Md: University Park Press; 1981:590–620.

23 Dubowitz V. Enzyme histochemistry of skeletal muscle: part 1, developing animal muscle; part 2, developing human muscle. *J Neurol Neurosurg Psychiatry*. 1965;28:516–524.

24 Haltia M, Berlin O, Schucht H, Sourander P. Postnatal differentiation and growth of skeletal muscle fibers in normal and undernourished rats: a histochemical and morphometric study. *J Neurol Sci*. 1978;36:25–39.

25 Cheek DB. Cited by: Widdowson EM. Changes in body composition growth. In: Davis JA, Dobbing J, eds. *Scientific Foundations of Paediatrics*. Baltimore, Md: University Park Press; 1981:338.

26 Widdowson EM. Changes in body composition during growth. In: Davis JA, Dobbing J, eds. *Scientific Foundations of Paediatrics*. Baltimore, Md: University Park Press; 1981:330–342.

27 Gauthier GF, Lowey S, Hobbs AW. Fast and slow myosin in developing muscle fibres. *Nature*. 1978;274:25.

28 Ovalle WK. The human muscle-tendon junction. *Anat Embryol (Berl)*. 1987;176:281–294.

29 Hurov JR. Soft-tissue bone interface: How do attachments of muscles, tendons, and ligaments change during growth? A light microscopic study. *J Morphol*. 1986;189:313–325.

30 Holder N. An experimental investigation into the early development of the chick elbow. *J Embryol Exp Morph*. 1977;39:115–127.

31 Fell HB, Canti RG. Experiments on the development *in vitro* of the avian knee joint. *Proc R Soc Lond (Biol)*. 1934;116:316–351.

32 Drachman DB, Sokoloff L. The role of movement in embryonic joint development. *Dev Biol*. 1966;14:401–420.

33 Murray PDF, Drachman DB. The role of movement in the development of joints and the related structures: the head and neck in the chick embryo. *J Embryol Exp Morphol*. 1969;22:349–371.

34 Schunke GB. The anatomy and development of the sacro-iliac joint in man. *Anat Rec*. 1938;72:313–331.

35 Walker JM. Age-related differences in the human sacroiliac joint: a histological study, implications for therapy. *Journal of Orthopaedic and Sports Physical Therapy*. 1986;7:325–334.

36 Gray DJ, Gardner E. Prenatal development of the human knee and the superior tibiofibular joints. *Am J Anat*. 1950;86:235–287.

37 McDermott LJ. Development of the human knee joint. *Arch Surg*. 1943;46:705–719.

38 Strayer LM Jr. Embryology of the human hip joint. *Clin Orthop*. 1971;74:221–240.

39 Andersen H. Histochemistry and development of the human shoulder and acromioclavicular joint with particular reference to the early development of the clavicle. *Acta Anat (Basel)*. 1963;55:124–165.

40 Andersen H, Bro-Rasmussen F. Histochemical studies on the histogenesis of the joints in human foetuses with special reference to the development of joint cavities in the hand and foot. *Am J Anat*. 1961;108:111–122.

41 Gardner E, Gray DJ. Prenatal development of the human shoulder and acromioclavicular joints. *Am J Anat*. 1953;92:219–276.

42 Gardner E, O'Rahilly R. The early development of the knee joint in staged human embryos. *J Anat*. 1968;102:289–299.

43 Gray DJ, Gardner E, O'Rahilly R. The prenatal development of the skeleton and joints of the human hand. *Am J Anat*. 1957;101:169–224.

44 Dee R. The innervation of joints. In: Sokoloff L, ed. *The Joints and Synovial Fluid*. New York, NY: Academic Press Inc; 1978;1:177–204.

45 Walker JM. Histological study of the fetal development of the human acetabulum and

labrum: significance in congenital hip disease. *Yale J Biol Med.* 1981;54:255–263.

46 Walker JM. Comparison of normal and abnormal human fetal hip joints: a quantitative study with significance to congenital hip disease. *J Pediatr Orthop.* 1983;3:173–183.

47 Walker JM, Goldsmith CH. Morphometric study of the fetal development of the human hip joint: significance for congenital hip disease. *Yale J Biol Med.* 1981;54:411–437.

48 Ralis Z, McKibbin B. Changes in shape of the human hip joint during its development and their relation to its stability. *J Bone Joint Surg [Br].* 1973;55:780–785.

49 Walker JM. Human fetal femoral head sphericity. *Clin Orthop.* 1980;147:301–304.

50 Harris NH. Acetabular growth potential in congenital dislocation of the hip and some factors upon which it may depend. *Clin Orthop.* 1976;119:99–106.

51 Almby B, Grevsten S, Lonnerholm T. Hip joint instability after the neonatal period, II: the acetabular growth potential. *Acta Radiol Diag (Stockh).* 1979;20:213–221.

52 Heikkilia E, Ryoppy S, Laihimo I. The management of primary acetabular dysplasia: its association with habitual side-lying. *J Bone Joint Surg [Br].* 1985;67:25–28.

53 Salter RB. Etiology, pathogenesis and possible prevention of congenital dislocation of the hip. *Can Med Assoc J.* 1968;98:933–945.

54 Felts JL. The prenatal development of the human femur. *Am J Anat.* 1954;94:1–44.

55 Watanabe RS. Embryology of the human hip. *Clin Orthop.* 1974;98:8–26.

56 Elftman H. Torsion of the lower extremity. *Am J Phys Anthropol.* 1945;2–3:255–265.

57 Stanisavljevic S. *Diagnosis and Treatment of Congenital Hip Pathology in the Newborn.* Baltimore, Md: Williams & Wilkins; 1964.

58 Staheli LT. Torsional deformity. *Pediatr Clin North Am.* 1986;33:1373–1393.

59 Cozen L. Knock-knee deformity in children. *Clin Orthop.* 1990;258:191–203.

60 Hsu RWW, Himeno S, Coventry MB, Chao EYS. Normal axial alignment of the lower extremity and load-bearing distribution at the knee. *Clin Orthop.* 1990;255:215–227.

61 Yagi T, Sasaki T. Tibial torsion in patients with medial-type osteoarthritic knee. *Clin Orthop.* 1986;213:177–182.

62 Walker JM. Congenital hip disease in a Cree-Ojibwa population: a restrospective study. *Can Med Assoc J.* 1977;116:501–504.

63 Warkany J. *Congenital Malformations: Notes and Comments.* Chicago, Ill: Year Book Medical Publishers Inc; 1971:992–997.

64 Bagnall KM, Harris PF, Jones PRM. A radiographic study of the human fetal spine, 1: the development of the secondary cervical curvature. *J Anat.* 1977;123:777–782.

65 Hooker D. Evidence of prenatal function of the central nervous system in man. In: Payton OD, Hirt S, Newton R, eds. *Scientific Basis for Neurophysiologic Approaches to Therapeutic Exercise.* Philadelphia, Pa: FA Davis Co; 1977:51–61.

66 Waugh KG, Mindel JL, Parker R, Coon VA. Measurement of selected hip, knee, and ankle joint motions in newborns. *Phys Ther.* 1983; 63:1616–1621.

67 Hoffer M. Joint motion limitation in newborns. *Clin Orthop.* 1980;148:94–96.

68 Haas SS, Epps CH Jr, Adams JP. Normal ranges of hip motion in the newborn. *Clin Orthop.* 1973;91:114–118.

69 Coon VA, Donato G, Houser C, Bleck EE. Normal ranges of hip motion in infants, six weeks, three months and six months of age. *Clin Orthop.* 1975;110:256–260.

70 Phelps E, Smith LJ, Hallum A. Normal ranges of hip motion of infants between nine and 24 months of age. *Dev Med Child Neurol.* 1985;27:785–792.

71 Watanabe H, Ogata K, Amano T, Okabe T. The range of joint motions of the extremities in healthy Japanese people: the difference according to age. *Nippon Seikeigeka Gakkai Zasshi.* 1979;53:275–291.

72 Drews JE, Vraciu JK, Pellino G. Range of motion of the joints of the lower extremities of newborns. *Physical and Occupational Therapy in Pediatrics.* 1984;4(2):49–62.

73 Reade E, Hom L, Hallum A, Lopopolo R. Changes in popliteal angle measurement in infants up to one year of age. *Dev Med Child Neurol.* 1984;26:774–780.

74 Dubowitz LMS, Dubowitz V. *The Neurological Assessment of the Preterm and Full-term Newborn Infant.* Philadelphia, Pa: JB Lippincott Co; 1981.

75 Boone DC, Azen SP. Normal range of motion in joint in male subjects. *J Bone Joint Surg [Am].* 1979;61:756–759.

Joint Mobilization for Children with Central Nervous System Disorders: Indications and Precautions

Susan R Harris
Beverley D Lundgren

Because clinicians are introducing joint mobilization into treatment programs for children with cerebral palsy, we felt that a review of the procedure and its scientific basis would be timely. The goals of the introductory section of this article are to define joint mobilization as it has been used for adults with musculoskeletal disabilities, to discuss various rationales for its effects, to describe contraindications and precautions for its use, and to discuss its efficacy as reported in the research literature. The latter part of the article deals with the use of joint mobilization for children with central nervous system (CNS) disorders. In an effort to understand precautions for the use of joint mobilization in children, musculoskeletal development will be described both for typically developing children and for children with spastic cerebral palsy. Indications for using joint mobilization techniques in children with spasticity will be outlined. Specific neurodevelopmental disabilities for which joint mobilization would be strongly contraindicated will be listed. Finally, future research directions in evaluating reliability of assessment of joint dysfunction and efficacy of joint mobilization in children will be discussed. [Harris SR, Lundgren BD. Joint mobilization for children with central nervous system disorders: indications and precautions. Phys Ther. 1991;71:890–896.]

Key Words: *Cerebral palsy, Joint mobilization, Manual therapy.*

Since the early 1970s, there has been a steady increase in the use of joint mobilization techniques by physical therapists.[1] The primary indication for use has been mechanical joint dysfunction in which there is restriction of joint play (accessory motion) leading to pain or limitation of active physiological movement.[2] Joint mobilization has most often been used in the evaluation and treatment of patients who have musculoskeletal disabilities of the spine and extremities. More recently, Cochrane[3] has suggested mobilization as an appropriate form of treatment for some of the joint restrictions that occur in children with cerebral palsy. The goals of the introductory section of this article are to define joint mobilization as used traditionally for adults with musculoskeletal disabilities, to discuss various rationales for its effects, to describe contraindications and precautions, and to discuss the efficacy of this treatment approach as reported in the research literature. The latter part of the article will deal with the applicability of joint mobilization for children with central nervous system (CNS) disorders.

Definitions

Used in its broadest sense, *joint mobilization* is a general term referring to any active or passive attempt to move a joint. As used in this article, the term is defined more specifically as any *passive* movement technique utilizing repetitive or oscillatory joint-play movements. Mobilization techniques are often graded as illustrated in Figure 1:

Grade 1: a small-amplitude movement performed at the beginning of the range.

Grade 2: a large-amplitude movement performed early in the range.

Grade 3: a large-amplitude movement performed to the end of the range.

Grade 4: a small-amplitude movement performed at the end of the range.[4]

SR Harris, PhD, PT, FAPTA, is Associate Professor, School of Rehabilitation Medicine, University of British Columbia, T325-2211, Wesbrook Mall, Vancouver, British Columbia, Canada V6T 2B5. Address all correspondence to Dr Harris.

BD Lundgren, BPT, PT, is Instructor, School of Rehabilitation Medicine, University of British Columbia, and is in private practice in Vancouver, British Columbia, Canada.

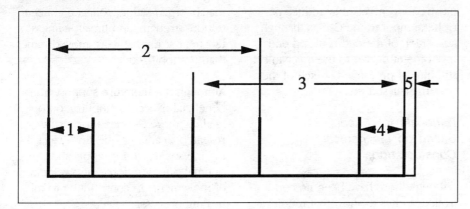

Figure 1. *Grades of joint-play movement. (Adapted with permission.[2])*

When these grades are used, techniques are performed slowly and rhythmically, making it possible for the patient to use voluntary muscle contraction to prevent the therapist from administering the technique[2,4–8]

Grade 5 (Fig. 1) refers to *manipulation*, which is defined as a small-amplitude, high-velocity thrust applied to a joint at the limit of the available range of motion (ROM) and done so quickly that the patient cannot prevent the movement from taking place. Manipulation represents a progression beyond mobilization by providing a quick stretch to the joint, often accompanied by a cracking sound.[4,8]

There has been no suggestion in the physical therapy literature that manipulation would be an appropriate form of treatment for children with CNS disorders; indeed, common practice recognizes manipulation to be contraindicated in cases of "physical involvement of the CNS."[9(p446)]

The reader should be aware, however, of these distinctions when considering the topic of joint mobilization. The term *manual therapy* will be used to refer to both mobilization and manipulation procedures.

Mechanical Joint Dysfunction

Dysfunction is a nonspecific term used to describe a deviation from normal. In the case of joint dysfunction, there is either deviation from the normal expected movement or pain accompanying the movement.[10] There are many different causes of mechanical joint dysfunction. For example, peripheral joint dysfunction can be due to capsular fibrosis, ligamentous adhesions, joint effusion, subluxation, and intra-articular derangement.[2] Spinal dysfunction has been related to disk lesions with or without nerve root involvement, zygapophyseal joint adhesions and derangements, segmental hypermobility, and subluxations.[4,8–11]

Not all types of joint dysfunction are appropriate for treatment by manual therapy. Careful evaluation of the type of dysfunction involves detailed assessment procedures.[5,8–11] The specific signs and symptoms of the patient enable the physical therapist to develop a diagnosis and determine suitability for treatment. Careful analysis of clinical features guides progression of treatment.

Manual therapy has been stated to be most effective when directed at "mechanical joint dysfunction in which there is restriction of accessory motion due to capsular or ligamentous tightness or adherence."[2(p91)] Assessment, therefore, includes testing of the accessory movements particular to that joint to determine the presence of pain or resistance, or both, to movement.[4,7] Resistance to movement is typically produced by either capsuloligamentous tightness (stiffness) or muscle activity (spasm).[7] The resistance produced by stiffness is described as being consistent in strength and position in the range of movement, whereas that produced by muscle spasm varies in response to the speed and method of the examination movement.[7] Skill and experience are required to appreciate these signs and symptoms when assessing the small movements associated with the peripheral and vertebral joints. The ability to reliably "feel" joint-play movements has been questioned by some authors[12] and supported by others.[13,14] A recent study by Jull and colleagues[13] confirmed the ability of a therapist to accurately diagnose cervical zygaphoseal joint syndromes using manual procedures, but additional studies are required in this area.

Rationale for the Effects of Mobilization

The mechanisms by which joint mobilization or manipulation "work" are not known, although many hypotheses have been proposed as our knowledge of articular and soft tissue neurology, biomechanics, and pathology has expanded. Although treatment rationales have been developed for the areas receiving the most research attention (ie, spinal mobilization and manipulation),[15] the proposed rationales for these effects can be applied to peripheral joints as well. Some of the possible mechanisms for these effects are described in the following paragraphs.

Neurophysiological Mechanisms for the Reduction of Pain and Muscle Spasm

Articular neurology has provided much of the background to understanding the effect of passive movement in modulating pain. The type I, II, and III mechanoreceptors located in joint capsules and ligaments are stimulated by active and passive joint movement.[16] Type IV nociceptors are completely inactive in normal situations, but are stimulated by excessive mechanical stress or by chemical irritants.[16] The gate-control theory postulated by Melzack and Wall in 1965[17] proposed that an afferent barrage from the joint receptors could modulate nociceptive afferent input by inhibition occurring primarily at the spinal cord level but influenced to some extent by higher centers.[15]

Passive mobilization techniques may be a means of activating type I and II mechanoreceptors, thereby reducing pain and reflex muscle spasm.[10] The type III mechanoreceptors (found only in capsules and ligaments of peripheral joints) may be activated by strong stretch or thrust techniques and may have an inhibitory effect on surrounding muscle.[10,16]

The gate-control theory has been criticized by Zusman, who contends that, in pain of spinal origin, manual therapy techniques applied at the end of the range of joint movement (ie, grades 3–5) effectively increase pain-free movement by two sequential mechanisms:

> The first of these is inhibition of muscle contraction by discharge produced in joint afferents with end of range passive joint movement. The second is a subsequent decrease in the overall level of peripheral afferent input.[15(p94)]

Zusman's contentions[15] have indirect support in the literature. Passive movement of a joint may inhibit reflex contraction of muscles both local and distant to the joint.[18] Studies on decerebrate cats confirm that the afferent activity produced by end-of-range passive movements at the knee and elbow joints has an inhibitory effect on reflex muscle contraction.[19,20] Such findings would lend support to the use of joint mobilization for children with spasticity.

End-of-range passive movements may reduce peripheral input to the CNS, thereby decreasing pain, in two ways. The first is via a temporary reduction in intra-articular pressure,[21,22] thought to be due to decreased tension on the joint capsule. This decrease in tension could be due either to fluid reduction within the joint space or to stretch of collagen fibrils.[23] Giovanelli-Blacker and colleagues[24] demonstrated a reduction in the intra-articular pressure in human apophyseal joints following passive oscillations performed at the

end range of joint movement. The second way in which end-of-range passive movements may reduce peripheral input to the CNS is through adaptation of the encapsulated endings of joint nerves to the mechanical stimulus of prolonged stretch of the periarticular soft tissue.[15,25,26]

Rationale for Effects Based on Mechanical Considerations

Although there have been no controlled studies to show that mobilization effectively restores ROM to hypomobile joints, there is literature that suggests mobilization may induce beneficial mechanical effects.[27–29]

When joint ROM is limited by capsular or ligamentous tightness or adherence, we believe that passive mobilization can be used to lengthen shortened structures or to rupture the adhesions. Paris[10] proposes that in order to have this effect, the mobilization must be performed at the limit of the joint's available range of movement, taking the tissue into the area of plastic deformation on the stress-strain curve, or, when adhesions are present, to the point of failure, causing rupture. Techniques presumably would have to be performed at the end of the range of movement (grades 3–5) for this effect. Secondary effects of improved mobility include beneficial effects on joint cartilage and intervertebral disks and improved blood and lymphatic flow.[30]

Studies comparing injured tissues (skin, tendons, ligaments) treated by immobilization with tissues treated by passive motion have demonstrated significant increases in cellularity, cell products, strength, and mobility in those tissues receiving passive motion.[30] Furthermore, Salter[31] has shown that injured articular cartilage treated by continuous passive motion improved markedly in the rate and extent of healing. A possible mechanism for this increased healing may be the improved nutrition of cartilage produced by movement. In their study of the effect of passive knee motion on the repaired medial collateral

ligaments of rabbits, Long and colleagues[32] demonstrated improved matrix organization, collagen concentration, strength, and linear stiffness of ligament scars that were moved rather than immobilized.

Although the literature supports the beneficial effects of mobilization on healing, there is a need for further research to answer questions regarding the specifics of its application (eg, optimal duration, force, and velocity of movement) in contributing to the healing process.

Rationale for Effects Based on Psychological Considerations

Psychological benefits of manual therapy that have been reported related to such factors as "the laying on of hands," reducing a pain-fear cycle, and the charisma of the clinician.[8,15] Wells[8] estimates the placebo effect to be in the neighborhood of 20% to 30%; this possibility must be considered in any critical analysis of joint mobilization efficacy and in the choice of therapeutic technique.

Contraindications and Precautions

In discussing peripheral joints, Hertling and Kessler[2] describe absolute contraindications to mobilization as bacterial infection, neoplasm, and recent fracture; relative contraindications are joint effusion or inflammation, arthroses, internal derangement, and general debilitation. Spinal mobilization, particularly spinal manipulation, has a potential for inducing serious damage to the central nervous system. Grieve lists the following absolute contraindications to mobilization of the spine[9(p445)]:

1. Malignancy involving the vertebral column.

2. Cauda equina lesions producing disturbance of bladder or bowel function.

3. Signs and symptoms of spinal cord involvement; involvement of more

than one spinal nerve root on one side or of two adjacent roots in one limb only.

4. Rheumatoid collagen necrosis of vertebral ligaments; the cervical spine is especially vulnerable.

5. Active inflammatory and infective arthritis.

6. Bone disease of the spine.

Conditions that require special care in treatment include the following: the presence of neurological signs, osteoporosis, spondylolisthesis, and the presence of dizziness that is aggravated by neck rotation or extension.[9] Documented cases in which spinal manipulation has produced consequences such as paraplegia, quadriplegia, and brain-stem thrombosis illustrate the potential danger of applying forceful techniques and emphasize the need for the clinician to proceed with skill, judgment, and caution.[33]

Application of Technique

In an effort to minimize risk to the patient, several important principles must be followed. The initial application of technique must be gentle. Assessment of the patient's signs and symptoms must occur continuously throughout the subsequent treatment. Any changes in these signs and symptoms must be used to monitor and guide treatment progression (ie, the therapist must continually monitor the response of the patient and of the joint being treated). The presence of pain or muscle spasm affects the application of the technique. Caution has been advised to avoid "pushing through" spasm when it is protecting the joint being treated.[6–8] The ability of the therapist to recognize the presence of muscle spasm while performing a small-amplitude accessory movement is therefore an essential safety factor.

Treatment techniques are chosen based on the spin, roll, and slide motions particular to the arthrokinematics of the joint and on the direction of the movement restriction.[2] As yet, the joint-play ROM has not been objectively quantified at each joint, making the grading of technique subjective. The grade of movement chosen for treatment is based on the effect desired and the irritability (ie, ease by which pain is provoked) of the joint being treated.[4–7] Grades 1 and 2 are used to treat pain; grades 3 to 5 are used to increase ROM.[4,7,10]

Efficacy of Joint Mobilization

The efficacy of any treatment modality is usually established through experimental research designs, such as clinical trials or single-subject research designs. Reviews of the literature and quantitative analyses of spinal mobilization and manipulation have concluded that efficacy has yet to be established reliably under controlled conditions.[34–36] There has been some evidence to support a small, short-term effect on pain[34–36] and a decrease in treatment visits when spinal manipulation is used.[36] In their meta-analysis on the efficacy of spinal manipulation and mobilization, Ottenbacher and Di Fabio[35] concluded that the effects of manipulation and mobilization were greater when provided in conjunction with other forms of treatment and were also greater within 1 month following therapy as compared with several months after treatment. This meta-analysis also showed that studies without random-assignment procedures were more likely to show effects in favor of the treatments than were more well-controlled studies.

Although the literature examining the efficacy of peripheral joint mobilization is extremely limited, there is some evidence to support its efficacy.[28,37] We believe that, as peripheral joint mobilization appears to be more widely used than spinal mobilization for children with cerebral palsy, there is clearly a need for additional research on the efficacy of peripheral mobilization for all types of patients.

In summary, although manual therapy is widely used and is thought to be an effective approach for treatment of pain and joint hypomobility, the scien-

tific evidence to support its efficacy is extremely limited (and nonexistent in pediatrics). The following section will explore the feasibility of using a technique designed for adults with orthopedic disorders on children with cerebral palsy and other CNS disabilities.

Joint Mobilization for Children with Central Nervous System Disorders

Even in the typically developing child, there is evidence to suggest that joint mobilization may be contraindicated. For the child with a CNS disorder, such as cerebral palsy, additional risk factors must be considered. To better understand both indications and precautions for use of mobilization in children, musculoskeletal development will be briefly described for both typically developing children and children with cerebral palsy.

Developmental Considerations

In the typically developing child, somatic muscle growth is stimulated by skeletal growth as a result of the increasing distance imposed on the muscle attachments as bone grows.[38] Thus, skeletal muscles "increase in length in parallel with, and apparently in response to, bone growth."[39(p543)] Such changes in muscle may develop if opposing muscles are paralyzed or weak, as in the case of the child with spastic cerebral palsy or in a child with spasticity (hypertonia) secondary to head injury. When the agonist muscle fails to grow normally, muscle contractures result.[40] Similarly, changes in muscle can have an effect on bones or joints (eg, muscle contractures will lead to a decrease in joint movement with possible subsequent conversion of part of the articular cartilage into fibrous tissue).[38]

Growth cartilage is present at three sites in the developing child: the epiphyseal plate, the joint surface, and the apophysis or tendon insertion (Fig. 2).[41] Injuries to each of these sites as a result of the repetitive stresses characteristic of some sports activities have been described in the

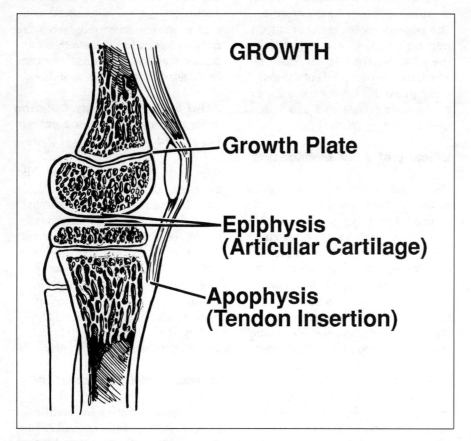

GROWTH

—— Growth Plate

—— Epiphysis
(Articular Cartilage)

—— Apophysis
(Tendon Insertion)

Figure 2. *Growth cartilage is present at three sites—the growth plate, the articular surface, and the apophysis—and is susceptible to overuse injury at each of these sites. (Adapted with permission.[41])*

literature.[41–43] During growth spurts in the typically developing child

... there can be a real increase in muscle-tendon tightness about the joints, loss of flexibility, and an enhanced environment for overuse injury.[41(p342)]

The epiphyseal growth plate has been reported to be particularly vulnerable to linear and torsional shears.[43]

Although muscle and bone growth are delayed in the involved limbs of children with cerebral palsy,[44] growth spurts presumably take place, because overall growth occurs. Research on normal and spastic mice, however, suggests that "spastic muscle grows more slowly than normal muscle in relation to bone growth."[45]

Clearly, the musculoskeletal development of children with congenital or acquired CNS injuries, particularly those that result in spasticity, is differ-

ent than that of typically developing children. Alterations in bone and muscle growth occur as a result of the effects of prolonged spasticity. According to Bleck,[46] contracture of the joint capsule occurs secondary to the immobility that results from spasticity.

Joint Mobilization in Children with Spasticity

Whereas capsular tightness may be the primary finding that indicates treatment by joint mobilization in persons with musculoskeletal disabilities, it is not the sole concern for the child with spastic cerebral palsy. When the associated findings of muscle shortening, hyperactive stretch reflexes, skeletal deviations, and muscle weakness are considered, the use of mobilization to enhance or restore joint mobility is not as straightforward. Further, clinicians must ponder the potential impact of applying repetitive mechanical forces to children. The

predisposition of immature growth plates to injury—particularly during growth spurts—suggests the need to be cautious when using joint mobilization on children.

Cochrane[3] has suggested that joint motion limitations in older children with long-standing hypomobility may be secondary to capsular tightening and adhesions. She proposed that joint mobilization, provided in conjunction with neurophysiological forms of therapeutic exercise, may be indicated for such children. Cochrane cautions, however, that

... capsular dysfunction may be difficult to differentiate from movement restriction caused by muscle tightness in the patient with spasticity.[3(p1108)]

She recommends that therapists become competent in assessing joints of individuals with and without orthopedic problems before trying to assess children who have neurologic deficits. In light of the complex problems associated with spasticity, such as hyperactive stretch reflexes, muscle shortening, and muscle weakness, we are in full agreement with Cochrane's suggestion.

In an overview of orthopedic manual therapy published in 1979, Cookson and Kent[4] described the treatment approaches of a number of the leading proponents of manual therapy—Cyriax, Kaltenborn, Maitland, and Mennell. Common to all of these approaches is the need for both "subjective" and "objective" evaluations before initiating treatment. The subjective evaluation is based predominantly on a pain model, with the examiner questioning the patient about the nature, location, and severity of the pain. The use of such a subjective evaluation for children with CNS disorders is problematic for two reasons. First, pain is not commonly an issue for children with cerebral palsy, except in some cases of hip subluxation or dislocation. It is doubtful that mobilization would be useful in such cases, because dislocation can be reduced only by surgery.[47] Second, many children with cerebral palsy are unable to communicate effectively because of speech impairments or mental retardation. Thus, a subjective evaluation is often not possible or may be unreliable. Failure to obtain a reliable subjective evaluation interferes with the therapist's ability to monitor response to treatment (ie, to determine whether treatment soreness has occurred).

In summary, the capsular restrictions that occur in joints of *older* children with spastic cerebral palsy may be indications for using joint mobilization procedures.[3] Caution, however, should be exercised. The technique that is recommended for a chronically tight joint is a vigorous grade 4 procedure.[48] As Cochrane has cautioned, however, care must be taken not to impose a quick stretch of the muscles surrounding the joint for fear of temporarily increasing spasticity.[3]

The presence of immature growth plates is another reason for caution. If joint mobilization were to be used for younger children or children undergoing growth spurts, for example, only gentle oscillations should be used to avoid the production of pain or reactive muscle spasm during treatment.

Central Nervous System Disorders for Which Joint Mobilization Is Contraindicated

Although a case can be made for cautious and conservative use of peripheral joint mobilization in older children with joint restriction secondary to spasticity, there are a number of neurodevelopmental disabilities for which joint mobilization and, particularly spinal manipulation, would be strongly contraindicated. Although physical therapists would likely not use joint mobilization in the presence of hypermobile joints, specific statements about the children for whom this treatment is contraindicated are warranted.

In the child with pure athetoid and ataxic forms of cerebral palsy, joints tend to be hypermobile.[49] Hypermobility of the spine in children with athetoid cerebral palsy may lead to cervical instability; researchers have

noted that "rapid and repetitious neck movements seem to accelerate the progression of cervical instability in athetoid CP patients."[50]

Another common neurodevelopmental disability in which joints are hypermobile secondary to lax ligaments is Down syndrome. In a report of 265 individuals with Down syndrome, 23% of the subjects had patellar instability leading to subluxation or dislocation and 10% had hip subluxation or dislocation.[51] Of even greater concern in Down syndrome is the presence of atlantoaxial instability, which has been reported in up to 15% of individuals with this disorder.[52]

Other, less common, neurodevelopmental disabilities, such as Prader-Willi syndrome, may be characterized by generalized hypotonia and hypermobile joints.[53] For these children as well, joint mobilization would be contraindicated. Many children with generalized development delay of unknown etiology also exhibit hypotonia and ligamentous laxity.

Future Research Directions in Joint Mobilization for Children with Central Nervous System Disorders

Cochrane[3] concluded that research on mobilization was warranted, both to document benefits and to determine precautions, for using joint mobilization for children with CNS deficits. In spite of that call for research more than 4 years ago, no published studies were located in the medical literature that addressed either precautions for or efficacy of joint mobilization in children.

Despite the lack of demonstrated efficacy for these procedures, short courses on joint mobilization in children continue to be offered throughout North America. A random perusal of continuing education courses advertised in *Physical Therapy* during the past 2 years revealed more than a dozen short courses on mobilization or manual therapy in the child with neurological involvement.

As Cochrane[3] has suggested, case studies should be conducted to document the outcomes of joint mobilization. Because children with spasticity and secondary joint hypomobility appear to be the candidates of choice for this procedure, case studies should be conducted by therapists who have been well trained in manual therapy, both in their entry-level education and in specific continuing education courses that strengthen baseline knowledge and skills.

Single-subject research designs, with replications across several subjects, would provide appropriate methodologies for assessing short-term and long-term effects of mobilization on ROM and minimization of contractures.[54,55] Randomized clinical trials, although difficult to conduct, could provide more generalizable answers about the efficacy of joint mobilization procedures. In addressing the effectiveness of this treatment modality, *functional* outcome measures should be used.[56] Clinical researchers will need to address the effect of mobilization not only on impairment but also on disability. For example, even if joint mobilization could be shown to increase isolated joint motions in the upper extremity, what effect would this have on the child's level of independence in eating or dressing?

In addition to examining the efficacy of these procedures, research is needed to evaluate the reliability of assessment techniques in differentiating the causes of movement restriction (ie, muscle tightness versus capsular restriction). In addition to studying children who have spastic cerebral palsy, mobilization for children who have chronic spasticity and joint restrictions resulting from traumatic brain injury should also be examined.

Conclusions

As has been true throughout the history of physical therapy, the fervor for adopting an innovative treatment technique, such as joint mobilization, has far exceeded the availability of scientific support for these procedures. Although there is limited research support for the use of mobilization in adults who have musculoskeletal disorders, there have been no published studies examining its efficacy for use in children with CNS disorders. Until such research is conducted and the results are disseminated, pediatric physical therapists should be cautious in their use of joint mobilization.

References

1 Ben-Sorek S, Davis CM. Joint mobilization education and clinical use in the United States. *Phys Ther.* 1988;68:1000–1004.

2 Hertling D, Kessler RM. *Management of Common Musculoskeletal Disorders: Physical Therapy Principles and Methods.* Philadelphia, Pa: JB Lippincott Co; 1990.

3 Cochrane CG. Joint mobilization principles: considerations for use in the child with central nervous system dysfunction. *Phys Ther.* 1987; 67:1105–1109.

4 Maitland GD. *Vertebral Manipulation.* Boston, Mass: Butterworth Publishers; 1986.

5 Cookson JC, Kent BE. Orthopedic manual therapy—an overview, part 1: the extremities. *Phys Ther.* 1979;59:135–146.

6 Cookson JC. Orthopedic manual therapy—an overview, part 2: the spine. *Phys Ther.* 1979;59:259–267.

7 Maitland GD. *Peripheral Manipulation.* Boston, Mass: Butterworth Publishers; 1977.

8 Wells PE. Manipulative procedures. In: Wells PE, Frampton V, Bowsher D, eds. *Pain Management in Physical Therapy.* East Norwalk, Conn: Appleton & Lange; 1988:181–217.

9 Grieve GP. Contra-indications to spinal manipulation and allied treatments. *Physiotherapy.* 1989;75:445–453.

10 Paris SV. Mobilization of the spine. *Phys Ther.* 1979;59:989–995.

11 Cyriax JH. *Textbook of Orthopaedic Medicine: Diagnosis of Soft Tissue Lesions.* 6th ed. Baltimore, Md: Williams & Wilkins; 1975:vol 1.

12 Matyas TA, Bach TM. The reliability of selected techniques in clinical arthrometrics. *Australian Journal of Physiotherapy.* 1985; 31:175–199.

13 Jull G, Bogduk N, Marsland A. The accuracy of manual diagnosis for cervical zygapophyseal joint pain syndromes. *Med J Aust.* 1988; 148:233–236.

14 Evans DH. The reliability of assessment parameters: accuracy of palpation technique. In: Grieve GP, ed. *Modern Manual Therapy of the Vertebral Column.* New York, NY: Churchill Livingstone Inc; 1986:498–502.

15 Zusman M. Spinal manipulative therapy: review of some proposed mechanisms and a new hypothesis. *Australian Journal of Physiotherapy.* 1986;32:89–99.

16 Wyke BD. The neurology of joints. *Annals of the Royal College of Surgeons of England.* 1967;41:25–50.

17 Melzack R, Wall PD. Cited by: Zusman M. Spinal manipulative therapy: review of some proposed mechanisms and a new hypothesis.

Australian Journal of Physiotherapy. 1986; 32:89–99.

18 Wyke BD. Articular neurology and manipulative therapy. In: Glasgow EF, Twomey LT, Scull ER, Kleynhans AM, eds. *Aspects of Manipulative Therapy.* Edinburgh, Scotland: Churchill Livingstone; 1985:72–77.

19 Baxendale RH, Ferrell WR. The effect of knee joint afferent discharge on transmission in flexion reflex pathways in decerebrate cats. *J Physiol (Lond).* 1981;315:231–242.

20 Baxendale RH, Ferrell WR. Modulation of transmission in forelimb flexion reflex pathways by elbow joint afferent discharge in decerebrate cats. *Brain Res.* 1981;221:393–396.

21 Levick JR. An investigation into the validity of subatmospheric pressure recordings from synovial fluid and their dependence on joint angle. *J Physiol (Lond).* 1979;289:55–67.

22 Nade S, Newbold PJ. Factors determining the level and changes in intra-articular pressure in the knee joint of the dog. *J Physiol (Lond).* 1983;338:21–36.

23 Wood L, Ferrell WR. Fluid compartmentation and articular mechanoreceptor discharge in the cat knee joint. *Q J Exp Physiol.* 1985; 70:329–335.

24 Giovanelli-Blacker B, Elvey R, Thompson E. Cited by: Zusman M. Spinal manipulative therapy: review of some proposed mechanisms and a new hypothesis. *Australian Journal of Physiotherapy.* 1986;32:89–99.

25 Grigg P, Greenspan BJ. Response of primate joint afferent neurons to mechanical stimulation of the knee joint. *J Neurophysiol.* 1977;40:1–8.

26 Millar J. Flexion-extension sensitivity of elbow joint afferents in the cat. *Exp Brain Res.* 1965;24:209–214.

27 Olson VL. Evaluation of joint mobilization treatment: a method. *Phys Ther.* 1987;67: 351–356.

28 Nicholson GG. The effects of passive joint mobilization on pain and hypomobility associated with adhesive capsulitis of the shoulder. *Journal of Orthopaedic and Sports Physical Therapy.* 1985;6:238–246.

29 Cibulka MT, Delitto A, Koldehoff RM. Changes in innominate tilt after manipulation of the sacroiliac joint in patients with low back pain. *Phys Ther.* 1988;68:1359–1363.

30 Frank C, Akeson WH, Woo SL-Y, et al. Physiology and therapeutic value of passive joint motion. *Clin Orthop.* 1984;185:113–125.

31 Salter RB. The biological effects of continuous passive motion. *J Bone Joint Surg [Am].* 1980;62:1232–1251.

32 Long ML, Frank C, Schachar NS, et al. The effects of motion on normal and healing ligaments. *Proc Orthop Res Soc.* 1982;7:43. Abstract.

33 Grieve GP. Incidents and accidents of manipulation. In: Grieve GP, ed. *Modern Manual Therapy in the Vertebral Column.* New York, NY: Churchill Livingstone Inc; 1986:873–884.

34 Di Fabio RP. Clinical assessment of manipulation and mobilization of the lumbar spine: a critical review of the literature. *Phys Ther.* 1986;66:51–54.

35 Ottenbacher K, Di Fabio RP. Efficacy of spinal manipulation/mobilization therapy: a meta-analysis. *Spine.* 1985;10:833–837.

36 O'Donoghue CE. Manipulation trials. In: Grieve GP, ed. *Modern Manual Therapy of the*

Vertebral Column. New York, NY: Churchill Livingstone Inc: 1986:849–859.

37 Moritz U. Evaluation of manipulation and other manual therapy: criteria for measuring the effect of treatment. *Scand J Rehabil Med.* 1979;11:173–179.

38 Sinclair D. *Human Growth After Birth.* 5th ed. Oxford, England: Oxford University Press; 1989.

39 O'Dwyer NJ, Neilson PD, Nash J. Mechanisms of muscle growth related to muscle contracture in cerebral palsy. *Dev Med Child Neurol.* 1989;31:543–552.

40 Bax MCO, Brown JK. Contractures and their therapy. *Dev Med Child Neurol.* 1985; 27:423–424.

41 Micheli LJ. Overuse injuries in children's sports: the growth factor. *Orthop Clin North Am.* 1983;14:337–360.

42 Zito M. Musculoskeletal injuries of young athletes: the new trends. In: Gould JA, ed. *Orthopaedic and Sports Physical Therapy.* 2nd ed. St Louis, Mo: CV Mosby Co; 1990:627–650.

43 Speer DP, Braun JK. The biomechanical basis of growth plate injuries. *The Physician and Sportsmedicine.* 1985;13:72–78.

44 Staheli LT, Duncan WR, Schaefer E. Growth alterations in the hemiplegic child. *Clin Orthop.* 1968;60:205–212.

45 Ziv I, Blackburn N, Rang M, Koreska J. Muscle growth in normal and spastic mice. *Dev Med Child Neurol.* 1984;26:94–99.

46 Bleck EE. The hip in cerebral palsy. *Orthop Clin North Am.* 1980;11:79–104.

47 Samilson RL, Tsou P, Aamoth G, Green WM. Dislocation and subluxation of the hip in cerebral palsy: pathogenesis, natural history and management. *J Bone Joint Surg [Am].* 1972;54:863–873.

48 Kessler RM, Hertling D. Cited by: Cochrane CG. Joint mobilization principles: considerations for use in the child with central nervous system dysfunction. *Phys Ther.* 1987;67:1105–1109.

49 Bobath K. *The Motor Deficit in Patients with Cerebral Palsy.* Lavenham, Suffolk, England: Lavenham Press; 1966:17–20, 47–51.

50 Ebara S, Harada T, Yamazaki Y, et al. Unstable cervical spine in athetoid cerebral palsy. *Spine.* 1989;14:1154–1159.

51 Diamond LS, Lynne D, Sigman B. Orthopedic disorders in patients with Down's syndrome. *Orthop Clin North Am.* 1981;12:57–71.

52 Pueschel SM, Scola FH. Epidemiologic, radiographic and clinical studies of atlantoaxial instability in individuals with Down syndrome. *Pediatrics.* 1987;80:555–560.

53 Fenichel GM. The newborn with poor muscle tone. *Semin Perinatol.* 1982;6:68–88.

54 Martin J, Epstein L. Evaluating treatment effectiveness in cerebral palsy. *Phys Ther.* 1976; 56:285–294.

55 Gonnella C. Single-subject experimental paradigm as a clinical decision tool. *Phys Ther.* 1989;69:601–609.

56 Harris SR. Efficacy of physical therapy in promoting family functioning and functional independence for children with cerebral palsy. *Pediatric Physical Therapy.* 1990;2:160–164.

Current Treatment Approaches in the Nonoperative and Operative Management of Adolescent Idiopathic Scoliosis

Idiopathic scoliosis is the most common type of lateral curvature of the spine, accounting for about 65% of adolescent patients with structural scoliosis. The treatment goal is to prevent moderate curves from becoming severe, because severe curves, in adults, may not only lead to serious medical and physical complications, but also cause significant cosmetic deformities. Fortunately, early detection, through school screening programs, has led to successful nonoperative management of idiopathic scoliosis. In those instances in which nonoperative management is not an option, surgical correction is available. Surgery prevents curve progression and offers the patient a significant correction of the cosmetic deformity. This article will review both treatment approaches in the management of adolescent idiopathic scoliosis. [Cassella MC, Hall JE. Current treatment approaches in the nonoperative and operative management of adolescent idiopathic scoliosis. Phys Ther. 1991;71:897–909.]

Key Words: *Curve progression, nonoperative, operative; Scoliosis.*

Michelina C Cassella
John E Hall

The word "scoliosis" is derived from the ancient Greek word, *Skolí-ōsis*, meaning a curve. In medicine, it means lateral curvature of the spine.[1] The spinal column, when examined in the sagittal plane, has normal anterior and posterior curvatures (lordosis and kyphosis, respectively). In the anteroposterior plane, a lateral curvature of over 10 degrees is usually abnormal. The purpose of this article is to review both operative and nonoperative treatment of adolescent idiopathic scoliosis.

Structural Versus Nonstructural Scoliosis

Scoliosis is either structural or nonstructural. A structural curve usually has a rotary component.[2,3] Clinically, a structural curve will not correct when the trunk is flexed forward and will not fully correct in a supine, bending radiograph. Conversely, a nonstructural curve has no rotary component and will usually straighten when the trunk is flexed forward. When viewed on radiographs, a nonstructural curve will often correct or overcorrect.[2] Some causes of nonstructural scoliosis are leg-length discrepancies, postural problems, muscle spasm (involuntary

muscle contraction), and spinal tumors. Nonstructural curves associated with muscle spasm and spinal tumors may even be exaggerated when the patient bends forward. This, however, causes pain, which is not a characteristic of other curves.

Classification

Structural scoliosis is classified by *magnitude, location, direction,* and *etiology.*[3] The Cobb method is the most widely accepted method of measuring curve magnitude (Fig. 1).[4] The location of a structural curve is determined by its apical vertebra, which is the spinal segment with the greatest degree of rotation (Fig. 2).[5] In structural scoliosis, the vertebral bodies rotate toward the convex side of the curve. The direction of a structural scoliosis is determined by the convex side of the curve. A structural curve is described by both the location of the apical vertebra and the direction

MC Cassella, BS, PT, is Associate Director, Department of Physical Therapy and Occupational Therapy Services, Children's Hospital, 300 Longwood Ave, Boston MA 02115 (USA), Physical Therapy Consultant to the Spinal Program, Children's Hospital, and Lecturer on Orthopaedic Surgery, Harvard Medical School, 25 Shattuck St, Boston, MA 02115. Address correspondence to Ms Cassella at the first address.

JE Hall, MD, is Orthopaedic Surgeon-in-Chief, Department of Orthopaedics, Children's Hospital, and Professor of Orthopaedic Surgery, Harvard Medical School.

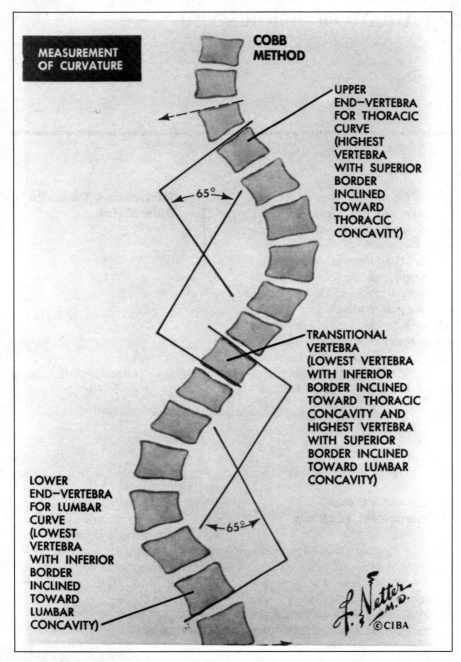

MEASUREMENT OF CURVATURE

COBB METHOD

UPPER END–VERTEBRA FOR THORACIC CURVE (HIGHEST VERTEBRA WITH SUPERIOR BORDER INCLINED TOWARD THORACIC CONCAVITY)

65°

TRANSITIONAL VERTEBRA (LOWEST VERTEBRA WITH INFERIOR BORDER INCLINED TOWARD THORACIC CONCAVITY AND HIGHEST VERTEBRA WITH SUPERIOR BORDER INCLINED TOWARD LUMBAR CONCAVITY)

LOWER END–VERTEBRA FOR LUMBAR CURVE (LOWEST VERTEBRA WITH INFERIOR BORDER INCLINED TOWARD LUMBAR CONCAVITY)

65°

Figure 1. *Cobb method of measurement.[4] (Reproduced with permission from Clin Symp. 1972;24[1].)*

(Tab. 1).[2] For example, if the apex is at T-8, with the convexity of the curve to the right, the curve is described as right thoracic.

Structural curves are further described as *major* and *minor* curves. An individual's major curve, by definition, is the largest curve and usually has the greatest degree of vertebral rotation of all the curves present. The minor curves are smaller and have lesser de-

grees of vertebral rotation. Minor curves are more flexible and usually develop to compensate for the major curve.[2,5]

Although there are many known causes of structural scoliosis, the most common type is idiopathic scoliosis, which occurs during the growing years.[6] Idiopathic scoliosis is categorized by age group: infantile (birth–3 years), juvenile (3–10 years), and

adolescent (>10 years). This classification indicates the age when the curve was diagnosed; however, age at diagnosis does not always coincide with the time the curve(s) first appeared.[7]

This article will focus on adolescent idiopathic scoliosis, which occurs in about 65% of adolescent patients with structural curves.[6] The term "idiopathic" means of unknown etiology. It is now known that idiopathic scoliosis is genetic in origin; however, the mechanism of development remains unknown. Current theories implicate neural mechanisms involving balance and coordination deficits as etiological factors.[8,9]

Early Detection and School Screening

Lateral curves are often first noticed by parents. Many times parents observe postural abnormalities when their children are wearing bathing suits, or a mother may detect an abnormality when hemming a pair of pants or a skirt. A comment often heard is: "I noticed a problem because I always have to alter her clothes so they will hang evenly."

Lateral curves are also detected by pediatricians during routine physical examinations. The majority of lateral curves, however, are detected in school screening programs. Screening programs began in the 1940s and have become widespread in the United States, Canada, and other countries.[7] School screening is currently mandatory in approximately one third of the schools in the United States. Screening programs are conducted on students aged 10 to 16 years (grades 5–9), because this is the age group of highest risk for adolescent idiopathic scoliosis.[7,10]

Much has been learned about the natural history of scoliosis from school screening programs. Most of the data generated from screening programs are predictive of prevalence rate. Prevalence rate refers to the proportion of a population with a disease or disorder and is ex-

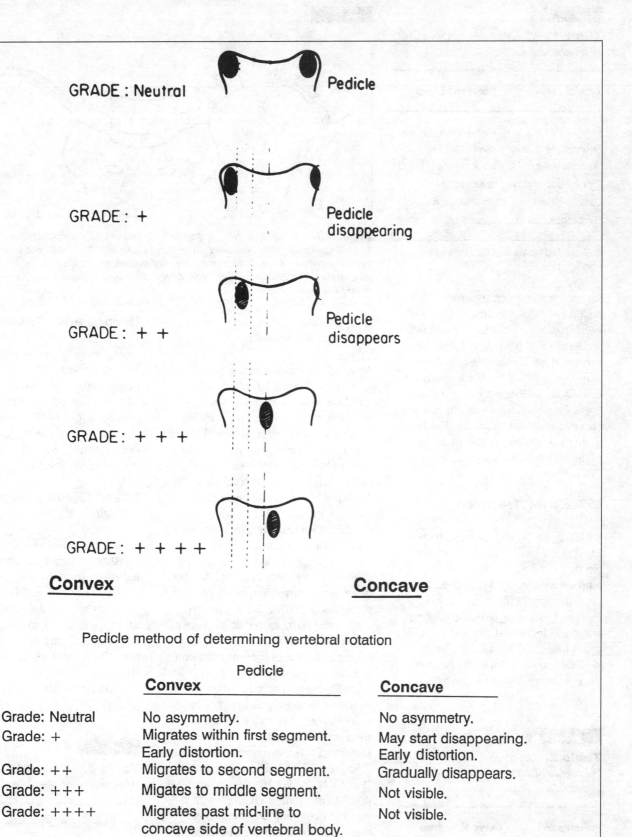

GRADE : Neutral — Pedicle

GRADE : + — Pedicle disappearing

GRADE : + + — Pedicle disappears

GRADE : + + +

GRADE : + + + +

Convex   **Concave**

Pedicle method of determining vertebral rotation

| | Pedicle | |
	Convex	Concave
Grade: Neutral	No asymmetry.	No asymmetry.
Grade: +	Migrates within first segment. Early distortion.	May start disappearing. Early distortion.
Grade: ++	Migrates to second segment.	Gradually disappears.
Grade: +++	Migates to middle segment.	Not visible.
Grade: ++++	Migrates past mid-line to concave side of vertebral body.	Not visible.

Figure 2. *Evaluation of vertebral rotation. (Reproduced with permission.[5])*

pressed as the number of cases per 1,000 individuals in the population.[11] Most studies reflect a preva-lence of 2% to 4% of the population for curves of at least 10 degrees. More important is the prevalence of curves greater than 20 degrees, be-cause children with remaining skel-etal growth and this degree of cur-

Table 1. *Classification of Curvatures by Anatomic Area*[a]

Type of Curve	Location of Apex
Cervical curve:	apex between C1–C6
Cervicothoracic curve:	apex at C7–T1
Thoracic curve:	apex between T2–T11
Thoracolumbar curve:	apex at T12–L1
Lumbar curve:	apex between L2–L4
Lumbosacral curve:	apex at L5–S1

[a]Reproduced courtesy of the Scoliosis Research Society.

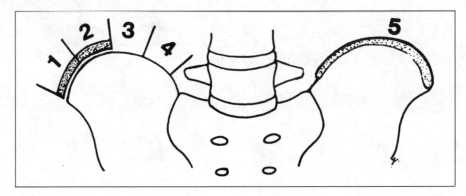

Figure 3. *Risser sign. Iliac epiphysis: ossification of the epiphysis usually starts at the anterior superior iliac spine and progresses posteriorly. The iliac crest is divided into four quarters, and the excursion or stage of maturity is designated as the amount of progression. The example shows 50% completion, indicating a Risser sign of 2. (Reproduced with permission.[7])*

vature may require treatment.[7] Based on most studies, it is considered that 1 to 3 children per 1,000 screened will have structural curves greater than 20 degrees. Nachemson,[12] using data from many studies, calculated a table showing the decreasing prevalence with increasing curve magnitude (Tab. 2). The female:male ratios appear to be dependent on curve magnitude (Tab. 3).[13]

Criteria for Treatment

Which children with positive findings for scoliosis will require treatment? No data exist as to which curves will tend to progress.[14,15] It is clear, however, that mild curves are very common and rarely progressive. Once a curve has increased beyond 30 degrees in a child with considerable skeletal growth remaining, progression is almost inevitable. Skeletal

growth is assessed by the Risser sign (Fig. 3) or by skeletal age.[16,17]

Although school screening programs have helped considerably to identify children with a potentially serious scoliosis, these programs have also caused many children with mild, nonprogressive curves to undergo unnecessary tests and evaluative procedures. One should be very careful in labeling a mild, nonprogressive curve as scoliosis because of the implication for the individual's future, with respect to health and life insurance.

In the past, the only definitive method of assessing curve progression was by roentgenogram. A child whose structural curve is diagnosed at 10 years of age could possibly have one or two roentgenograms every 6 months until the end of skeletal growth, as indicated by radiographic analysis.[17] Alternatives to roentgenography that do not require exposure to radiation are moiré shadow photography (Fig. 4) and the Integrated Shape Investigation System (ISIS) topographical scanning system (Fig. 5). Both alternatives have made it possible to monitor children with mild structural curves without exposing them to unnecessary radiation.[18–20] A roentgenogram is necessary only if there is a significant change in the moiré pattern or ISIS contour.

Nonoperative Treatment

In our view, there is little doubt among experts that a 25- to 30-degree curve in a growing child with documented progression by roentgenogram will require treatment.[7,12] Controversy remains, however, about the effectiveness of nonoperative regimens.[21]

Lateral Electrical Surface Stimulation

Lateral electrical surface stimulation consists of stimulating the paraspinal musculature on the convex side of the major curve. The technique requires nightly application of intermittent electrical stimulation by use of surface electrodes.[22] The indications for lateral electrical surface stimulation are essentially the same as those for orthotic treatment: skel-

Table 2. *Relationship Between Prevalence of Idiopathic Scoliosis and Magnitude of Curve*[a]

Prevalence	Curve Magnitude
2–3%	>10 degrees
0.3–0.5%	>20 degrees
0.2–0.3%	>30 degrees

[a]Reproduced with permission.[12]

Table 3. *Relationship Between Curve Magnitude and Female:Male Ratio*[13]

Curve Magnitude (°)	Female:Male Ratio
6–10	1:1
11–20	1.4:1
>21	5.4:1
Curves under treatment	7.2:1

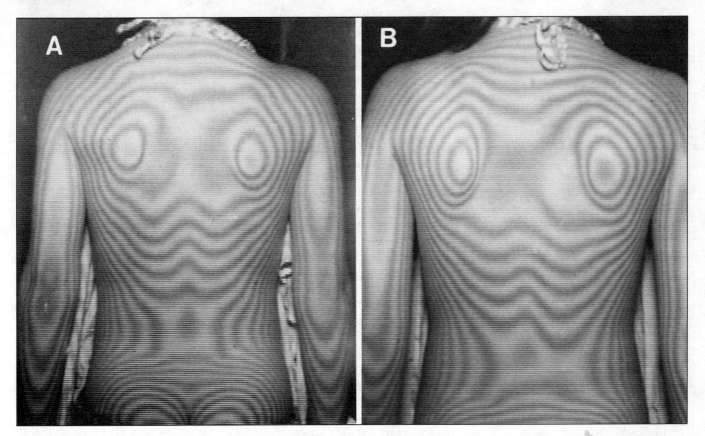

Figure 4. *Moiré topography, a noninvasive, photogrammetric technique using shadow patterns as contours to assess surface asymmetry[20]: (A) relative symmetric contour; (B) asymmetric contour. (Courtesy of Department of Orthopaedics, Children's Hospital, Boston, Mass.)*

etal immaturity, a structural curve(s) of 25 to 40 degrees, and documenting progression of the curve(s).[23] This treatment is appealing to children because they have the stimulation at night, while sleeping, and are therefore free from having to wear a brace during the day.

Although early studies using lateral electrical surface stimulation appeared promising, the results of this treatment in recent years, have been disappointing.[21,23] Sullivan et al[23] reported on 142 patients who were treated by the Scolitron method of lateral electrical surface stimulation. One hundred fourteen of the patients (80.1%) were compliant with the treatment, which was continued until skeletal maturity, as determined by radiography. A curve progression of 10% was considered a failure. With this criterion, 56% were classified as failures, 27% as successes, and 17% as undetermined because treatment was not completed. Noncompliant patients were included with the failures. The authors concluded that this method

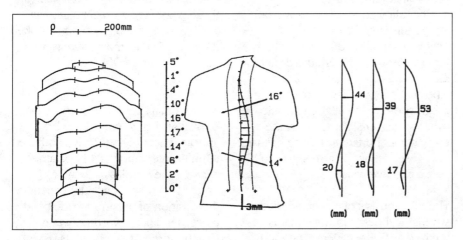

Figure 5. *Integrated Shape Investigation System (ISIS), a noninvasive, automated stereophotogrammetric technique that utilizes computer imaging and measures contours in the transverse, frontal, and sagittal planes.[21] Contour patterns of a patient with a right thoracolumbar structural scoliosis. (Courtesy of Department of Orthopaedics, Children's Hospital, Boston, Mass.)*

could not be considered an alternative to bracing.

Orthotic Management

In the skeletally immature child, the use of orthoses is the most widely accepted method of nonoperative treatment for progressive curves greater than 25 degrees. The use of braces to stop the progression of structural curves dates back to the time of Hippocrates.[3] From the 4th century until the early part of the 20th century, spinal deformities were treated with forcible horizontal traction and leg distraction in suspension, corsets, casts, and a variety of braces.[3,7] The brace, however, that established the role of orthoses in effective curve control is the Milwaukee brace (MWB), developed by Blount and Schmidt in 1946.[24] This brace was originally designed as a postoperative means of spinal support to substitute for the distraction plaster jacket. The MWB, however, has been used successfully in the nonoperative management of scoliosis since the mid-1950s.[3,24]

The MWB consists of a customized pelvic girdle taken from a plaster cast of the asymmetric spine. A metal superstructure, which initially served as a distractive force, is then attached to the pelvic girdle. The lateral corrective pads are applied slightly below the apex of the curve in the thoracic region and at the apex of the curve in the lumbar region. The lumbar pads are located within the pelvic girdle. The thoracic pads are secured onto the superstructure. The superstructure extends to the occiput posteriorly and to throat level anteriorly.[24]

The MWB was the brace of choice until the early 1970s when the low-profile, Boston Bracing System (BBS) was designed by Hall and Miller.[25,26] The development of the BBS led to a variety of bracing approaches for management of adolescent idiopathic scoliosis without the use of a superstructure. Variants of the BBS are referred to as either low-profile or thoracolumbar-sacral (TLSO) orthoses.[27]

Long-term follow-up studies using the MWB indicate that the brace is most successful in halting the progression of moderate curves.[28] Because moderate curves respond better to a lateral force than to a distractive force, a brace that would eliminate the metal superstructure and still provide lateral correction might be more cosmetically acceptable to children. The BBS provides this alternative.

Both the MWB and the BBS adhere to the principles of providing active and passive correction through pelvic stabilization, together with a system of lateral corrective forces to facilitate remodeling of the vertebral column. Each brace uses pressure pads, with relief or void areas opposite the pressure pads. The most effective method of curve control is to apply a direct force at the apex of the curve; however, because the vertebral column is not accessible, corrective forces must be applied indirectly.[7,24] This corrective force is applied via the ribs in the thoracic spine and via the paraspinal muscles overlying the transverse processes in the lumbar spine. In the lumbar spine, the lateral force is applied at the apex of the curve; however, because of the downward slope of the ribs in the thoracic spine, the lateral corrective force is applied to the rib attached to the vertebra below the apex. In order to achieve the best application of corrective forces, the vertebral column must be controlled and not allowed to move away from the posterolateral corrective pads. This is accomplished by controlling lumbar lordosis through the design of the pelvic girdle.[3] The overall goal of a bracing program is to prevent curve progression and to align the trunk over the sacrum. Whichever brace is used, it is important to realize that the brace itself is merely a shell to support corrective pads.

The BBS consists of a prefabricated symmetrical pelvic module that is customized to fit the patient. The modules are available in 22 sizes and fit 85% of all patients requiring braces. Structural curves with apices at T-7 and below have been successfully treated using this brace without a su-

perstructure.[29] The lateral corrective pads are located within the module. The BBS has the advantage of improved cosmesis and rapid fabrication. An experienced orthotist can fabricate a brace in about 2 hours.

The BBS is actually a system of braces using different modules for different levels of curves (Fig. 6).[30] In order for the bracing program to be successful, the patient must

1. Be willing to wear the brace for the prescribed number of hours per day until skeletal growth is completed, as determined by a left hand and wrist roentgenogram.[27]

2. Have a well-fitting brace that has been fabricated using the roentgenogram as a blueprint. A bracing facility with orthotists who adhere to design specifications and are experts in brace fabrication is essential.[30]

3. Try to resume a normal lifestyle while wearing the brace, so that the brace becomes a natural part of daily life. This goal may not be possible for insecure adolescents.

Until the late 1980s, patients were instructed to wear the brace 23 hours per day. Recent studies by Emans et al[29] and Bassett et al,[31] however, noted similar success rates between patients who were fully compliant and those who were partially compliant with wearing the brace the prescribed 23 hours. Today, most patients are instructed to wear the brace 16 to 18 hours per day.

A preliminary report by Price et al[32] of patients using a nighttime brace appears encouraging. They conducted a multicenter study of 139 patients wearing the Charleston bending brace. This brace holds the patient in the position of maximum side-bend correction and is worn only at night. One hundred fifteen patients (83%) showed improvement or less than a 5-degree change in curvature. Twenty-four patients (17%) demonstrated an increase in curvature of greater than 5 degrees. Only 44 patients, however,

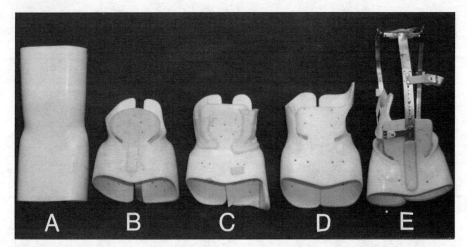

Figure 6. *Boston braces: (A) Module from which the brace is fabricated (comes in 22 sizes); (B) Boston lumbar brace, for lumbar curves (apex at L2–4 and lumbosacral curves; (C) Boston thoracolumbar brace, for thoracolumbar curves (apex at T12-L1) and low thoracic curves (apex at T10–11), (D) Boston thoracic brace, for thoracic curves with apex at T-8 and below and for double curves when the upper curve has its apex at T-8 or below; (E) Boston brace with superstructure, for thoracic curves with apex above T-8 and double curves when the upper curve has its apex at about T-8. (Courtesy of Department of Orthopaedics and the National Orthotics and Prosthetics Corp (NOPCO), Children's Hospital, Boston, Mass.)*

completed the treatment program. Based on these findings, use of this type of brace appears promising, although further investigation with longer follow-up will be necessary.[32]

We believe that successful orthotic management of children with idiopathic scoliosis depends on the following factors: proper curve selection, patient/family commitment and education, and a dedicated team of professionals committed to a successful bracing program. Patients undergoing treatment must be examined at regular intervals (eg, 3 months, 6 months, or more frequently if there are problems) to monitor the effects of treatment.

Team Approach

A treatment team consisting of an orthopedic surgeon, an orthotist, a nurse, and a physical therapist, who monitor this patient population in a clinical setting, makes the long-term management of these patients not only successful but also very rewarding. Patients and their families gain knowledge and support from the professional team as well as from other children and families undergoing sim-

ilar treatment. The clinician, however, should not attempt to minimize the social impact on the adolescent of wearing a brace and appearing "different" from peers during this crucial period.

Each member of the treatment team plays an important role in the success of the bracing program. In our experience, the orthopedic surgeon performs a clinical assessment, interprets the radiographic findings, and discusses a treatment plan with the patient and family. The orthotist measures the patient and fabricates and fits the brace. The nurse coordinates the clinic, instructs the patient in brace application and skin care, and provides the patient with a schedule for adjusting to the brace. The physical therapist performs a comprehensive assessment, interprets the results, and designs an individual exercise program based on the findings. Each team member provides a great deal of emotional support to both the patient and family throughout the course of treatment. A highly motivated, enthusiastic team can have a very positive influence on both patients and families.

Physical Therapy Management

The role of exercise in the nonoperative management of adolescent idiopathic scoliosis is controversial.[33] There have been attempts to correct structural curves with vigorous exercises alone, stressing active derotation of the spine.[34]

Lovett devoted an entire section of his 1907 text *Lateral Curvature of the Spine and Round Shoulders*[35] to the appropriate role of exercises. Although Lovett was a strong supporter of the use of exercises in conjunction with the nonoperative approach to the management of adolescent idiopathic scoliosis, he did state,

> It is obviously unreasonable to expect free standing gymnastic exercises to straighten marked or severe curves or to change the shape of distorted bones.[35(p120)]

Lovett further stated,

> The purely gymnastic treatment of severe structural scoliosis is today being largely pursued by two classes of persons. First, by irresponsible masseurs and medical gymnasts who hold as a tradition that gymnastic exercises are curative or at least helpful in scoliosis and, second, by competent surgeons who do not believe in corsets or supports.[35(pp120–121)]

Today, most experts agree that exercise alone will not affect the progression of a structural scoliosis. There is agreement, however, that a selective exercise program in conjunction with bracing treatment is beneficial.[36,37]

Prior to the initiation of an exercise program, the patient should have a comprehensive assessment, which includes the following measures:

1. *Posture*—inspection of the patient's natural, relaxed posture in the anterior, posterior, and lateral views.

2. *Leg length*—measurement of leg lengths, both real (measured from the anterior superior iliac crest to the medial malleolus) and apparent (measured from the umbilicus to the medial malleolus). These measurements are used to deter-

mine the presence of leg-length discrepancies that might affect postural alignment and brace fit.

3. *Range of motion (ROM)*—with emphasis on areas that could have a negative effect on brace fit such as the hip flexor, hamstring, tensor fasciae latae, and low back muscles and the trunk and shoulder girdle.

4. *Muscle strength*—with emphasis on the abdominal musculature.

5. *Breathing pattern*—essential especially if the patient has a history of asthma or any other respiratory disorder.

6. *Functional activity levels*—to establish a baseline, in order to assist the patient in returning to prebracing activity levels.

Designing a realistic, individual therapeutic exercise program targeting areas with positive findings can be instrumental in assisting the patient with brace compliance. If the brace fits well and the patient can resume physical activities, he or she is more likely to wear the brace the prescribed number of hours.

The purpose of the exercise program is to help the patient:

1. Develop postural awareness with the ability to maintain corrected alignment not only while wearing the brace but also at the completion of the bracing program.

2. Maintain proper respiration and chest mobility.

3. Maintain muscle strength, especially in the lower and oblique abdominal muscles.

4. Maintain joint ROM and spinal flexibility.

5. Resume prebracing levels of functional activity. Teaching the patient how to move, walk, run, and perform activities while wearing the brace helps the patient to achieve this goal.

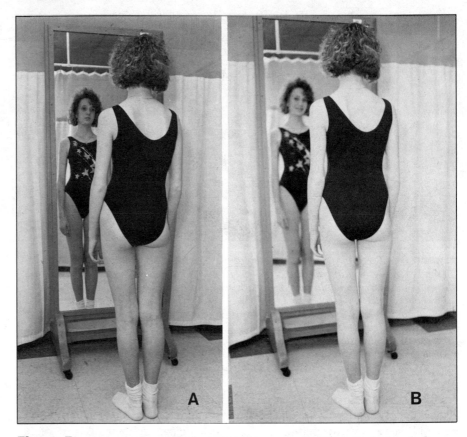

Figure 7. *Patient with a right thoracolumbar scoliosis performing postural alignment: (A) incorrect alignment; (B) correct alignment. (Courtesy of Department of Physical Therapy, Children's Hospital, Boston, Mass.)*

In order for the bracing program to be successful, the brace must fit properly. Thus, if a patient has muscle tightness in structures that directly affect brace alignment and fit, appropriate exercises to alleviate this tightness should be implemented. For example, one of the main bracing principles is to reduce lumbar lordosis in an effort to stabilize the pelvis.[38] This is accomplished by building lumbar flexion into the pelvic module, allowing only 15 degrees of lumbar lordosis in most modules.

If a patient has tightness in the iliopsoas muscle, as indicated by a positive Thomas test, this tightness will have an adverse effect on postural alignment in the brace.[39] When the patient attempts to stand upright while wearing the brace, he or she must compensate for the hip flexor tightness by either flexing the knee or extending the upper back over the posterior-superior borders of the brace. This compensatory extension results in a flattening of the thoracic spine that could lead to hypokyphosis.

One of the major goals of the bracing program is to align the trunk over the sacrum. Therefore, teaching the patient correct postural alignment, both with the brace on and with the brace off, is a significant part of the physical therapy program. Often, patients with structural curves are unaware of their asymmetrical posture. In our experience, when patients who are poorly aligned are placed in proper anatomical alignment, the statement is frequently made: "I feel crooked." Establishing normal alignment, both during and after the bracing program, is an ongoing challenge. Use of a mirror to assist the patient in achieving postural awareness and alignment is very helpful (Fig. 7).

Compliance with exercise programs designed to complement brace wearing varies widely.[29] We have observed that patients generally appear to be compliant during the period in which they are initially adjusted to wearing the brace. Once they are fully accustomed to the brace and have resumed normal activities, however, compliance appears to diminish. We believe that patients tend to resume their exercise program when it is time to be weaned from the brace. At this time, they will often comment that their back "feels tired." During this period, they are usually taught vigorous abdominal muscle strengthening exercises.

An important factor to emphasize to both patients and parents is the overall goal of the bracing program, which is *prevention* of further progression of the curve(s) rather than *complete correction* of the scoliosis. Long-term results of bracing indicate that curve magnitudes recorded at the completion of the bracing program usually are the same as those recorded at the beginning of bracing (Fig. 8).

Despite the best efforts on the part of the patient, the family, and the treatment team, children with structural curves who meet the criteria for bracing do not respond positively and will require surgical intervention.[29] Fortunately, the majority of patients with moderate, progressive curves, who meet the criteria for bracing and are enrolled in a comprehensive bracing program, will have a successful result and avoid surgery.

Operative Management

Patients with curves that exceed 40 degrees when the patients are still growing and those with curves that are in excess of 50 degrees after the end of growth are candidates for surgical correction.[40] The indications for surgical correction in the adult are somewhat more complex than in the growing child and involve such additional factors as late progression, pain, and decreasing respiratory function.

When nonoperative management fails in a child with idiopathic scoliosis, operative management must be considered, depending on the age of the

child. If the child has early-onset idiopathic scoliosis and fails to respond to nonoperative management, then a decision must be made whether to operate on the front of the spine as well as the back. Because of the camshaft phenomenon (as described by Jean Dubousset and colleagues,[41] posterior fusion in a young child (under 10 years of age) will result in tethering the posterior elements. The anterior vertebral bodies will continue to grow, causing increased rotation and curvature by the end of growth.

The eventual success of any correction will depend on the quality of the spinal fusion. It is essential that there be a meticulous dissection of the spine, an adequate resection of the facet joints, a thorough decortication of the posterior elements wherever possible, and some form of supplemental bone graft.

The traditional aims of surgical management of spinal deformities are (1) to straighten the spine as much as possible consistent with safety; (2) to balance the trunk of the pelvis; and (3) to stabilize the spine by arthrodesis, which will maintain the correction.

The actual percentage of correction is less important than the balancing and stability of the spine and the attention to the correction of the spine in three dimensions, including rotation.

For many years, the standard instrumentation has been the Harrington set, consisting of both distraction and compression rods (Fig. 9).[42] The compression rods are used in kyphosis and are contraindicated if the patient has a flat back or thoracic lordosis. Supplemental sublaminar or spinous process wiring has increased the correction and the stability obtained with the use of Harrington instrumentation.[42] This instrumentation is still in wide use in many parts of the world. All of the modifications that have been made to the original Harrington instrumentation have been toward helping to correct the rib hump and obtaining more stability so that less external immobilization will be required.

The Cotrel-Dubousset instrumentation, introduced in the United States in 1984, is designed to rotate the spine to obtain correction of the rib hump and to establish a normal sagittal contour with the proper amount of thoracic kyphosis and lumbar lordosis (Fig. 10).[43] The Cotrel-Dubousset set is more stable because of the introduction of cross-linking, using an apparatus to link the two rods to make the system stable in rotation as well as in lateral bending and compression.

Many new types of instrumentation, such as the Texas Scottish-Rite Hospital system, have been developed based on the Cotrel-Dubousset principles and have introduced such advantages as an improved cross-linking apparatus with all open hooks to allow for easier insertion. It must be emphasized, however, that it is more important to adhere to the principles of surgical correction and spine fusion than to dwell on the type of instrumentation used.

Long-term follow-up of patients who have had spinal fusion as adolescents or young adults has shown that it is more important to pay attention to the sagittal contour.[44] Many patients whose lumbar lordosis has been obliterated by the use of a straight Harrington rod have developed a problem known as the flat back syndrome. These patients have great difficulty standing erect because of collapse of the disks below the level of fusion. When they attempt to maintain erect posture, they must either lean forward or flex their knees. The new systems, which allow retention of the normal lumbar lordosis, should minimize this complication in the future.

Other potential complications, such as neurologic problems up to and including paraplegia, are fortunately rare. Their prevention is aided by the use of intraoperative monitoring of spinal cord function and intraoperative wake-up tests.[45]

Physical Therapy Management

The preoperative assessment includes the following measures:

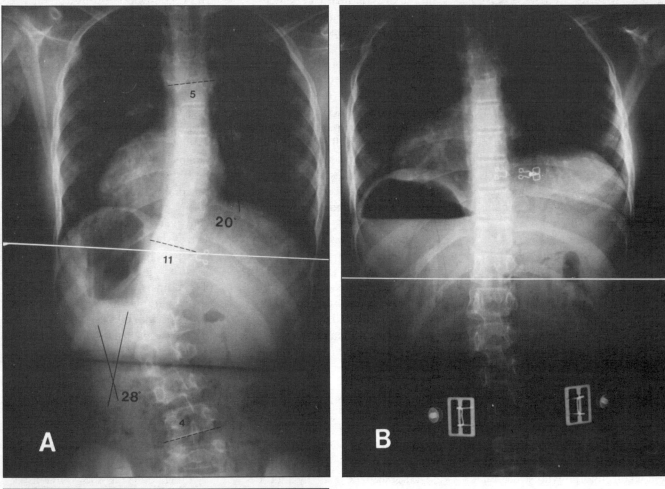

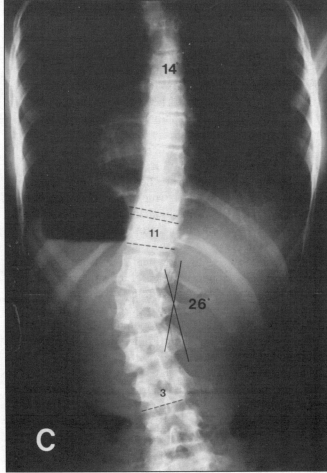

Figure 8. *Posterior/anterior radiographic view of a patient with a right thoracic, left lumbar structural scoliosis treated with a Boston brace: (A) structural curve at the start of treatment with brace off; (B) same curve 2 years into brace wearing; (C) same curve 2 years after the completion of brace treatment. (Courtesy of Department of Orthopaedics, Children's Hospital, Boston, Mass.)*

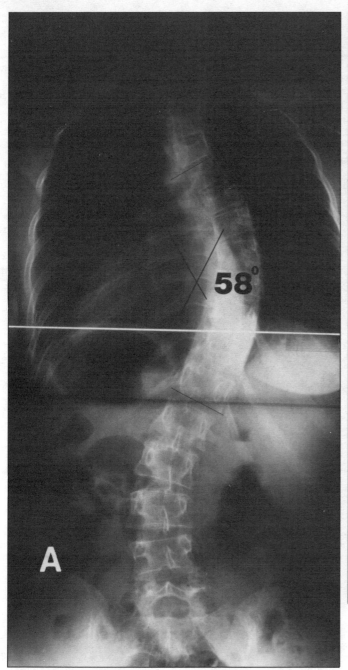
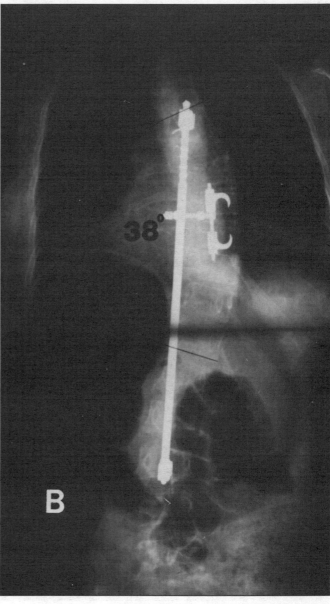

Figure 9. *Posterior/anterior radiographic view of a patient with a right thoracic, left lumbar scoliosis treated with a spinal fusion using Harrington rod fixation. (A) preoperation; (B) postoperation. (Courtesy of Department of Orthopaedics, Children's Hospital, Boston, Mass.)*

1. *Posture*—inspection and documentation of postural abnormalities in the anterior, lateral, and posterior views.

2. *Range of motion*—with emphasis on limitations in the lower extremities that may affect the patient's ability for early postoperative mobilization such as tightness of the hamstring muscles, hip flexors, and heel cords.

3. *Leg length*—measurement of both real and apparent leg lengths. If the patient has a real leg-length discrepancy and wears a prescribed shoe lift, this measure will be needed for postoperative ambulation.

4. *Muscle strength*—a detailed muscle examination is performed to establish a baseline. Significant areas of weakness are summarized and highlighted so that they will not be attributed to postoperative complications.

5. *Respiratory function*—with emphasis on lateral costal expansion and diaphragmatic breathing. This mea-

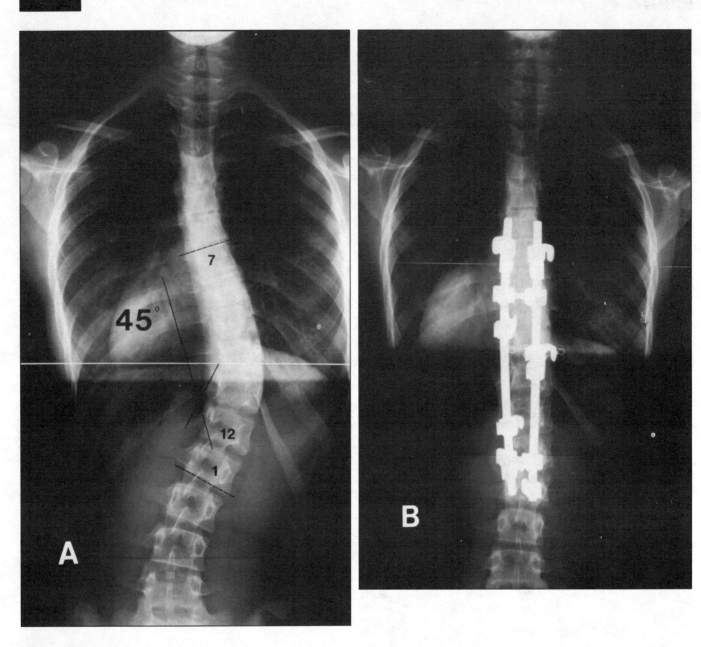

Figure 10. *Posterior/anterior radiographic view of a patient with a right thoracolumbar structural scoliosis treated with a spinal fusion using Cotrel-Dubousset instrumentation: (A) preoperation; (B) postoperation. (Courtesy of Department of Orthopaedics, Children's Hospital, Boston, Mass.)*

sure is particularly important if the patient has a history of asthma or any other respiratory disorders.

Preoperative therapy includes deep-breathing training and instruction in deep, effective coughing. Techniques of postural drainage are reviewed with and explained to the patient in the event of any respiratory postoperative complications. In addition, the patient is shown how to log roll and come to a sitting position.

The primary postoperative goal is early mobilization to prevent postoperative complications. Once again, a team treatment approach is emphasized. The physician, nurse, and physical therapist work together to assist the patient in achieving this goal. Patients are encouraged to breathe deeply and to cough both frequently and effectively. Lower-extremity exercises are indicated only if the patient is having difficulty with early mobilization. Usually, patients are able to sit up in a chair the first postoperative

day. External support (ie, a bivalved plastic clamshell brace) may or may not be necessary. Most patients are able to independently ambulate within 4 to 7 postoperative days.

Improved surgical techniques[43] allow for both early mobilization and a shorter hospital stay (about 7–10 days, at the present time, if there are no complications). Operative management of idiopathic scoliosis remains complex, however, and it is clear that further research into etiology is essential in order to prevent the development of idiopathic scoliosis rather than having to resort to extreme measures such as surgery and prolonged bracing to correct it.

Summary

Although the management of adolescent idiopathic scoliosis has improved over the last several years, the treatment remains a very extensive process. Nonoperative and operative regimens are major events for both the patients and their families. The treatment team should never underestimate the effect of treatment on patients and families. Sensitivity, support, honesty, and communication of accurate information are the key ingredients toward successful treatment.

Acknowledgments

We gratefully acknowledge the helpful advice and comments of Alice M Shea, ScD, PT, Associate for Research and Education, Department of Physical Therapy and Occupational Therapy Services, Children's Hospital, Boston, Mass. Our appreciation is expressed for the photographs taken by James Koepfler, Biomedical Photographer, Department of Orthopaedics, Children's Hospital.

References

1 *Webster's New Universal Unabridged Dictionary, Delux.* 2nd ed. New York, NY: Simon & Shuster; 1983.

2 Terminology Committee, Scoliosis Research Society. A glossary of scoliosis terms. *Spine.* 1976;1:57–58.

3 Moe JH, Bradford DS, Winter RB, Lonstein JE. *Scoliosis and Other Spinal Deformities.* Philadelphia, Pa: WB Saunders Co; 1978.

4 Cobb JR. *Outline for the Study of Scoliosis: Instructional Course Lectures, The American Academy of Orthopaedic Surgeons.* Ann Arbor, Mich: JW Edwards Co; 1948;5:261–275.

5 Nash CL Jr, Moe JH. A study of vertebral rotation. *J Bone Joint Surg [Am].* 1969;51:223–229.

6 Riseborough EJ, Hendron JH. *Scoliosis and Other Deformities of the Axial Skeleton.* Boston, Mass: Little, Brown & Co Inc; 1975.

7 Bradford DS, Lonstein JE, Moe JH, et al. *Moe's Textbook of Scoliosis and Other Deformities.* 2nd ed. Philadelphia, Pa: WB Saunders Co; 1987.

8 Riseborough EJ, Wynne-Davies R. A genetic survey of idiopathic scoliosis in Boston, Massachusetts. *J Bone Joint Surg [Am].* 1973;55:974–982.

9 Yamada K, Yamamoto H, Nakagawa Y, et al. Etiology of idiopathic scoliosis. *Clin Orthop.* 1984;184:50–57.

10 Lonstein JE, Bjorklund S, Wanninger MH, et al. Voluntary school screening for scoliosis in Minnesota. *J Bone Joint Surg [Am].* 1982;64:481–488.

11 Lonstein JE. Natural history and school screening for scoliosis. *Orthop Clin North Am.* 1988;19:227–237.

12 Lonstein JE. Risk of progression of idiopathic scoliosis in skeletally immature patients. *Spine: State of the Art Reviews.* 1978;1:181–193.

13 Rogala EH, Drummond DS, Gurr J. Scoliosis: incidence and natural history, a prospective epidemiological study. *J Bone Joint Surg [Am].* 1978;60:173–176.

14 Lonstein JE, Carlson JM. The prediction of curve progression in untreated idiopathic scoliosis during growth. *J Bone Joint Surg [Am].* 1984;66:1061–1071.

15 Weinstein SL. Idiopathic scoliosis: natural history of curve progression—symposium on epidemiology, natural history and nonoperative treatment of idiopathic scoliosis. *Spine.* 1986;11:780–783.

16 Risser JG. The iliac apophysis: an invaluable sign in the management of scoliosis. *Clin Orthop.* 1958;11:111–119.

17 Greulich WW, Pyle ST. *Radiographic Atlas of the Skeletal Development of the Hand and Wrist.* 2nd ed. Stanford, Calif: Stanford University Press; 1950.

18 Moreland MS, Pope MH, Armstrong GWD. *Moiré Fringe Topography and Spinal Deformity.* New York, NY: Pergamon Press Inc; 1981.

19 Koepfler JW. Moiré topography in medicine. *J Biol Photogr.* 1983;51:3–9.

20 Turner-Smith AR, Shannon TML, Houghton GR, Knopp DA. *Assessing Idiopathic Scoliosis Using a Surface Measurement Technique: Surgical Rounds for Orthopaedics.* Oxford, England: Orthopaedic Engineering Centre; 1988:52–58.

21 Axelgaard J, Brown JC. Lateral surface stimulation for the treatment of progressive idiopathic scoliosis. *Spine.* 1983;8:242–260.

22 Farady JA. Current principles in the nonoperative management of structural adolescent idiopathic scoliosis. *Phys Ther.* 1983;63:512–523.

23 Sullivan JA, Davidson R, Renshaw TS, et al. Further evaluation of the Scolitron treatment of idiopathic adolescent scoliosis. *Spine.* 1986;11:903–906.

24 Blount WP, Moe JH. *The Milwaukee Brace.* Baltimore, Md: Williams & Wilkins; 1973.

25 Hall JE, Miller ME, Cassella MC, et al. *Manual for the Boston Brace Workshop.* Boston, Mass: Department of Orthopaedics, Children's Hospital; 1976.

26 Watts HG, Hall JE, Stanish W. The Boston bracing system for the treatment of low thoracic and lumbar scoliosis by use of a girdle without superstructure. *Clin Orthop.* 1977;126:87–92.

27 Redford JB. *Orthotics Etcetera.* 2nd ed. Baltimore, Md: Williams & Wilkins; 1980.

28 Carr WA, Moe JH, Winter RB, et al. Treatment of idiopathic scoliosis in the Milwaukee brace: long-term results. *J Bone Joint Surg [Am].* 1980;62:599–612.

29 Emans JB, Kaelin A, Bancel P, et al. The Boston bracing system for idiopathic scoliosis: follow-up results in 295 patients. *Spine.* 1986;11:792–801.

30 *Manual for the Boston Brace Course.* Boston, Mass: Department of Orthopaedics, Children's Hospital; 1989.

31 Bassett GS, Bunnell WP, MacEwen GD. Treatment of idiopathic scoliosis with the Wilmington brace. *J Bone Joint Surg [Am].* 1986;68:602–605.

32 Price CT, Scott DS, Reed FE, Riddick MF. Nighttime bracing for adolescent idiopathic scoliosis with the Charleston bending brace: preliminary report. *Spine.* 1990;15:1294–1299.

33 Lonstein JE, Winter RB. Adolescent idiopathic scoliosis: nonoperative treatment. *Orthop Clin North Am.* 1988;19:239–246.

34 Klapp B. *Das Klapp'sche Kriechverfahren.* Stuttgart, Federal Republic of Germany: Georg Thieme Verlag; 1966.

35 Lovett RW. *Lateral Curvature of the Spine and Round Shoulders.* Philadelphia, Pa: P Blakiston's Son & Co; 1907.

36 Blount WP, Bolinske J. Physical therapy in the nonoperative treatment of scoliosis. *Phys Ther.* 1967;47:919–925.

37 Miyasaki RA. Immediate influence of the thoracic flexion exercise on vertebral position in Milwaukee brace wearers. *Phys Ther.* 1980;60:1005–1009.

38 Lindh M. The effect of sagittal changes on brace correction of idiopathic scoliosis. *Spine.* 1980;5:26–36.

39 Thomas HO. *Diseases of the Hip, Knee and Ankle Joints with Their Deformities, Treated by a New and Efficient Method.* Liverpool, England: T Dorr & Co; 1876.

40 Weinstein SL, Ponseti IV. Curve progression in idiopathic scoliosis. *J Bone Joint Surg [Am].* 1983;65:447–455.

41 Dubousset J, Herring A, Shufflebarger H. The crankshaft phenomenon. *J Pediatr Orthop.* 1989;9:541–550.

42 Harrington PR. Treatment of scoliosis, correction and internal fixation by spine instrumentation. *J Bone Joint Surg [Am].* 1962;44:591–610.

43 Cotrel Y, Dubousset J. New segmental posterior instrumentation of the spine. *Orthop Trans.* 1985;9:118. Abstract.

44 Kostuik JP. Treatment of scoliosis in the adult thoracolumbar spine with special reference to fusion to the sacrum. *Orthop Clin North Am.* 1988;19:371–381.

45 Hall JE, Levine CR, Sudhir KG. Intraoperative awakening to monitor spinal cord function during Harrington instrumentation and spine fusion. *J Bone Joint Surg [Am].* 1978;60:533–536.

Physical Therapy Management of Patients with Juvenile Rheumatoid Arthritis

Juvenile rheumatoid arthritis (JRA) is the most common pediatric rheumatic disease and is a leading cause of childhood disability. Physical therapists play a crucial role in the treatment of these children and serve as essential members of the interdisciplinary treatment team. An understanding of the etiology and background of this disease is critical to appropriate evaluation, goal setting, and treatment planning. This review article will provide an overview of the epidemiology, immune system pathophysiology, and clinical characteristics of JRA. Physical therapy principles of care, evaluation procedures, and treatment techniques will be covered in depth. In addition, common orthopedic manifestations and their management, including surgical approaches, will be discussed. [Rhodes VJ. Physical therapy management of patients with juvenile rheumatoid arthritis. Phys Ther. 1991;71:910–919.]

Key Words: *Arthritis, rheumatoid arthritis; Orthopedics, general; Pediatrics, treatment.*

Valerie J Rhodes

Juvenile rheumatoid arthritis (JRA) is the most common pediatric rheumatoid disease in North America and a major cause of childhood disability.[1] Up to 25% of children with JRA have unremitting disease, which may lead to contracture and deformity,[2] and approximately 10% will enter adulthood with severe functional disabilities.[1] Significant visual impairment may also occur as a consequence of this illness, secondary to iridocyclitis, a chronic eye inflammation affecting the iris and ciliary body.

Etiology, Incidence, and Clinical Manifestations

Although the cause of JRA is unknown, the disease is thought to have a multifactorial etiology; possibly an infectious agent triggers a genetically predisposed autoimmune response, which results in joint inflammation.[1,3]

There have been several epidemiologic studies that have attempted to determine the incidence of JRA. Recent data from the Mayo Clinic show an incidence of 13.9 cases per 100,000 individuals per year and a prevalence of 113.4 cases per 100,000 individuals.[1] A 1986 Finnish study[4] estimated that the incidence is 19.6 cases per 100,000 individuals per year. Most recently, Andersson-Gore and Fasth[5] presented data from Göteborg, Sweden, that showed an incidence of 11 cases per 100,000 individuals per year and a point prevalence (number of total cases at a given point in time) of 82 cases per 100,000 individuals. Juvenile rheumatoid arthritis affects girls 2:1 over boys.[1,3] There are three distinct modes of onset in JRA, however, and sex ratios are strongly affected by onset type.[1,3,6] The American College of Rheumatology's criteria for classification of JRA are listed in the Appendix.[1]

Certain manifestations of JRA differ from those of adult rheumatoid arthritis (RA). Systemic disease is more common in children with JRA than in adults with RA. Unlike adult RA, chronic eye inflammation (iridocyclitis) may be a symptom of JRA. In children with JRA, there is predominantly large joint involvement and frequent cervical spine anklyosis. Typical wrist and hand deformities in children with JRA include wrist subluxation and radial deviation with ulnar deviation of fingers. In adults with RA, wrist ulnar deviation with finger radial deviation is the usual pattern. Additionally, rheumatoid factor (RF), an abnormal immune complex in the blood, is seen in fewer than 15% of young children with JRA, but is seen in 80% to 85% of adults with RA.[3]

VJ Rhodes, MPH, PT, is Senior Physical Therapist, Newington Children's Hospital, 181 Cedar St, Newington, CT 06111 (USA).

Pathophysiology

Inflammation occurs naturally within the body as part of the immune system's defense against disease and trauma. Antigens (bacteria, viruses, and other foreign substances) are initially processed by macrophages and mononuclear cells. Cellular chemicals, such as cytokines, attract the humoral (B cell) and cellular (T cell) arms of the immune response. These lymphocytes may then work in concert or independently to immobilize the antigen. B cells produce specific antibodies that may attach to the antigen, attract complement proteins, and form immune complexes. These complexes may then activate other components of the inflammatory system, including phagocytic neutrophils, kinins, and proteolytic enzymes.

In the development of inflammatory arthritis, either immune complexes or a putative antigen invades the synovium, initiating the cascade of inflammatory events. Lymphocytes lose their ability to distinguish between antigens and healthy tissue. Lysosomal enzymes and collagenase released into the joint fluid destroy synovial membrane cells.

Synovial proliferation results from the inflammatory reaction, creating a mass, or pannus, that can then overlie the articular surface and soften and weaken the cartilage. Destruction of the bone can occur at the articular margins through blood vessel foramina.[7] Effusion and synovial thickening lead to increased intra-articular pressures. Surrounding soft tissues undergo fibrosis and contracture. Uncontrolled disease may lead to joint fibrosis or even bony ankylosis.

After bone destruction has occurred, the synovial membrane and periarticular tissues contain products of bone and cartilage destruction. This contamination may further contribute to synovial and periarticular fibrosis, as well as direct involvement of tendons with adhesions and contracture.[6] Readers wishing further information regarding pathogenesis should refer

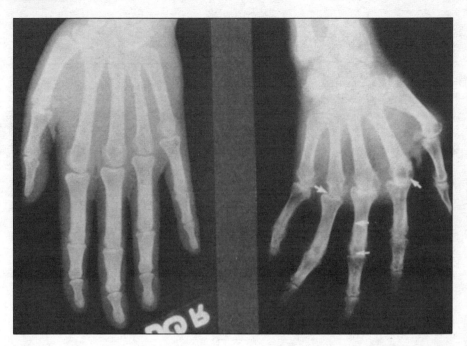

Figure 1. *Radiographs of normal hand (left) and arthritic hand (right). (Arrows denote loss of normal axial alignment.) (From Arthritis Health Professions Teaching Slide Collection,[9] copyright 1980. Used with permission of the Arthritis Foundation.)*

to chapter 2 of Cassidy and Petty's *Textbook of Rheumatology.*[1]

Radiologic Changes in the Rheumatoid Joint

The following changes may be noted by observing radiographs of affected joints: (1) opaque-looking bone, suggesting osteoporosis; (2) decreased joint space, suggesting erosion of cartilage (Fig. 1); (3) variations in bony outline, indicating bone cysts, erosions, or spurs; and (4) loss of normal axial alignment of adjoining bones.[8] Cartilage loss may be seen by magnetic resonance imaging before appearing on radiographs. There may be hypertrophy, accelerated growth, or irregular growth of bone around an involved joint, probably attributable to an increased blood supply secondary to inflammation. Premature fusion of epiphyses also commonly occurs.[1–3,8]

Characteristics of the Three Onset Types

There are three distinct onset types of JRA. Because the course of the disease, as well as the prognosis, varies among the onset types, it is very important to understand the differences among them.

Systemic-onset JRA, also known as Still's disease, accounts for 10% of all cases and occurs throughout childhood, with a 1:1 female-to-male sex ratio. Clinical findings may include an intermittent spiking fever, which may be as high as 104°–105°F, and a fleeting rash of pale erythematous macules is present in the majority of patients.[1,3] The rash appears on the trunk and proximal extremities and less commonly on the distal extremities (Fig. 2). The rash may recur for months or years, even in the absence of other signs of disease activity. Systemic symptoms may include pericarditis, hepatosplenomegaly, and lymphadenopathy. Laboratory findings may include anemia, an increased white blood cell count, and an elevated erythrocyte sedimentation rate, a measure of inflammation. Most children with Still's disease develop chronic polyarthritis. Approximately half those diagnosed with systemic-onset JRA have a progressive increase in the number of joints involved, and

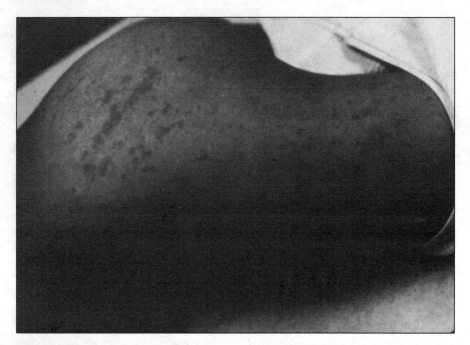

Figure 2. *Rash of systemic-onset juvenile rheumatoid arthritis.*

they eventually have moderate to severe disability.[1]

Polyarticular JRA, the second subtype, occurs in 40% of all children with JRA. It occurs throughout childhood, peaking at 1 to 3 years of age, with the female-to-male ratio being 3:1.[1] Clinical findings include acute or insidious symmetrical arthritis of the upper and lower extremities, with more than four joints involved. There is an absence of systemic symptoms. Laboratory findings include an elevated erythrocyte sedimentation rate and may include a positive rheumatoid factor.[1,3] Children with rheumatoid factor-positive polyarticular JRA have a poor prognosis, with a greater possibility of erosive arthritis. Their arthritis more closely resembles adult RA, with frequent findings of subcutaneous nodules attached to the tendon sheaths of periarticular structures.

The third subgroup of JRA is known as *pauciarticular JRA*, or *oligoarticular JRA*, with four or less joints involved. This type occurs in 50% of all children with JRA. It usually occurs in children under 10 years of age, peaking at 1 to 2 years of age, with the male-to-female ratio being 5:1.[1] In pauciarticular JRA of the lower extremities, involvement is often asymmetrical. The knee is the most commonly affected joint, followed by the ankle and the elbow.[9] Laboratory findings include an elevated sedimentation rate and may include a positive antinuclear antibody (ANA) blood test. The presence of immunoglobulins, which act against nuclear cellular material, results in ANAs. In pauciarticular ANA-positive JRA, the child is at high risk for development of iridocyclitis, a chronic eye inflammation. Iritis may lead to impaired vision: 15% to 30% of children with iritis will eventually develop functional blindness.[1] Iridocyclitis is treated with ophthalmologic corticosteroid preparations and pupil-dilating drops, which prevent scarring of the pupil and iris.

The prognosis in pauciarticular arthritis is good. Few joints are affected, and functional disability is uncommon. In addition, a greater

percentage of these children have early remission.[1]

Principles of Care in Juvenile Rheumatoid Arthritis

The treatment program for children with JRA must be individualized. A team approach that involves the family and child as key members is ideal. Professionals who may become involved with the child include pediatric rheumatologists, nurses, physical therapists, occupational therapists, social workers, psychologists, ophthalmologists, orthopedists, orthotists, dietitians, and cardiologists. The goals of team management are to decrease joint inflammation, relieve pain, achieve or maintain an optimal level of function, and educate the patient and family as to the course of the disease and the care required.

Principles of care include a long-term program supervised by a rheumatologist, adequate rest and good health habits, an exercise program directed by a physical therapist, medications to control joint inflammation, and school support and intervention where needed.

Medications play a major role in the management of the patient with JRA. The drugs of choice are the anti-inflammatories, which include salicylates (aspirin) and other nonsteroidal anti-inflammatory drugs such as ibuprofen and naproxen. These drugs provide symptomatic relief of pain, stiffness, and swelling. They act, in part, by interfering with prostaglandin synthesis in the inflammatory process.[1,3]

The second-line drugs are called remitting agents, or slow-acting or disease-modifying antirheumatic drugs, because they are believed to interfere with the autoimmune process itself.[3] These drugs include gold salts, hydroxychloroquine (Plaquenil®*), D-penicillamine, and sulfasalazine. Immunosuppressive drugs, such as methotrexate, and corticosteroids have selected roles in management.[1,3] Experimental therapies include intravenous immune globulin and biologic

---

*Winthrop Pharmaceuticals, 90 Park Ave, New York, NY 10016.

agents such as specific targeted (monoclonal) antibodies.[10,11]

Principles of exercise and activity are of primary importance to physical therapists working with children with JRA. The Affiliated Children's Arthritis Centers of New England have developed physical therapy standards for the care of children with chronic arthritis. This program, funded by a Bureau of Maternal and Child Health and Resources Development Special Projects of Regional and National Significance (SPRANS) grant, consists of a network of 13 tertiary pediatric institutions located throughout the six New England states. Readers should consult these standards for ongoing guidance in the assessment, problem and goal identification, and treatment planning for children who have JRA.[12] Generally, children with arthritis are encouraged to participate in age-appropriate physical activities, with limitations imposed only if the child experiences discomfort during or following an activity.

Physical therapists should remember that normal joint function cannot be maintained in the absence of motion and weight bearing.[13] Additionally, I believe that in young children who continue to mature motorically, physical exploration is essential for the acquisition of balance, coordination, perceptual skills, and self-confidence. Modifications of activities may be necessary, such as restricting gymnastic activities (eg, tumbling), for children with severe wrist disease or cervical spine involvement or limiting contact sports in children with extensive arthritis.[14] Such restrictions may be necessary to prevent exacerbation of inflammation or to avoid injury or fracture at a joint with limited mobility.

Children and their families should be educated in basic joint protection techniques. Static flexion positions should be avoided. When at rest, involved joints should be maintained in an extended position. Total body weight should not be placed on non–weight-bearing joints if these joints are affected; activities such as cartwheels,

handstands, chin-ups, and rope climbing should be avoided.[14] Joint stress can be minimized in the upper extremities by carrying items close to the body and by using both hands; stress can be decreased in the fingers by using the palms of the hands for carrying items and for turning doorknobs, faucet handles, and lids. When ankles or metatarsals are involved, shoes with heels are to be avoided in order to prevent excessive stress on metatarsal heads as well as to maintain length of the Achilles tendons.

Physical Therapy Evaluation

Physical therapy evaluation begins with a baseline examination. Serial reevaluations are used to chart the progress of the disease and the effect of treatments, including medications and physical therapy. Because there is no single measure of disease activity, assessment of pain, swelling, range of motion (ROM), muscle strength (as determined by manual muscle testing), and mobility are critical in determining the overall benefits of team treatment and are essential in goal setting and treatment planning.

The first element of the evaluation should be the patient history. Information, such as the presence and duration of morning stiffness, should be obtained. Additionally, the patient's (and parents') perception of pain and fatigue are noted. Information is gathered about the child's independence in activities of daily living, functional mobility at home and in school, and endurance throughout the day. The child's ability to participate in physical education, sports, and recreational activities is discussed. Any specialized equipment, splinting, or exercise programs already in place are observed and evaluated.

Next, an examination of the spine and lower-extremity joints is performed (upper-extremity joints as well, if the child is not also seen by an occupational therapist). Joints are evaluated for the presence of effusion, synovial thickening, heat, and redness. Swelling of the hip is not easily detected unless the child is thin. Knee swelling

is most commonly seen over the medial superior and lateral aspects of the patella. Swelling can be detected at the knee by the use of "patellar tap" and "bulge" signs. The patellar tap is performed by stabilizing and slightly distracting the patella by the use of the thumb and forefinger proximally. The other forefinger is used to press quickly and firmly down on the patella. The patellar tap is positive if a rush of fluid is felt escaping from under the patella. The bulge sign is seen by firmly "milking" fluid away from the anatomical depression medial to the patella, then pushing gently against the patella laterally. If fluid is seen to refill the depression, an effusion is believed to be present. Therapists are cautioned regarding the use of girth measurements to assess swelling at the knee. Bony overgrowth of the femoral condyles commonly accompanies knee arthritis; therefore, even in the absence of effusion, an involved knee may be larger circumferentially than an uninvolved knee, if measured at the joint line. If girth measurements are taken, they are best performed proximal to the superior patellar border, above any effusion, to avoid the effect of bony overgrowth.

Ankle effusions are seen most frequently around the malleoli and dorsum of the joint.[3] If swelling is present, the normal indentation between the anterior tibial tendon and the medial malleolus is lost. When the tarsal area is inflamed, swelling appears over the dorsum of the foot.[3] Swelling in the metatarsophalangeal joints can be assessed through observation and palpation, although this swelling may be difficult to detect. Swelling is often assessed using a three-point scale: 1+ =minimal, 2+=moderate, and 3+ =severe.

Pain is first evaluated by asking the child about pain at rest. Pain on motion and weight bearing is then assessed. Tenderness is differentiated from pain in that tenderness is determined by deep palpation of the tissue about the joint.[3]

Measurement of ROM of the spine and lower extremities is then performed by the use of goniometry.[15] Linear measures, such as the Schöber test of lumbosacral mobility and the incisor gap, are also helpful.[1] The Schöber test is performed, with the child in a standing position, by measuring 5 cm below and 10 cm above a surface landmark (eg, a line between the dimples of Venus). The patient then flexes forward maximally, and the change in the linear measurement is recorded. Normal values are available for comparison.[1] The incisor gap, a measure of temporomandibular joint mobility, is assessed by recording the distance between upper and lower incisors. The distinction between true joint limitation and muscle tightness should be made. When assessing joint ROM, care must be taken to place any two-point muscle in a shortened position over one of the joints.[3] For example, knee flexion is measured with the child in a supine position, as opposed to a prone position, in which knee flexion could be limited by rectus femoris muscle tightness. Ankle dorsiflexion is measured during knee flexion, as opposed to during knee extension, to eliminate the effects of gastrocnemius muscle shortening on ROM.

A muscle examination includes manual muscle testing, observation of muscle atrophy, and measurement of thigh and calf girth to determine whether the effect is asymmetrical. If a child is too young to participate in manual muscle testing, the child's ability to perform within the developmental sequence may give an indication of weakened areas.

A postural assessment is completed from anterior, sagittal, and posterior views. Postural deviations are noted, including the presence of scoliosis (structural versus functional), forward head, rounded shoulders, scapular "winging," lordosis, kyphosis, and pelvic obliquity. Additional postural deviations/deformities common to JRA include femoral anteversion, genu valgum, tibial torsion, pes cavus or valgus, hallux valgus, and hammertoes.[16] Possible leg-length discrepancies are noted, because such discrep-

ancies are common with unilateral knee arthritis.

Gait is usually assessed by observation. Using gait laboratory analysis, Lechner and colleagues[16] found significantly decreased velocity, cadence, and stride length in their subjects with JRA as compared with a group of children without JRA. The anterior pelvic tilt of the subjects with JRA was significantly increased throughout the gait cycle. Hip extension at terminal stance and ankle plantar flexion at toe-off were significantly decreased. Gait assessment should include observation of walking on level surfaces, stairs, and inclines, as well as assessment of distance that can be covered and the use of any assistive devices.

Functional mobility must be assessed on the basis of the following four measures: (1) proficiency, or the child's ability to independently complete a task from beginning to end; (2) movement quality, or the need to substitute muscle groups, revert to a lower developmental pattern, or use two hands or other body parts to assist in completion of a task; (3) speed of performance; and (4) endurance, or the ability to perform multiple repetitions of an activity.[12] An example of pediatric functional assessment tools that are used for the JRA population is the Pediatric Evaluation of Disability Inventory (PEDI).[17] Currently undergoing normalization for ages birth through 7 years, this tool evaluates the areas of self-care, mobility, and social functions, as well as caregiver assistance required and modifications needed.

Several investigators have attempted to develop assessment tools for use specifically with the JRA population. These instruments include a modified version of the adult Arthritis Impact Measurement Scales (AIMS)[18]; the Newington Children's Hospital JRA Evaluation, a movement quality-oriented developmentally based tool for use in children 1 to 10 years of age[19]; and the Juvenile Arthritis Functional Assessment Scale,[20] a task-oriented, timed assessment aimed at children 7 to 18 years of age. For discussion of the reliability and validity

of the AIMS, the reader should refer to Coulton et al.[18] The Juvenile Arthritis Functional Assessment Scale has an internal reliability of .85 (Cronbach's coefficient of alpha) and a convergent validity of .40 between score and total number of joints involved. A functional mobility assessment should include evaluation of developmental milestones and gross motor skills, bed/mat mobility, transfer abilities, and wheelchair mobility, if appropriate.

The child should also be assessed for splinting needs. Splints are indicated for joint contractures that are unresponsive to exercise. Lower-extremity splints are usually resting splints used at night and at nap times. The most commonly required lower-extremity splint is for knee extension. This type of splint is required because of the frequency of knee joint involvement in all subtypes of JRA, the weakening of the quadriceps femoris muscle mechanism in the presence of knee swelling,[21] and the tendency for the knee joint to be flexed for comfort. Nighttime splinting of ankles to prevent heelcord shortening and in-shoe orthotic devices to correct forefoot or hindfoot deviations may also be helpful.[12]

Finally, the need for adaptive equipment is noted. This equipment may include a raised toilet seat, tub transfer seat, grab bars, ambulation aids, or a wheelchair.

Physical Therapy Techniques

The physical therapy program must be individualized for each child. In acute phases of JRA, the goal of treatment is to prevent loss of motion, disuse atrophy, and osteoporosis with loss of activities of daily living and functional mobility. During this time, appropriate treatment techniques include measures to provide comfort; active, active-assistive, and passive ROM exercises (no vigorous stretching); isometric exercises; and contract/relax techniques.[12] Care should be taken to avoid excessive fatigue; rest is felt to be important when recovering from a flare of the disease. Therapeutic activities should not increase the child's symptoms, and painful exercises are to be avoided.

During chronic phases of JRA, goals need to be modified. The careful addition of progressive resistive exercises is permitted as long as an increase in symptoms (eg, pain, stiffness, swelling) does not occur. The child's activity level is gradually increased as tolerated. General conditioning programs such as swimming and bicycling are encouraged.

Various physical therapy modalities may be helpful in easing joint symptoms, especially stiffness and protective muscle spasm in acute stages of the disease. Moist heat in the form of a tub bath or shower, whirlpool, hot packs, or warm swimming pool appears to be beneficial. A paraffin bath can be used for hands or feet. Retaining body warmth overnight through use of warm pajamas or a heated water bed or sleeping bag can help to minimize morning stiffness.[14] Deep heating techniques, such as ultrasound or diathermy, are not recommended.[22] In addition to concern about the effects of these modalities on the epiphyseal plate in growing children, deep heating techniques may increase joint inflammation. The use of cold in the form of ice massage or cold packs can also decrease joint pain by providing local anesthesia; however, in my experience, most children with arthritis prefer heat.

Another useful method, if a patient has one or two very painful joints, is transcutaneous electrical nerve stimulation (TENS). This modality may provide enough pain relief to allow active or active-assistive exercise during a flare of JRA in order to maintain joint ROM. I have also found TENS to be very effective for use in early mobilization postoperatively. When TENS is used, the patient should be old enough to communicate discomfort and not be fearful of the procedure.

During any stage of the disease, biofeedback may be helpful in increasing joint ROM by providing information to the patient regarding correct muscle activation and by encouraging optimal effort. In already restricted joints, biofeedback may be necessary to obtain correct movement without muscle substitution and to overcome spasm.

Gait training in children with JRA should seek to minimize or eliminate observed deviations. This may be done through postural training; weight-bearing activities; and attention to symmetry, form, and cadence.[12] Primary deformities, such as femoral anteversion or genu valgum, may lead to secondary problems such as tibial torsion or pes cavum. Orthotic management may assist in easing areas of painful pressure and providing proper alignment.

Assistive devices may be used as training aids for short-term rehabilitation following surgery or to sustain independent ambulation in a patient with severe involvement. The assistive device should maintain good postural alignment. In the child with multiple joint involvement, care must be taken not to place the upper extremities in positions that may exacerbate the child's symptoms (eg, pain, stiffness, swelling). The use of a platform attachment for a walker or a crutch is a good alternative to abnormal weight-bearing stresses on the wrist and hand.

Improving functional mobility is a key goal of rehabilitation. Ongoing mobility and transfer assessments are essential. In my view, normal, age-appropriate motor patterns are the guide for training; however, modifications may sometimes be necessary. For example, excessive work on half-kneel-to-stand transitions or reciprocal stair climbing may be inappropriate in the presence of severe knee inflammation.

To assess aerobic fitness, Jasso and colleagues[23] compared the physical work capacity of children with JRA, as determined by measurement of maximal oxygen uptake, with that of children without JRA. The 16 children with JRA were found to be significantly less fit than their age-matched controls. Jasso and associates concluded that the amount of physical work that children with JRA are able to accomplish is related to the severity of their articular disease. This research also established that children with JRA have a problem in maintaining normal levels of physical fitness.

At Newington Children's Hospital (Newington, Conn), we conducted a study of aerobic exercise in children with JRA (VJ Rhodes, L Zemel; unpublished data; 1987). The purpose of the study was to determine whether aerobic capacity, as measured by maximal oxygen uptake, could be increased through training without adverse effects on involved joints or overall physical status. Seven subjects, aged 4 to 18 years, underwent 20 minutes of aerobic in-pool training three times weekly for 12 weeks, and six age-matched controls participated in a nonaerobic pool exercise program for the same duration and frequency. Although we were unable to demonstrate a statistically significant difference in maximal oxygen uptake (prestudy mean of 28.7 mL/kg/min; poststudy mean of 27.5 mL/kg/min) in the subjects involved in the aerobic exercise program, we did show a significant decrease in resting heart rate (decrease in means from 118 to 104 bpm). All children stayed well during the study period, without deterioration in selected variables of interest, including joint count (a measure of ROM and swelling),[24] sedimentation rate, and morning stiffness. This research indicates the need to consider nonstressful means of aerobic conditioning in a pool or on a bicycle when designing exercise programs for children with JRA. Improving physical fitness does not need to be time-consuming. Harkcom and colleagues[25] found that as little as 15 minutes of exercise three times a week is sufficient to improve aerobic capacity in women with RA.

Orthopedic Management

Orthopedic manifestations of JRA are common, in that the hip joint is involved in 10% to 38% of children with JRA.[26] Within 1 year of onset of disease, the hips of 9% of all children with JRA are affected.[27] Figure 3 dem-

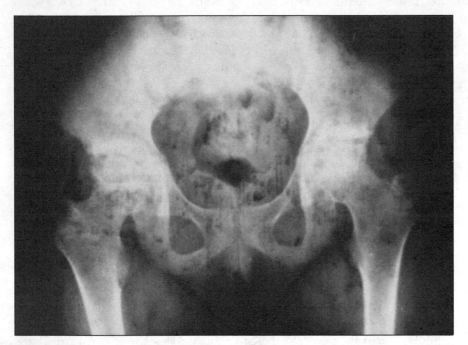

Figure 3. *Radiograph showing severe hip disease in child with juvenile rheumatoid arthritis. Note loss of joint space and cartilage, with irregular articulating surfaces.*

onstrates the results of severe hip disease, including loss of joint space and cartilage and irregular articulating surfaces. Typical hip deformities include hip flexion contractures and loss of hip extension, abduction, and rotation. Hip movement may be painful at end ranges and with weight bearing.

Prone lying for at least 20 minutes daily is used to prevent or minimize hip flexion contracture.[15] Occasionally, an abduction orthosis may be prescribed to prevent adduction contractures. The length of the iliotibial band should be monitored by use of serial Ober's tests.[15] Acute synovitis of the hip may be relieved by skin traction, applied with the pull toward abduction, to distract and rest the joint.[7] Prolonged sitting at a desk or in a wheelchair increases the likelihood of losing ROM. A tricycle or bicycle may also be used to maintain ROM and muscle strength if ambulation becomes difficult.

If soft tissues surrounding the hip joint become contracted, surgical releases may be indicated to restore ROM. Adductor and psoas muscle tenotomies are most often performed, with success noted in increasing ROM and relieving pain.[7] Joint integrity, however, must be present. In hips with significant deterioration, with loss of joint space and irregular articular surfaces, nothing will be gained by soft tissue release. Espada et al[28] have shown a marked drop in flexion contractures and an improvement in joint motion up to the first 3 years postsurgery. They concluded that soft tissue release is a beneficial option in preserving alignment and function in hip and knee flexion deformities affecting patients with JRA.

Indications for total hip arthroplasty in children with JRA include marked functional impairment or severe disabling pain.[29] Several authors[7,30–32] have described successful outcomes in hip replacement surgery in this population. Custom-made or special miniature prostheses are required by as many as 50% of all children with JRA; these devices can be specially fabricated using computerized tomography linked with a computer-driven lathe.[29] Component wear is usually not a significant problem because of the small stature of children with JRA, although loosening is the most common reason for failure of prostheses.[29]

Postoperative physical therapy care for the patient with total hip arthroplasty includes an emphasis on early mobilization, with ambulation (with partial weight bearing on the operated hip) beginning as early as the

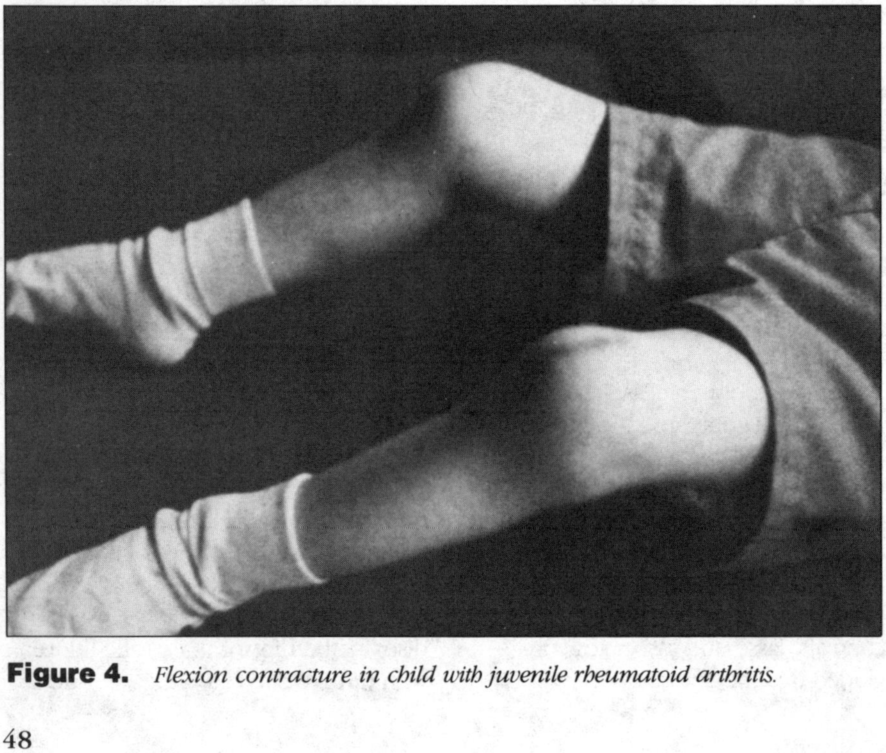

Figure 4. *Flexion contracture in child with juvenile rheumatoid arthritis.*

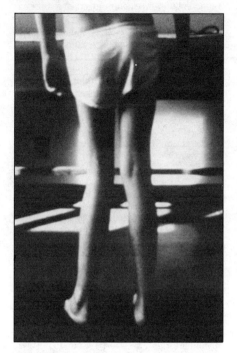

Figure 5. *Leg-length discrepancy in child with juvenile rheumatoid arthritis.*

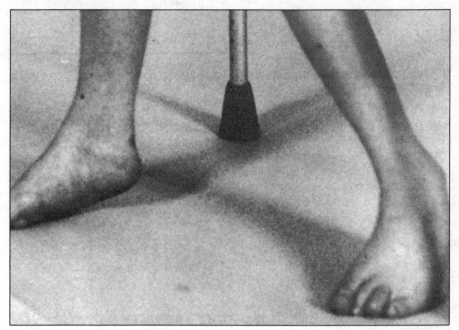

Figure 6. *Equinovarus deformity.*

second day. A positioning program teaches avoidance of hip adduction/external rotation and flexion beyond 90 degrees for 6 weeks following surgery because of risk of subluxation. Hyperextension is not permitted, an abductor pillow is used in bed and while sitting, and a raised toilet seat and chair are used for ease of transfer. Exercises include active and active-assistive hip flexion and extension and active hip abduction exercises in a supine position.[33]

Common knee joint problems include effusion with flexion contracture (Fig. 4) and quadriceps femoris muscle atrophy, valgus deformity, and leg-length discrepancy (Fig. 5). The leg-length discrepancy is often secondary to asymmetric knee arthritis, leading to overgrowth of the affected side attributable to stimulation of the growth plate by chronic inflammation.[15] Treatment emphasizes maintaining knee extension and quadriceps femoris muscle strength. Placement of pillows under the knees

should be avoided. Bicycling and swimming may be helpful in maintaining muscle strength and ROM.

Knee flexion contractures are usually managed conservatively by nighttime extension splinting or short-term serial casting. Dynamic splinting, such as the use of Dynasplints™[†] to achieve knee flexion or extension, can be used to reduce contractures that do not respond to static splinting (splinting with the joint held in one position without allowing free motion). Skin traction may also be helpful.[9] Because of muscle spasm or contracture, the tibia frequently moves backward relative to the femur, leading to a tightened anterior cruciate ligament. Hamstring muscle releases are advised early to prevent such contractures and subluxation; as movement is regained, the joint is better nourished and larger articular surfaces make contact. This can lead to healing if the disease remits.[7]

Leg-length discrepancy may be monitored by serial orthoroentgenograms. If necessary, an epiphysiodesis may

be performed to halt overgrowth of the longer limb.[7] Leg-length discrepancy is often treated with shoe lifts to maintain postural alignment. A partial epiphysiodesis or osteotomy may be necessary to correct genu valgum deformity. For some patients, Ilizarov instrumentation can correct leg-length discrepancies or valgus deformities.[34]

Knee synovectomy can be performed to remove overgrown, inflamed synovium and relative joint inflammation.[35] Although the synovium will eventually grow back, this can be a useful procedure to relieve pain and may assist in gaining motion. Some authors,[7,35] however, disagree on the procedure's overall effectiveness in this young population.

Total knee arthroplasty is indicated for older children with JRA for preservation of ambulation and is effective in reducing pain and increasing functional mobility. Postoperatively, a knee immobilizer is used, with isometric quadriceps femoris muscle strengthening and active-assistive ROM beginning on the second day and ambulation on the third day. Continuous passive motion machines are often used to restore mobility. The goal of this approach is

---

[†]Dynasplint Systems Inc, 6655 Amberton Dr, Ste A, Baltimore, MD 21227.

to achieve 90 degrees of knee flexion and full active extension by the 14th day postoperatively.[36]

Ankle and foot deformities also occur in children with JRA. In severe cases of the disease, an equinovarus deformity may be seen (Fig. 6). This condition may necessitate surgical correction of calcaneal deformity (such as a Dwyer osteotomy) and soft tissue releases for correction of alignment. In milder cases, valgus or pronated feet are often apparent. Shoe inserts or custom-molded orthoses may be useful in improving weight-bearing position. Heel cups may be indicated for painful heel spurs. Metatarsal bars may be used in shoes to relieve pressure from painful metatarsal heads. Another common foot deformity is hallux valgus with hammertoes. Custom-molded shoes may be indicated for painful deformities such as these, which are not responsive to a more conservative orthotic approach.

Conclusions

Physical therapists play a vital role in the care and management of children with JRA throughout the course of the disease. The physical therapist's serial evaluations can provide a barometer of disease activity, assisting the rheumatologist in decision making. Goal setting should be comprehensive and address all problem areas, which may include ROM, strength, pain, posture, aerobic conditioning, gait, and functional mobility. Physical therapy plays a crucial role in the team management of children with JRA. Components of this program include center-based treatment, as well as home exercises and guidelines for joint protection; positioning; and appropriate recreational activities. The physical therapist also participates in postoperative management of surgical interventions, which may include soft tissue releases, synovectomies, epiphysiodeses, arthrodeses, and joint replacements. Understanding the many facets of JRA, including the effects of exercise and activity, is important in attaining optimal functional outcomes for these patients.

Appendix. *American College of Rheumatology Criteria for Classification of Juvenile Rheumatoid Arthritis (JRA)*

1. Age of onset less than 16 years.
2. Presence of arthritis in one or more joints defined as swelling or effusion, or, in the absence of swelling, by the presence of at least two of the following:

    Limitation of range of motion

    Tenderness or pain on motion

    Increased heat
3. Duration of disease of at least 6 weeks.
4. Type of onset in the first 6 months characterized as one of the three onset types of JRA.
5. Exclusion of other rheumatic or viral diseases that may mimic JRA.

Acknowledgments

I thank Dr Lawrence Zemel for his support as teacher and friend and for his technical assistance in writing this article. I also thank Mary Gail Horelick, JD, MS, PT, and Joan Page, MA, PT, for their support and editorial assistance and Eleanor Fox for typing the manuscript.

References

1 Cassidy JT, Petty RE. Juvenile rheumatoid arthritis. In: *Textbook of Rheumatology*. 2nd ed. New York, NY: Churchill Livingstone Inc; 1990: chaps 1–3, 5.

2 Schaller JG. Chronic arthritis in children. *Clin Orthop*. 1983;182:79–89.

3 Brewer EJ, Giannini EH, Pearson DA. *Juvenile Rheumatoid Arthritis*. Philadelphia, Pa: WB Saunders Co; 1982: chaps 1, 2, 10, 17.

4 Kunnmo I, Kallio P, Pelkonen P. Incidence of arthritis in urban Finnish children. *Arthritis Rheum*. 1986;29:1232.

5 Andersson-Gore B, Fasth A. Incidence and prevalence of juvenile chronic arthritis: a 5-year prospective population survey. Presented at the Third International Pediatric Rheumatology Conference; March 1991; Park City, Utah.

6 Ansell BM, Wood P. Prognosis in juvenile chronic polyarthritis. *Clin Rheum Dis*. 1976;2:397.

7 Swann M. The surgery of juvenile chronic arthritis. *Clin Orthop*. 1990;259:83–91.

8 Ansell BM. Joint manifestations in children with juvenile chronic polyarthritis. *Arthritis Rheum*. 1977;20:204–206.

9 *Arthritis Health Professions Teaching Slide Collection*. Atlanta, Ga: Arthritis Foundation; 1980.

10 Silverman E, Isacovics E, Schneider R, et al. Effect of intravenous gamma globulin on immunoglobulin production in systemic onset juvenile arthritis. *Arthritis Rheum*. 1988;31:527.

11 Burmester GR, Horneff G, Emmrich F, Kalden JR. Immunomodulatory treatment of rheumatoid arthritis with an anti-CD4 (anti-helper T cell) monoclonal antibody. Podium presentation at the annual meeting of the American College of Rheumatology; 1990; Seattle, Wash.

12 DeNardo BS, Rhodes VJ, Gibbons B, et al. *Physical Therapy Standards of Care for Children with Chronic Arthritis*. Boston, Mass: The Affiliated Children's Arthritis Centers of New England; 1990.

13 Kiviranta I, Jurvelin J, Tammi M, et al. Weight bearing controls glycosaminoglycan concentration and articular cartilage in the knee joints of young beagle dogs. *Arthritis Rheum*. 1987;30:801–808.

14 Scull SA, Dow MB, Athreya BH. Physical and occupational therapy for children with rheumatic diseases. *Pediatr Clin North Am*. 1986;33:1053–1077.

15 Scull S. Juvenile rheumatoid arthritis. In: Tecklin JS. *Pediatric Physical Therapy*. Philadelphia, Pa; JB Lippincott Co; 1989:216–236.

16 Lechner DE, McCarthy CF, Holden MK. Gait deviations in patients with juvenile rheumatoid arthritis. *Phys Ther*. 1987;67:1335–1341.

17 Haley S, Faas RM, Coster WJ, et al. *Pediatric Evaluation of Disability Inventory*. Boston, Mass; New England Medical Center; 1989.

18 Coulton CJ, Zborowky E, Lipton J, Newnan J. Assessment of the reliability and validity of the arthritis impact measurement scales for children with juvenile arthritis. *Arthritis Rheum*. 1987;30:819–824.

19 Rhodes VJ, Pumphrey KF, Zemel L. Development of a functional assessment tool for children with juvenile rheumatoid arthritis. *Arthritis Rheum*. 1988;31(suppl 4):S151. Abstract.

20 Lovell DJ, Howe S, Shear E, Hartner S. Development of a disability measurement tool for juvenile rheumatoid arthritis. *Arthritis Rheum*. 1989;32:1390–1395.

21 DeAndrade JR, Grant C, Dixon AS. Joint distension and reflex muscle inhibition in the knee. *J Bone Joint Surg [Am]*. 1965;47:313–322.

22 Koch B. Rehabilitation of the child with joint disease. In: Molnar GE, ed. *Pediatric Rehabilitation*. Baltimore, Md: Williams & Wilkins; 1985:233–271.

23 Jasso MS, Protas EJ, Giannini EH, Brewer EJ. Physical work capacity (PWC) in juvenile rheumatoid arthritis (JRA) patients and healthy children. Presented at the Annual Meeting of the American Rheumatism Association/American Health Planning Association; 1986; New Orleans, La.

24 Weinblatt ME, Coblyn JS, Fox DA, et al: Efficacy of low-dose methotrexate in rheumatoid arthritis. *N Engl J Med*. 1985;312:818–822.

25 Harkcom TM, Lampman RM, Banwell BF, Castor CW. Therapeutic value of graded aerobic exercise training in rheumatoid arthritis. *Arthritis Rheum*. 1985;28:32–39.

26 Isdale IC. Hip disease in juvenile rheumatoid arthritis. *Ann Rheum Dis*. 1970;29:603–638.

27 Ansell BM: Introduction. In: Arden GP, Ansell BM, eds. *Surgical Management of Juve-*

nile Chronic Polyarthritis. New York, NY: Grune & Stratton Inc; 1978:1–7.

28 Espada G, Alvarez MM, Gagliardi S. Long-term results of soft tissue release surgery for hips and knees in juvenile chronic arthritis (JCA). Presented at the Third International Pediatric Rheumatology Conference; March 1991; Park City, Utah.

29 Scott RD. Total hip and knee arthroplasty in juvenile rheumatoid arthritis. *Clin Orthop.* 1990;259:83–91.

30 Lachiewicz PF, McCaskill B, Inglis A, et al. Total hip arthroplasty in juvenile rheumatoid

arthritis: two-to-eleven-year results. *J Bone Joint Surg [Am].* 1986;68:502–508.

31 Ruddlesdon C, Ansell BM, Arden GP, Swann M. Total hip replacement in children with juvenile chronic arthritis. *J Bone Joint Surg [Br].* 1986;68:218–222.

32 Gudmundsson GH, Harving S, Pilgaard S. The Charaley total hip arthroplasty in juvenile rheumatoid arthritis patients. *Orthopedics.* 1989;12:385–388.

33 *University of Connecticut Health Center Multidisciplinary Total Hip Replacement Proto-*

col. Farmington, Conn: University of Connecticut Health Center.

34 Ilizarov GA. The principles of the Ilizarov method. *Bull Hosp Jt Dis Orthop Inst.* 1988;48(2):1–11.

35 Rydholm U, Elborgh R, Ranstam J, Schröder A. Synovectomy of the knee in juvenile chronic arthritis. *J Bone Joint Surg [Br].* 1986;68:223–228.

36 Carmichael E, Chaplin DM. Total knee arthroplasty in juvenile rheumatoid arthritis: a seven-year follow-up study. *Clin Orthop.* 1986;210;192–200.

Prosthetic Management of Children with Limb Deficiencies

David E Krebs
Joan E Edelstein
Maureen A Thornby

Children with amputations present challenging management problems. Surgical management, prosthetic fitting options, and training regimens have progressed substantially over the past several decades. Clinicians should be familiar with the available technological options to provide children with amputations the best possible care. The plethora of small components available for lower- and upper-limb prostheses indicates the desirability of managing juvenile patients in an interdisciplinary, specialized clinical setting where the advantages and disadvantages of prosthetic options can be related to the particular needs and wishes of each young client and the client's family. Although prostheses are not anatomical avatars, careful appliance prescription and training, coordinated with the child's growth and developmental changes, can optimize the benefits the child derives from the prosthesis. [Krebs DE, Edelstein JE, Thornby MA. Prosthetic management of children with limb deficiencies. Phys Ther. 1991;71:920–934.]

Key Words: *Amputations, children/prosthetics; Orthotics/splints/casts, general; Pediatrics, equipment.*

Children with amputations are not miniature adults. Only in the last three decades have children with limb deficiencies been served by specialized pediatric clinics; many clinics were established following the 1950s' thalidomide disaster in Europe.[1] The prosthetic clinic team should be cognizant not only of the current needs of juvenile patients with limb reductions, but also of the long-term, adult sequelae that may result from current prosthetic management choices. For example, if a childhood limb deficiency is treated by early distal surgical amputation, the effect of prosthesis-imposed forces on the limb segments and spine as well as eventual mature limb length must be considered.[2] Treatment options for children should be chosen on the basis of anticipated function, comfort, and appearance, and the psychological and physiological needs of children should be weighed against compromise to their eventual function.[3]

The purpose of this article is to review the clinical factors specific to children with amputations. Although the literature is replete with anecdotal and case reports, few systematic data are available on the nature of the clinical problem. Most published information is based on small and perhaps unrepresentative samples. We will begin by describing the juvenile population, then briefly describe the most common prosthetic options, and finally summarize current training considerations. In this article, we will consider persons under 21 years of age whose limb reductions are from surgical or congenital causes.

Epidemiologic Factors

Because the population of children with amputations is diverse and because no standard data-collection efforts are required of health facilities treating children with amputations in the United States, no comprehensive characterization of this population is available. Nevertheless, the following section provides an overview of the epidemiologic factors influencing

DE Krebs, PhD, PT, is Associate Professor, Graduate Program in Physical Therapy, MGH Institute of Health Professions, 15 River St, Boston, MA 02018-3402 (USA). Address all correspondence to Dr Krebs.

JE Edelstein, MA, PT, is Associate Professor of Clinical Physical Therapy, Columbia University, 630 W 168th St, New York, NY 10032.

MA Thornby, MA, PT, is in private physical therapy practice and is a doctoral student in the Department of Physical Therapy, School of Education, Health, Nursing, and Arts Professions, New York University, New York, NY 10003.

This work was supported in part by NIH Grant R01-AR40029 (Dr Krebs).

prosthetic management of children with amputations. Because most pediatric limb deficiencies are from congenital causes and because many children with congenital amputations have multiple limb involvement, these epidemiologic factors often direct clinical decisions.

Prevalence

The National Center for Health Statistics and other agencies estimate that about one tenth of 1% of the US population have a "major limb reduction" (ie, more than a missing toe or part of a finger) and that 13% of these individuals are younger than 21 years of age.[4,5] Therefore, the estimated prevalence of major pediatric amputation in the United States is 32,500. Congenital loss accounts for the majority of pediatric limb reductions; however, trauma, tumor, and other diseases, in descending order, are the causes for most postnatal pediatric amputations.[5,6]

Incidence

The only published report examining the incidence of pediatric amputations in North America was completed several years ago, so its conclusions may be outdated compared with current amputation incidence.[6] That census was limited to 4,105 children with limb deficiencies treated at specialty clinics. Thus, it is not known to what extent that census reflects the total North American population. Given these limitations, however, the rate of new cases treated by the pediatric clinics was about 17% of the total caseload, with three fifths of these 17% being children with congenital limb reductions.[6] Applying this rate to federal population estimates suggests that the United States would likely experience 5,525 new cases of childhood amputations per year, with about 3,315 of these amputations being congenital. Sampling estimate errors and childhood deaths may explain the numeric discrepancies between the incidence and prevalence data.

Characteristics

The population of children with amputations differs from the population of adults with amputations in several ways. Few childhood amputations are caused by the vascular disorders so prevalent among older persons, and, unlike adults, most children with amputations have upper-limb deficiency. In treating children, decisions should emphasize developmental function and avoidance of related residuum (formerly called the "stump") anomalies such as terminal spike and distal bone overgrowth,[1] rather than residuum care and length preservation.

Congenital anomalies are taxonomically diverse and are classified as being either *transverse*, in which all skeletal elements distal to the level of loss are absent, or *longitudinal*, in which some distal skeletal elements remain.[7] Transverse deficiencies resemble surgical amputations, although there is no scar. Longitudinal deficiencies are more variable. For example, in fibular absence—a rather common lower-limb longitudinal deficiency—the foot may be intact, but often the fourth and fifth rays may be missing, with tarsal abnormalities and a markedly bowed tibia.

Among the most challenging lower-limb anomalies are proximal femoral focal deficiency (PFFD), which includes a foreshortened femur and a reasonably normal tibia, fibula, and foot, resulting in severe reduction in limb length, and phocomelia, in which the foot is articulated with the pelvis. In both anomalies, the pelvis is abnormally formed. Comparable longitudinal deficiencies appear in the upper limb, particularly absence of the ulna.[7]

Level of deficiency and residuum characteristics. Although most adult patients have unilateral lower-limb amputations, fully 20% of children with amputations have bilateral, quadrimembral, or trimembral reductions—many of these reductions include complex congenital anomalies such as PFFD.[6] Cosmetic considerations notwithstanding, acceptable

surgical (such as the Van Nes rotation-plasty) and conservative management and expert rehabilitative care can enable these children to be quite functional.[8,9] Although a given limb reduction is usually fitted prosthetically similarly to that of an adult amputation of the same level, both prosthetic and surgical options should be carefully discussed with the child's parents, and, if possible, with the child.[2,3] Conversion of a congenital anomaly to a more proximal amputation through surgery should be undertaken only after all members of the clinic team have participated in the decision. Consideration should be given to the potential limb length, current and future prosthetic options, and cosmetic and functional expectations of the child and family. Rarely are postsurgical joint stiffness and healing major factors; children virtually always regain full joint mobility, and, because few such residua have vascular impediments to healing, wound recovery is usually prompt.

Of the children most frequently seen in pediatric amputation clinics, most have left upper-limb deficiency, and most of these children have below-elbow reductions.[6] Nearly one quarter of all children with amputations have below-elbow deficiencies; all except 13% of these children have had congenital anomalies (Fig. 1). Therefore, physical therapists who work with such children should become familiar with upper-limb treatment options.[6]

Approximately 7% of all children with amputations have three or more limb reductions. Children with congenital amputations and those with very early surgically acquired, bilateral upper-extremity amputations often learn to feed and otherwise care for themselves by developing "prehensile toes" (as one of our patients referred to his ability to use his feet as most of us use our hands). Children with trimembral amputations, and especially those with quadruple amputations, however, invariably need special assistive devices. Technology is rapidly enhancing the ability of these individuals to be more independent. Nonspecialist therapists should seek assist-

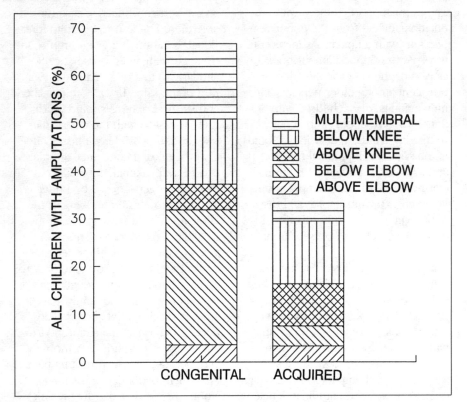

Figure 1. *The rate and composition of the two major subgroups of children with amputations, congenital (usually in utero limb reductions) and acquired (postperinatal amputations), differ substantially. About two thirds of all children with amputations have congenital etiologies, and most of them have below-elbow deficiencies; the latter are most frequently associated with prenatal teratogens. By contrast, acquired amputations occur most frequently in the lower limb and are most frequently caused by malignancies and machinery-related trauma. Data from Table 3 of Krebs and Fishman[6] have been recombined such that below-knee amputations include all transverse deficiencies distal to the knee, including ankle and foot reductions, whereas above-knee amputations include all through-the-knee and proximal reductions; similar logic is followed for upper-limb data.*

ance from pediatric amputation centers to help these patients achieve their full potential with current technological options.[10]

If the residuum contains vestigial articulations and epiphyseal growth plates, it is critically important to observe the distal end for bone overgrowth. Bony overgrowth can eventually cause skin penetration in cases in which the initial symptoms (eg, sharp and clearly located pain) and signs (eg, a palpable and irregular stiff spike immediately subcutaneous to the distal-most surgical flap or congenital residuum end) are ignored. Controversy exists concerning the utility of firm prosthetic contact, such as that provided by distal end-bearing sockets, for treating or preventing

bony overgrowth. Recent evidence suggests that appositional bone growth from the periosteal residuum is a causative agent in both congenital and acquired (postpartum) osseous spikes.[11] Until conclusive evidence emerges on the effects of mechanical stimulation in general, and distal contact in particular, on the genesis of residuum overgrowth, we believe that end-bearing and mechanical loading of the remaining epiphyses contribute to the long-term well-being of the residual limb.

Age. About two thirds of all pediatric limb reductions are due to perinatal (usually congenital) events. The remaining third occur over the first two decades of life. About half of all children seeking care for the first time at

a typical amputation specialty clinic are less than 3 years old. About 16% of children with congenital amputations do not receive such care until they are about to begin school.[6] We believe clinicians need to be more proactive in identifying young patients who may benefit from early prosthetic fitting.

Gender, side, and etiology. More boys (59%) than girls (41%) comprise the population of children with amputations, regardless of age. Overall, most limb reductions occur on the body's left side (Fig. 2); this sinistral predilection can be explained in part by congenital teratologic side-specificity.[11] Teratogens also probably explain the excess peril to boys prenatally,[12,13] but excessive risk-taking and poor parental supervision account for many gun-related, farm,[14] and railway[15] acquired amputations. Such data highlight the important role physical therapists can play in preventing accidental amputations.

Boys account for well over half of amputations in which the etiology is cancer, including the most common carcinoma among children: osteosarcoma.[16] Most carcinoma-related limb reductions occur in the second decade of life. New treatment methods can be used to address the desire of appearance-conscious adolescents for nonprosthetic limb salvage. Options include *en-bloc* resections, in which a major portion of the femur is replaced with an endoprosthesis, and rotationplasty.[9] *En-bloc* salvage procedures would seem to offer superior appearance, because the natural external shape and size of the thigh is retained, and reasonable performance, because the natural knee is preserved. Few data, however, have been reported to support this supposition. Indeed, the operative risks attendant to pediatric surgery should always be a part of the many considerations guiding surgical management options.

Prostheses and Prescription Options

Children's prosthetic needs are dictated by their small size and physical

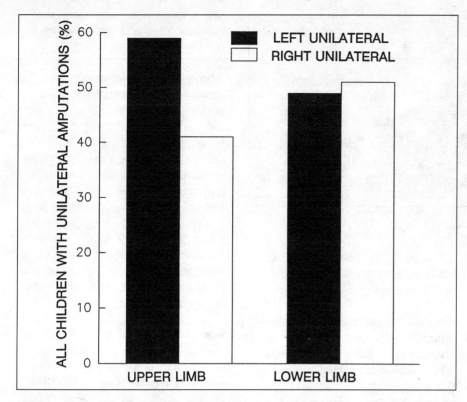

Figure 2. *The number of left- and right-side amputations differs insignificantly among lower-limb reductions, but left-limb deficiencies substantially predominate among children with unilateral upper-limb amputations. The reason for the left and right upper-limb disparities is unknown, but is speculated to be related to the genetic predisposition of certain genome positions to prenatal damage. Note that although right (ie, usually dominant side) traumatic amputations from farm and other machinery might be expected to far exceed left upper-limb reductions, these data[6] belie that expectation.*

and psychosocial growth and development. Parental concerns also affect prosthetic prescription. Some families are primarily interested in disguising the amputation, particularly upper-limb reductions. Personal financial resources play a key role in prescription, especially when private insurance and public funding are meager. A list of commercial vendors of prosthetic components is provided in the Appendix.

Lower-Limb Prostheses

Children with acquired below-knee amputations or congenital transverse deficiencies at the below-knee level wear prostheses having four elements: (1) a foot-ankle assembly, (2) a shank, (3) a socket, and (4) a suspension. A modified below-knee prosthesis is also used by patients with some congenital longitudinal deficiencies, such as fibular hemimelia, which are functionally comparable to below-knee amputations.[17]

Ankle-foot assemblies. Infants are given flat solid-ankle cushion heel (SACH) assemblies[*,†]; this simple foot provides a stable standing base and, when the infant walks, flat initial contact. By 1.5 years of age, nearly all nondisabled toddlers can contact the floor with the heel[18,19] and progress with a heel-toe transition; with a basic prosthetic foot, the pediatric amputee should be able to perform similarly.

The smallest commercial prosthetic foot is 9 cm (3.5 in) long, equal to a juvenile size 1 shoe, and is suitable for an infant approximately 4 months old. This foot has an external keel and a smooth distal border. The 10-cm (4-in) SACH assembly is available with an internal keel and molded toes. The SACH feet are durable, inexpensive, and lightweight. The smallest Syme's model of the SACH foot is somewhat longer (14 cm [5.5 in]).

For school-aged children and adolescents, energy storing-releasing feet are used. They have flexible keels, which bend upon loading in early stance to store energy and recoil in late stance to release energy. This feature affords the wearer more spring when walking, running, and jumping. The smallest components are 12 cm (4.7 in) long; they are the "STored ENergy" (STEN)* (Fig. 3), Flex-Foot[‡] (Fig. 4),[20] and Flex-Walk[‡] (Fig. 4) feet. The new split-toe option of the Flex-Foot greatly improves maneuvering over rough terrain and hills. The smallest child's model of the Seattle LightFoot[§] (Fig. 5) is 13 cm (5 in) long, and that of the SpringLite[‖] is 14 cm long.

Initially, a prosthetic foot may be aligned anteriorly relative to the socket to promote stability. As the wearer gains confidence, the alignment can be altered to favor mobility.

Shanks. The remainder of the below-knee prosthesis is custom-made, regardless of the size of the patient. The shank, connecting the foot and the socket, may be an endoskeletal or exoskeletal device. Exoskeletal devices are usually carved from wood and then covered with a protective plastic coating. Exoskeletal

*Kingsley Manufacturing Co, 1984 Placentia Ave, Costa Mesa, CA 92628.

†Otto Bock Orthopedic Industries Inc, 300 Xenium Ln, Plymouth, MN 55422.

‡Flex-Foot Inc, 27071 Cabot Rd, Ste 106, Laguna Hills, CA 92653.

§Model and Instrument Development Co, 861 Poplar Pl S, Seattle, WA 98144.

‖SpringLite, 1006 W Beardsley Pl, Salt Lake City, UT 84119.

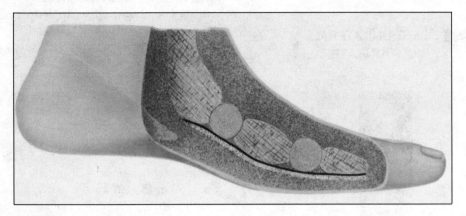

Figure 3. *"STored ENergy" (STEN) prosthetic foot.*

constructions are relatively inexpensive, resist abrasions, are durable, and cannot be saturated by urine from young children who are not toilet trained. An endoskeletal shank consists of an aluminum and steel, or ultralightweight carbon-fiber or titanium, central pylon. Endoskeletal devices are covered with foam rubber shaped to match the contralateral limb; the rubber may not be durable enough for children who engage in vigorous games.

Below-knee sockets. These sockets are molded of rigid plastic, usually polyester laminate, with a liner of polyethylene foam. The socket should contact the entirety of the amputation limb to maximize sensory feedback and to ensure that moderate pressure is applied to the distal end of the residuum, thereby preventing circulatory and dermatologic disorders. Even in the presence of skin grafts, children can generally tolerate more distal loading than can adults.[21]

The socket must be aligned in greater abduction and flexion to complement the infantile gait pattern, which lacks bimodal knee flexion/extension movement until the child is 2 years of age.[18] Young children with amputations walk with excessively flexed knees and hips during the stance phase.[19] Prostheses for toddlers should be aligned to accommodate the wide walking base and external hip rotation that persist in children until they are 3 years of age.[19]

Below-knee prosthetic suspensions. Suspension can be achieved in several ways. A baby may require a supracondylar cuff joined to an anterior elastic strap, which, in turn, buckles to a waist belt or harness.[17] The strap maintains the prosthesis in place even when the wearer reverts to crawling. Some toddlers need a harness to counteract attempts at unsupervised undressing. As the skeleton matures, the femoral epicondyles become more prominent, making supracondylar or supracondylar/suprapatellar suspensions good choices. The supracondylar/suprapatellar suspension, in particular, decreases pistoning and enhances gait stability, even for children with an absent fibula or a short residual limb.[22] The one-piece construction eliminates the risk of losing the supracondylar device's medial suspension wedge.[23] Teenagers often opt for an elastic sleeve in place of the cuff or to augment supracondylar suspension; the sleeve provides suspension that is advantageous during athletics and creates a smooth silhouette under snug clothing. Suction, particularly with the Silicone Suction Socket, maximizes security. The wearer rolls a silicone sock over the amputation limb. The sock has a distal metal ring that is secured to the

medial and lateral socket walls with a transverse rod.[24] Thigh corset suspension is rarely necessary, unless the anatomic knee is unstable or the child has Van Nes rotationplasty.[9,25]

Above-knee components. The above-knee prosthesis has five components, two of which—the foot and the shank—are essentially the same as for the below-knee appliance. Recently introduced endoskeletal shank systems include the Otto Bock aluminum and steel endoskeletal modular system[†] designed for children 2 to 14 years of age who weigh less than 40 kg (99 lb). The Endolite system,[#] manufactured of carbon fiber and titanium, is lighter, but appreciably more expensive, than the aluminum and steel components.

Knee units. An infant's first prosthesis may lack a knee unit and have an ischial bearing socket mounted on a pair of side bars above a foot.[26] The creative prosthetist can fashion a pair of plastic overlap knee hinges or use small hinges intended for a below-elbow prosthesis.

For school-aged wearers, knee units, with or without a stabilizing mechanism, are manufactured as small as 24 cm (9.5 in) in circumference at the calf, with the knee bolt 6.5 cm (2.5 in) wide. Active preteenagers and adolescents often use hydraulic and pneumatic knee units, in which frictional control of knee swing adjusts automatically to changes in walking or running velocity.

Above-knee sockets. Plastic total-contact sockets are essential for virtually all children with amputations, whether infants in diapers or adolescents who perspire profusely while engaged in strenuous activities. "Ischial socket contours," which have a narrower width than in the anteroposterior dimension, are used by many children, whereas other children use quadrilateral sockets, which are narrower in the anteroposterior dimension. Regardless of shape, the flexible polyethylene socket in a carbon-fiber reinforced frame is appropriate for children.[27] The thin socket is comfort-

---

#afi Endolite, 2480 W 82nd St, Hialeah, FL 33016.

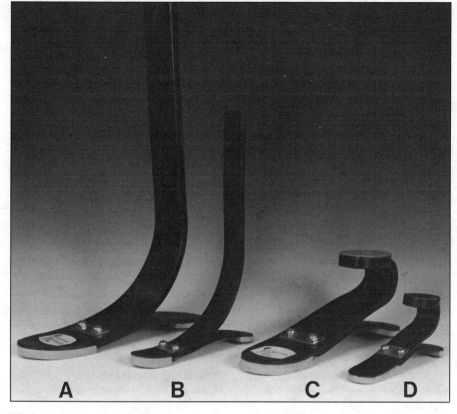

Figure 4. *Flex-Foot and Flex-Walk components: (A) adult Flex-Foot, (B) child Flex-Foot, (C) adult Flex-Walk, (D) child Flex-Walk.*

able, dissipates heat well, yields to the chair seat when the wearer sits, and conforms to changes in muscle contour when the wearer walks. In addition, the flexible polyethylene clings to the skin to enhance suspension and is translucent, enabling clinicians to visualize fit. The socket is very easy to adjust to accommodate for growth.[27]

Above-knee prosthetic suspensions. Very young patients usually need a combination of suction and some form of auxiliary suspension, typically a Silesian bandage, to retain the prosthesis on soft subcutaneous tissue. Toddlers may require the continued use of a Silesian bandage to aid reapplication of the prosthesis when there is accidental loss of suction. By age 6 years, children can use full suction suspension, which eliminates the necessity of straps around the torso.[25] Although some clinicians do not recommend total suction suspension until the patient is 14 years of age, believing there may be problems with independent donning,[28] in our experience, children as young as 5 years of age can manage prostheses with flexible sockets, suction suspension, and a Silesian bandage.[27]

Prostheses for children with congenital deformities. Children with hip anomalies, such as PFFD, often require a funnel-shaped socket to provide full contact. The distal end of the socket is similar to that for the child with surgical amputation. If the foreshortened PFFD limb has not been revised surgically, however, the socket may accommodate the anatomic foot. The anatomic foot is plantar flexed to minimize the bulkiness of the thigh section of the prosthesis. Ordinarily, a Silesian bandage is attached. The patient with unilateral phocomelia can wear a modified hip disarticulation prosthesis or, depending on the strength of the foot, a variant above-knee prosthesis; in both instances, the foot aids suspension and prosthetic control.[26] Several youngsters with bilateral amelia or phocomelia or with sacral agenesis have been fitted successfully with a modified reciprocating gait orthosis.[29]

Adjustments for growth. Adjustments for growth should be anticipated at the time of prosthesis prescription to extend the life of the prosthesis and reduce both expense and office visits, which disrupt school and home routines. In addition to these adjustments, children's prostheses are replaced more frequently than those for adults because the young wearers' greater activity takes its toll on movable components and the external finish. Growth occurs in spurts, particularly in infancy and in preadolescence, necessitating a new prosthesis every 1 to 2 years.[30] Persistent redness of the skin and a tissue roll over the edge of the socket are signs of tightness. Maintaining the prosthesis equal to the length of the sound limb is important to prevent the patient from walking with excessive lateral trunk bending. Purchasing larger shoes so that the sound foot can be fitted properly is another event signaling the need to revise the prosthesis. For the individual with bilateral amputations, the impetus for lengthening prostheses often comes from the youngster's concern about conforming to one's peers or being taller than younger siblings. Frequent inspection of the amputation limb is required to determine when adjustment or a new prescription is needed. We recommend quarterly clinic visits for young patients, although in our experience,

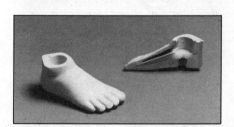

Figure 5. *Seattle LightFoot Child's Play component.*

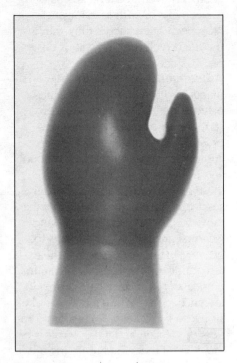

Figure 6. *Passive mitten terminal device.*

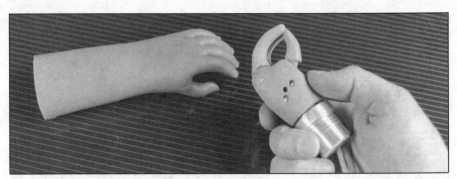

Figure 7. *Child's myoelectric hand and glove.*

adolescents generally do not require more than semiannual examination.

Approximately a third of lower-limb growth occurs at the proximal femoral epiphysis[31]; consequently, most of the limb length will be below the socket. Exoskeletal shanks can be lengthened by prosthetists, who section the shanks near the ankle unit and insert shims of appropriate thickness. Ordinarily, the girth of the shank is not increased. Annual calf growth is normally only 0.3 cm for children between 2 and 6 years of age and 0.2 cm for 7- to 10-year-olds.[32] Endoskeletal shanks are lengthened by substituting longer piping for the outgrown pylon. By the time the shank needs lengthening, a new cosmetic cover will be required to replace the old, often damaged, cover. Alternatively, for both types of shank, a 1-cm (0.5-in) insert can be placed in the shoe on the prosthetic side.

Socket length and circumference can be increased in several ways. When the prosthesis is fabricated, two concentric sockets can be nested in the outer socket, with the inner sockets removed as the amputation limb grows. Extra liners can be used in the same manner. Both approaches, however, require that the new prosthesis be relatively bulky. In addition, because the amputation limb does not grow uniformly, the final socket version may not fit precisely. A socket with an adjustable section held by several straps[33] is another option. The ideal arrangement involves a flexible socket that can readily be modified. The polyethylene above-knee socket can be heated to be reshaped as much as 4 cm (1.5 in) on the lateral aspect. The rigid frame is constructed with a thick lamination proximally and 2-cm (0.7-in) polyurethane filler distally. The prosthetist can grind away material as the child grows.[27]

Prosthetic foot size should keep pace with the anatomic foot, which for children 4 to 14 years of age, grows approximately one size per year.[32] The ipsilateral knee will be more difficult to flex if the child walks with a small prosthetic foot inside a large shoe.

Upper-Limb Prostheses

Most upper-limb prostheses include a terminal device (TD), which replaces the missing hand, a wrist unit, and a custom-made socket. Depending on the mode of TD control, the prosthesis may also include an individually fashioned harness and a cable system.

Terminal devices. The tiniest TD resembling a hand is the passive mitten** (Fig. 6), 8.6 cm (3.4 in) in circumference across the "metacarpophalangeal joints," suitable for infants approximately 6 months old. Although it disguises the amputation, the pink or brown mitten does not provide for unilateral prehension, nor does it allow the baby to stabilize the limb on a crib rail to pull up to stand. The device is replaced when the child is ready for active prosthetic control.[34] The smallest passive hand is 10.2 cm (4 in) in circumference at the "knuckles" and is covered with a glove, manufactured in nine colors approximating skin tones.

The smallest voluntary-opening, cable-operated hand is 5 cm (2 in) wide, intended for children 2 to 6 years of age.[35] At the hand's minimum spring setting, it does not close tightly over paper; at its maximum setting, pinch force is so great that the wearer must exert substantial force on the harness to open the hand.[36]

Children 18 months of age have been fitted with myoelectrically controlled hands†† (Figs. 7, 8), 5 cm wide,[37] although there is no convincing support for fitting prior to 2.5 years of age.[38] This battery-powered component eliminates the need for harnessing and provides greater grasp force than do cable-operated hands, but the

---

**Hosmer Dorrance Corp, 561 Division St, Campbell, CA 95008.

††Liberty Mutual Research Center, 71 Frankland Rd, Hopkinton, MA 01748.

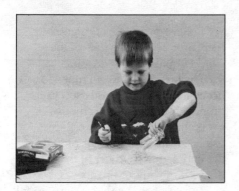

Figure 8. *Boy wearing below-elbow myoelectric prosthesis.*

myoelectric unit is heavier and more fragile than passive or cable-operated TDs. A very small child will have to wear the battery in a chest or waist holster if space in the forearm shell between the distal end of the socket and the proximal end of the hand is insufficient to house the battery. Some patients with very short residual limbs complain about the distal weight. All prosthetic hands, whether myoelectric or body-powered, require a glove, which matches the wearer's skin color and protects any mechanism in the component. The gloves tear and stain easily and require constant upkeep.

Hook TDs enable infants to appreciate bimanual prehension. When the toddler is 12 to 15 months old, a cable is added to the TD to prepare for independent activation.[39,40] The smallest voluntary-opening model—the Hosmer Dorrance infant's 12P hook** (Fig. 9)—is 7 cm (2.7 in) long and has a pink or brown plastic covering. Pinch force is regulated by the number of rubber bands worn on the hook; increasing closing force increases the harness force needed to open the hook. The smallest voluntary-closing hook, the Anatomically Designed-Engineered Polymer Technology (ADEPT) hook[‡‡] (Fig. 10), is tan and of similar size to the Hosmer Dorrance infant's 12P hook; grasp depends on the amount of

force exerted on the cable at the harness. One report[41] suggested that fitting a voluntary-closing hook at 6 months of age improves gross motor development.

An intermediate TD design provides the prehensile capability of a hook with a more anthropomorphic contour. One such device—the Child Amputee Prosthetics Project (CAPP) voluntary-opening TD** (Fig. 11)—is manufactured in two sizes: The smaller device is 0.5 cm longer than the smallest hook and is available in brown and pink. Other options for young patients include electric switch-controlled hands and hooks** (Fig. 12) and an electric prehension actuator, which can be used with any voluntary-opening TD.

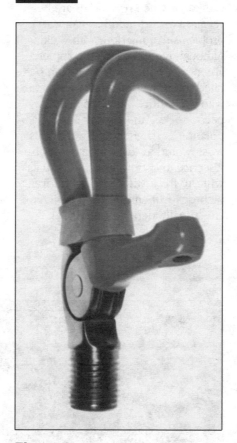

Figure 9. *Infant's 12P voluntary-opening hook.*

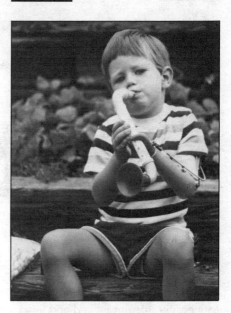

Figure 10. *Boy wearing below-elbow prosthesis with Anatomically Designed-Engineered Polymer Technology (ADEPT) voluntary-closing hook.*

Wrist units. The TD is screwed into a wrist unit, which provides passive pronation and supination. Two commercially available units** also enable the child to palmar flex the TD.

Proximal components. The socket, harness, and cable system of prostheses are custom-made. The flexible polyethylene socket in a rigid frame has been used for all levels, from wrist disarticulation to above-elbow, although older-style laminated sockets are also popular.[42]

Above-elbow prosthetic components. The above-elbow prosthesis is composed of a TD, wrist unit, forearm section, elbow unit, socket, harness, and cable system. The forearm section may be custom-made or manufactured as part of the elbow unit. The smallest elbow units are 5.1 cm (1.5 in) in diameter. The simplest model has a fraction joint, whereas the more complex type has a cable that permits locking the elbow at the desired angle. Electric switch-controlled elbows[§§] (Fig. 13) manufactured for toddlers respond to minimum force on a push or pull activator, but are appreciably heavier than simpler models.[37]

[‡‡]Therapeutic Recreation Systems Inc, 1280 28th St, Boulder, CO 80303.

[§§]Variety Ability Systems Inc, 3701 Danforth Ave, Scarborough, Ontario, Canada M1N 2G2.

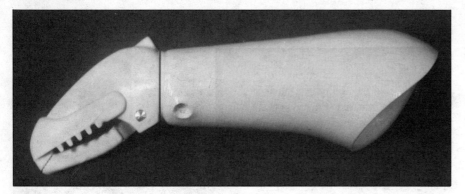

Figure 11. *Child Amputee Prosthetics Project (CAPP) voluntary-opening terminal device.*

Adjustments for growth. Progressively larger TDs and forearm sections must be supplied to maintain symmetry between the amputated and intact limbs. Wrist units are available in small, medium, and large sizes. The below- or above-elbow socket can be enlarged in ways similar to those used with lower-limb prostheses.[42–44]

Other Appliances

The pediatric patient may benefit from other appliances at various ages. Toddlers with unilateral lower-limb amputations generally manage independent walking, but, like nondisabled toddlers, may ride in a stroller to traverse long distances. The child with bilateral lower-limb deficiencies may need to use a wheelchair until proficiency with the prostheses is gained, or when prostheses are being repaired or the child has medical problems that interfere with walking. Although individuals with complete absence of both lower limbs can be fitted with a pair of prostheses or with two artificial limbs joined to a pelvic socket, the energy cost of ambulation is so great and walking is so slow and awkward that, by adolescence, most of these individuals will opt for a wheelchair. Children with quadrimembral limb deficiencies usually depend on special crutches[45] and adaptive equipment for daily activities.[46]

We believe prostheses designed for recreation should be part of the child's equipment. Many pursuits, such as bicycling and running, do not necessitate special prostheses. Children with unilateral leg amputations generally ski without a prosthesis, using ski poles with small rudders at the end. Similarly, most of these children swim without prostheses; however, waterproof prostheses are useful at the beach or water's edge. Several recreational TDs (Fig. 14) are manufactured, including the Super Sport flexible mitt[‡‡] for gymnastics and appliances for bowling, holding ski poles, using a baseball mitt, and managing golf clubs and cameras.

Prosthetic Training

The fundamental differences between adults and children with amputations—growth, responsibility, and functional needs—make pediatric prosthetic training a complex process of assessment, training, and intermittent upgrading of functional activities suited to the child's stage of development. The rehabilitation process must also focus on maintaining prosthetic durability and function.[47]

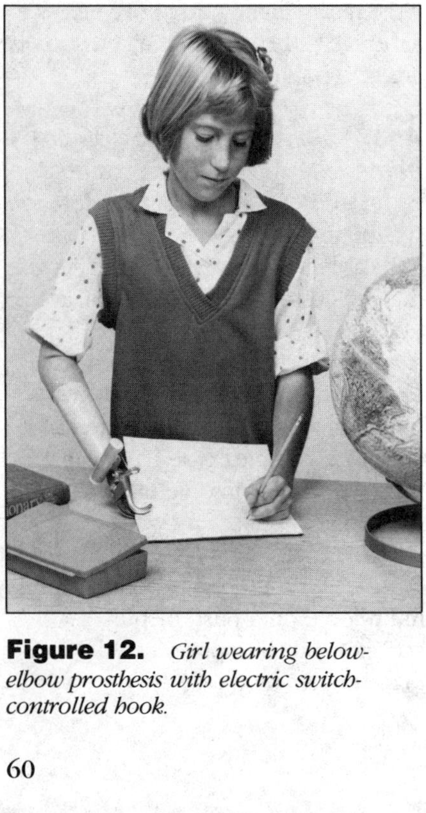

Figure 12. *Girl wearing below-elbow prosthesis with electric switch-controlled hook.*

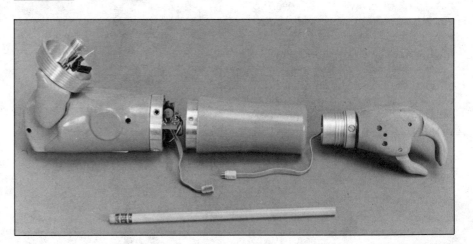

Figure 13. *Electric switch-controlled elbow and hand intended for above-elbow or shoulder disarticulation prosthesis.*

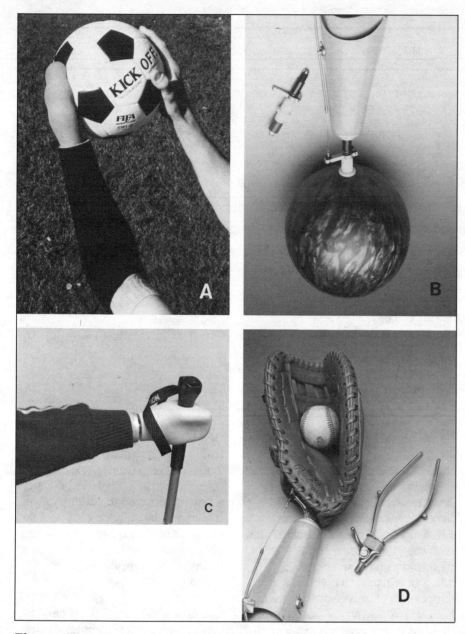

Figure 14. *Recreational terminal devices: (A) Super Sport, (B) bowling attachment, (C) ski hand, (D) baseball glove attachment.*

establish trust and a reciprocal working relationship.[51] Providing accurate and current information to the family about the child's prosthesis and prosthetic management will enable the family to participate constructively in decision making and to encourage prosthetic use at home.[52,53]

Age of Fitting

Lower limb. Developmental readiness is an important consideration when fitting children with lower-extremity amputations. There is little functional need for a prosthesis prior to standing at about 6 months of age.[28] The first fitting generally occurs when the child shows interest in pulling to a standing position (ie, at about 6–9 months of age), which is presumed to assist the developmental progression toward independent ambulation.[28,47,49,54]

Children with bilateral lower-limb deficiencies move independently, using their arms and residual limbs. Low "stubbies" (short, nonarticulated pegs with rocker-bottom distal ends), however, aid postural stability for up-

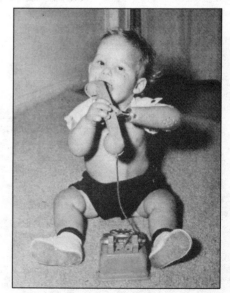

Figure 15. *Infant holding telephone receiver with passive prosthesis. (From Setoguchi Y, Rosenfelder R, eds, The Limb-Deficient Child, 1982.[28] Courtesy of Charles C Thomas, Publisher, Springfield, Ill.)*

Role of Parents in Rehabilitation

Whether the patient is born with a limb deficiency or acquires an amputation during childhood, successful pediatric rehabilitation requires the intensive interaction and cooperation of parents.[48] Parental attendance at and participation in therapy sessions are vital to the child's welfare. Parents should be taught how and when to assist their child, and they should be provided with a home program that enhances prosthetic wearing tolerance and emphasizes activities important to fostering prosthetic use.[48,49] Rehabilitation also includes teaching parents to operate, care for, and maintain the prosthesis.[28,47,50] Parents of children with acquired amputations should be provided a postoperative and preprosthetic program of residuum care and exercises for maintaining range of motion (ROM) and strength.[28,47]

Therapists must incorporate parents' needs and expectations in order to

Table. *Normal Developmental Skills That Can Be Incorporated into Prosthetic Therapy Regimens*

Birth to Age 1 Year	Age 1–3 Years	Age 3–6 Years
Brings hands together	Builds tower of two cubes	Alternates feet ascending stairs
Grasps rattle	Walks, seldom falling	Jumps from bottom step
Reaches for objects, brings objects to mouth	Seats self in small chair, climbs into adult chair	Rides tricycle, using pedals
Transfers object hand to hand	Imitates stroke with a crayon	Feeds self well
Rolls over	Dumps pellet from a bottle	Puts on shoes
Bangs and shakes rattle	Holds and opens jar	Throws ball overhead
Puts feet to mouth	Carries out two-step directions	Hops on one foot
Sits independently	Pulls toys on a string	Washes and dries hands and face
Creeps and pulls to a standing position	Holds and cuts paper	Brushes teeth
Feeds self cracker	Feeds self, in part, with spilling	Skips, alternating feet
Walks with one hand held	Runs well without falling	Stands on one foot
Stands alone, momentarily "cruises"	Walks up and down stairs	Catches ball two-handed
Creeps upstairs	Kicks large ball	Dresses and undresses without assistance
Puts pellet in bottle	Pulls on simple garment	Prints letters
Plays "pat-a-cake"	Jumps up and down	Walks on line backward, heel to toe
	Walks backward	Ties shoelaces
	Unbuttons large buttons	

right ambulation. By increasing the height of the stubbies as balance improves,[47,50] the child is encouraged to perform standing activities.[47]

Children with an acquired amputation can be fitted with a prosthesis immediately following wound healing for effective early rehabilitation.[53] The temporary pylon equalizes leg length and allows gait acquisition to proceed.[47,50]

Upper limb. Although many authorities[47,49,51–53,55,56] advocate early prosthetic fitting to improve prehensile skill and prosthetic acceptance, recent studies[57,58] indicate no relationship between early fitting and prosthetic skill or spontaneous use of prosthetic devices among children with unilateral below-elbow amputations. A better rationale for early fitting is that it enables the infant to use both arms for gross motor developmental tasks, such as prone propping, creeping, coming to sitting position, and pulling to standing position, and consequently that equalizing limb length

should provide a functional advantage for development.[47,48,51,52]

Fitting should commence when independent sitting is achieved.[28,47–49,52,53,59] In this stage of development, about 6 to 8 months of age, nondisabled children begin to use their hands to explore and manipulate objects. Although the infant is too young to learn to operate a TD,[28] a passive device to hold objects inserted by an adult will draw the child's attention to the prosthesis (Fig. 15).[28,47,48,52,53]

Children with bilateral upper-extremity amputations, although delayed in achieving developmental milestones,[52,60] learn to compensate with the head, trunk, and legs to attain gross motor skills such as sitting and pulling to a standing position.[52] Because foot function is essential to their development,[55] prosthetist specialists generally agree to fit these children later than children with unilateral amputations, based on their needs and abilities and when a prosthesis can be used effectively for light grasping activities.[28,48,52]

Determination of the readiness of children with unilateral or bilateral amputations to use a cable-activated or myoelectric TD is based on the following criteria: the ability to follow two-step directions, an attention span of 5 to 10 minutes, an interest in bimanual activities, and the ability to perform the TD control motions.[28,49,52]

Children with multiple limb deficiencies present greater complexities for rehabilitation. Each child's development readiness and abilities, as well as functional need for prostheses, should guide the timing of fitting the first prosthesis.[28,48,52]

Developmental Approach to Treatment

Because treatment should be coordinated with normal growth and development,[28,47–49,52] some relevant developmental skills from birth to 6 years of age[61] that can be incorporated into the intervention services are listed in the Table.

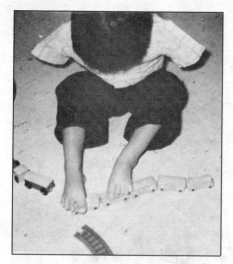

Figure 16. *Child with bilateral upper-extremity amputations attaining prehension with his feet. (From Setoguchi Y, Rosenfelder R, eds, The Limb-Deficient Child, 1982.[28] Courtesy of Charles C Thomas, Publisher, Springfield, Ill.)*

Preprosthetic program. Observation of the infant's level of development and the interaction between parent and child during the therapist's initial evaluation enables the therapist to plan activities suited to the child's age and stage of development, regardless of site and level of limb deficiency.[28,52] A preprosthetic program consisting of ROM activities to increase mobility of the limbs and trunk, a general strengthening program using positioning to assist the child in maintaining postural stability against gravity, and stimulating equilibrium reactions to foster the balance required for trunk control will help prepare the child for maximal independent functioning with and without a prosthesis.[48,60] Development activities, including rolling, crawling, kneeling, standing, and falling, can be incorporated into a mat exercise program.[47] Following visits at regular intervals prior to the initial prosthetic fitting will enable the therapist to monitor the child's development and prepare the child and family for a prosthesis.[28,51,52,60]

For children with bilateral upper-limb deficiency, treatment typically focuses on opportunities for tactile exploration.[47,52] Although the child will de-

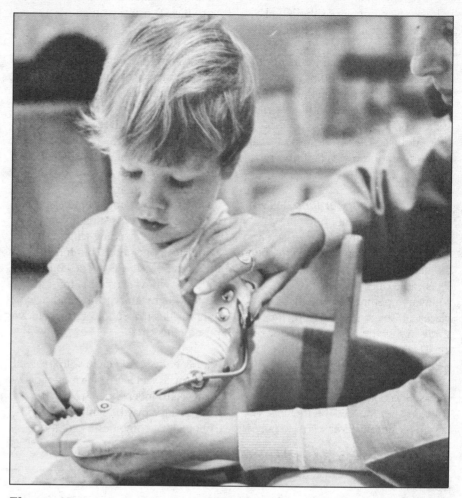

Figure 17. *Therapist passively moves child's arm to open prosthetic terminal device. (From Setoguchi Y, Rosenfelder R, eds, The Limb-Deficient Child, 1982.[28] Courtesy of Charles C Thomas, Publisher, Springfield, Ill.)*

velop tactile awareness through the feet without formal training, this skill can be enhanced by keeping the feet uncovered, placing toys on the floor for grasping by the toes, and providing a variety of objects for learning to differentiate different textures, shapes, and weights (Fig. 16).[55,59]

Common principles. Once the definitive prosthesis is received by a child, both a mechanical and a functional evaluation should be completed to determine whether the prosthesis fits correctly and the components work properly and to ensure that the materials and construction are satisfactory.[28,51,52] Treatment often consists of games and play activities to stimulate use of the prosthesis.[47,48,54,56,59]

Initial training: lower limb. Training children with lower-extremity amputations through play activities in an open area with tables and chairs of varying heights encourages getting up and down from the floor, "cruising" (walking along furniture), and standing and playing.[28,47,50] Placing toys that require bimanual manipulation at various positions on a table allows the child to develop weight shifting and balance in standing (Fig. 17).[28,47]

Gait training requires knowledge of the gait pattern typical of the child's age.[18,47,62] The nondisabled child demonstrates characteristic gait differences from year to year, with an adult pattern evidenced by age 5 years.[18] Exercises that are believed to activate innate motor patterns appropriate for the age-specific gait pattern expected should be incorporated into the training program.[62] Many children with below-knee amputations, both unilateral and bilateral, do not require assistive devices for independent ambulation[47]; however, initial training with crutches using a four-point gait enables the therapist to emphasize a reciprocal gait pattern and heel-strike at foot contact.[18,47] For the very young child, doll carriages and pushcarts can be used temporarily as ambulatory aids.[28,47]

Initial training: upper limb.

Initial training of TD activation for the child with an upper-extremity amputation focuses on teaching the child to open the hand or hook TD. If the prosthesis is cable operated and has a voluntary-opening TD, the therapist places an object in the TD, then passively moves the child's arm to open the TD (Fig. 18).[28] This is followed by helping the child open the TD actively, close it on an object, and then release the object.[28,49,52] For the voluntary-closing TD, the therapist first moves the wearer's arm to put tension on the cable to close the hook. The child is then guided to close the TD actively on an object and relax to open the book. When the child successfully learns the control motions of the TD, training is directed toward activities of daily living.[50] All activities should promote a problem-solving approach through trial and error.[28,52] Developmentally appropriate activities combining play and the activities of daily living should provide the child with a variety of gross and fine motor exercises.[63] Allowing the child ample time to perform the activity, assisting only when necessary, and avoiding fatigue should stimulate spontaneous and functional use of the prosthesis.[48] The child with an above-elbow prosthesis must also be provided with reaching and placing activities that require active elbow positioning.[28,49,52]

Although the young child with bilateral deficiencies can learn activities-of-daily-living skills, independent prosthetic performance may be limited.[47,48,55] Training that combines use of the feet

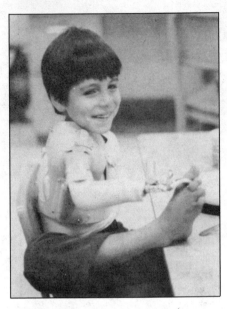

Figure 18. *Child with bilateral upper-extremity amputations using feet and prostheses for activities of daily living. (From Setoguchi Y, Rosenfelder R, eds, The Limb-Deficient Child, 1982.[28] Courtesy of Charles C Thomas, Publisher, Springfield, Ill.)*

Appendix. *Commercial Vendors of Prosthetic Components*

Lower-Limb Prosthetic Components

Kingsley Manufacturing Co, 1984 Placentia Ave, Costa Mesa, CA 92628 (SACH,[a] STEN[b] feet)

Otto Bock Orthopedic Industries Inc, 300 Xenium Ln, Plymouth, MN 55422 (SACH feet, endoskeletal system)

Flex-Foot Inc, 27071 Cabot Rd, Ste 106, Laguna Hills, CA 92653 (Flex-Foot, Flex-Walk feet)

Model and Instrument Development, 861 Poplar Pl S, Seattle, WA 98144 (Seattle LightFoot)

SpringLite, 1006 W Beardsley Pl, Salt Lake City, UT 84119 (SpringLite foot)

afi Endolite, 2480 W 82 St, Hialeah, FL 33016 (Endolite endoskeletal system)

United States Manufacturing Co, 180 N San Gabriel Blvd, Pasadena, CA 91107 (knee units)

Ohio Willow Wood Co, 15441 Scioto-Darby Rd, Mount Sterling, OH 43134 (knee units)

Mauch Laboratories Inc, 3035 Dryden Rd, Dayton, OH 45439 (hydraulic knee units)

Upper-Limb Prosthetic Components

Hosmer Dorrance Corp, 561 Division St, Campbell, CA 95008 (passive mittens, passive hands, voluntary-opening hands and hooks, CAPP[c] terminal devices, electric switch-controlled hands and elbows)

Liberty Mutual Research Center, 71 Frankland Rd, Hopkinton, MA 01748 (myoelectric hands)

Variety Ability Systems Inc, 3701 Danforth Ave, Scarborough, Ontario, Canada M1N 2G2 (myoelectric and electric switch-controlled hands and elbows)

Therapeutic Recreation Systems Inc, 1280 28th St, Boulder, CO 80303 (ADEPT[d] hook, Super Sport, and other recreational devices)

---

[a]SACH=solid-ankle cushion heel.

[b]STEN="STored ENergy."

[c]CAPP=Child Amputee Prosthetics Project.

[d]ADEPT=Anatomically Designed-Engineered Polymer Technology.

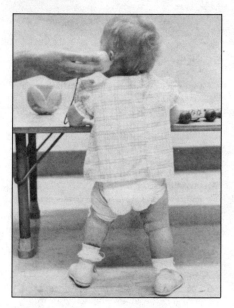

Figure 19. *Example of prosthesis that is too long, as noted by excessive abduction of left lower extremity. (From Setoguchi Y, Rosenfelder R, eds, The Limb-Deficient Child, 1982.[28] Courtesy of Charles C Thomas, Publisher, Springfield, Ill.)*

and the prostheses will help maximize independence (Fig. 19).[48] The preschooler often needs assistive clothing and toileting and other hygienic devices to enhance functional independence.[47,48] With the absence of arms for protection, the child needs to learn to fall safely.

Continued training considerations. With growth and maturity, higher-level purposeful activities are incorporated into the program. Functional needs change with age. Play activities, such as painting, tool use, paper cutting, and simple games with cards or checkers, improve the basic upper-extremity motor skills. Lower-extremity games that incorporate kicking, walking backward and sideways, purposeful walking, climbing, and running enhance functional ambulation.[28,47,49,50,54] Training should eventually incorporate all adolescent and adult activities of daily living (eg, tying a necktie, fastening a brassiere) and vocational skills.

Summary

Physical characteristics determine the range of prosthetic management options available to each child, and epidemiologic factors are important in allocating health resources. Experienced multidisciplinary treatment teams are required to treat all except those children with the least complex limb reductions. Current surgical management, prosthetic fitting options, and training regimens have progressed substantially over the past several decades, and clinicians involved in the care of children with amputations should be familiar with recent technological options to provide the best possible care. The plethora of small components available for lower- and upper-limb prostheses emphasizes the desirability of managing juvenile patients in an interdisciplinary clinic setting where the relative advantages and disadvantages of prosthetic options can be related to the needs and wishes of each young patient. Although prostheses may never be the avatars of normal limbs, they can enhance the child's functional abilities. Prosthetic training, coordinated with normal growth, parental participation, and developmental expectations, can enable the young patient to achieve maximum function.

Well-founded advice is probably the most important contribution clinicians provide to children with limb deficiencies. With well-fitting prostheses, many children will teach themselves the functional skills they need to provide their current needs. Experienced clinicians, however, can offer advice on how current choices affect future function.

References

1 Gillespie R. Deformities and amputation surgery in children. In: Kostuik JP, Gillespie R, eds. *Amputation Surgery and Rehabilitation: The Toronto Experience*. New York, NY: Churchill Livingstone Inc; 1981:105–136.

2 Pozo JL, Powell B, Andrews BG, et al. The timing of amputation for lower limb trauma. *J Bone Joint Surg [Br]*. 1990;72:288–292.

3 Turgay A, Sonuvar B. Emotional aspects of arm or leg amputation in children. *Can J Psychiatry*. 1983;28:294–297.

4 Goldberg RT. New trends in the rehabilitation of lower extremity amputees. *Rehabil Lit*. 1984;45:2–11.

5 Davies EJ, Friz BR, Clippinger FW. Amputees and their prostheses. *Artif Limbs*. 1970;14:19–48.

6 Krebs DE, Fishman S. Characteristics of the child amputee population. *J Pediatr Orthop*. 1984;4:89–95.

7 Day HJB. Nomenclature and classification in congenital limb deficiency. In: Murdoch G, Donovan RG, eds. *Amputation Surgery and Lower Limb Prosthetics*. Oxford, England: Blackwell Scientific Publications Ltd; 1988:271–278.

8 Murray MP, Jacobs PA, Gore DR, et al. Functional performance after tibial rotationplasty. *J Bone Joint Surg [Am]*. 1985;67:392–399.

9 Cammisa FP, Glasser DB, Otis JC, et al. The Van Nes tibial rotationplasty: a functionally viable reconstructive procedure in children who have a tumor of the distal end of the femur. *J Bone Joint Surg [Am]*. 1990;72:1541–1547.

10 Lee KS, Thomas DJ. *Control of Computer-Based Technology for People with Physical Disabilities: An Assessment Manual*. Toronto, Ontario, Canada: University of Toronto Press; 1990.

11 Cary JM, Thompson RG. Planning for optimum function in amputation surgery. In: American Academy of Orthopaedic Surgeons. *Atlas of Limb Prosthetics: Surgical and Prosthetic Principles*. St Louis, Mo: CV Mosby Co; 1981;24–46.

12 Hay S. Sex differences in the incidence of certain congenital malformations: a review of the literature and some new data. *Teratology*. 1971;4:277–286.

13 Kricker A, Elliott JW, Forrest JM, McCredie J. Congenital limb reduction deformities and use of oral contraceptives. *Am J Obstet Gynecol*. 1986;155:1072–1078.

14 Hansen RH. Major injuries due to agricultural machinery. *Ann Plast Surg*. 1986;17:59–64.

15 Thompson GH, Balourdas GM, Marcus RE. Railyard amputations in children. *J Pediatr Orthop*. 1983;3:443–448.

16 Lane JM, Hurson B, Boland PJ, et al. Osteogenic sarcoma: ten most common bone and joint tumors. *Clin Orthop*. 1986;204:93–110.

17 Kruger LM. Congenital limb deficiencies: lower limb deficiencies. In: American Academy of Orthopaedic Surgeons. *Atlas of Limb Prosthetics: Surgical and Prosthetic Principles*. St Louis, Mo: CV Mosby Co; 1981:522–552.

18 Wyatt MP. Gait in children. In: Smidt GL, ed. *Gait in Rehabilitation*. New York, NY: Churchill Livingstone Inc; 1990:157–184.

19 Sutherland DH. *Gait Disorders in Childhood and Adolescence*. Baltimore, Md: Williams & Wilkins; 1984.

20 Edelstein JE. Prosthetic feet: state of the art. *Phys Ther*. 1988;68:1874–1881.

21 Aitken GT, Pellicore RJ. Introduction to the child amputee. In: American Academy of Orthopaedic Surgeons. *Atlas of Limb Prosthetics: Surgical and Prosthetic Principles*. St Louis, Mo: CV Mosby Co; 1981:493–501.

22 Hauge AL, Eckhardt AL, Campbell P. Evaluation of the patellar-tendon-supracondylar prosthesis for children. *Inter-Clinic Information Bulletin*. 1971;11:1–6.

23 Lyttle D. Suspension of the below-knee prosthesis: comparison of supracondylar cuff and brim. *J Assoc Child Prosthet Orthot Clin.* 1987;22:79–80.

24 Fillauer CE, Pritham CH, Fillauer KD. Evolution and development of the Silicone Suction Socket (3S) for below-knee prostheses. *J Prosthet Orthot.* 1989;2:92–103.

25 Kruger LM, Hayes R. Lower limb prosthetic management. In: American Academy of Orthopaedic Surgeons. *Atlas of Limb Prosthetics: Surgical and Prosthetic Principles.* St Louis, Mo: CV Mosby Co; 1981:581–594.

26 Day HJB. Prosthetic management of congenital lower limb deficiency. In: Murdoch G, Donovan RG, eds. *Amputation Surgery and Lower Limb Prosthetics.* Oxford, England: Blackwell Scientific Publications Ltd; 1988: 291–294.

27 Fishman S, Edelstein JE, Krebs DE. Icelandic-Swedish-New York above-knee prosthetic sockets: pediatric experience. *J Pediatr Orthop.* 1987;7:557–562.

28 Setoguchi Y, Rosenfelder R, eds. *The Limb-Deficient Child.* Springfield, Ill: Charles C Thomas, Publisher; 1982.

29 Ekus L, Kruger L, Ferguson N. A reciprocation prosthesis for a patient with sacral agenesis. *Inter-Clinic Information Bulletin.* 1984;19:76–79.

30 Blakeslee B. *The Limb Deficient Child.* Berkeley, Calif: University of California Press; 1963:21.

31 Moseley CF. Growth. In: Lovell WW, Winter RB, eds. *Pediatric Orthopaedics.* Philadelphia, Pa: JB Lippincott Co; 1978:29–30.

32 Krebs DE. Orthotic implications of lower-limb growth. *Inter-Clinic Information Bulletin.* 1982;18:1–10.

33 Watts HG, Carideo JF, Marich MS. Variable-volume sockets for above-knee amputees: managing children following amputation for malignancy. *Inter-Clinic Information Bulletin.* 1982;18:11–14.

34 Tooms RE: The amputee. In: Lovell WW, Winter RB, eds. *Pediatric Orthopaedics.* Philadelphia, Pa: JB Lippincott Co; 1978:999–1053.

35 Krebs DE, Lembeck W, Fishman S. Acceptability of the NYU #1 child size hand. *Arch Phys Med Rehabil.* 1988;69:137–141.

36 Patton JG. Upper-limb prosthetic components for children and teenagers. In: Atkins DJ, Meier RH, eds. *Comprehensive Management of the Upper-Limb Amputee.* New York, NY: Springer-Verlag New York Inc; 1988:99–120.

37 Sauter WF. Electric pediatric and adult prosthetic components. In: Atkins DJ, Meier RH, eds. *Comprehensive Management of the Upper-Limb Amputee.* New York, NY: Springer-Verlag New York Inc; 1988:121–136.

38 Sorbye R. Upper-limb amputees: Swedish experiences concerning children. In: Atkins DJ, Meier RH, eds. *Comprehensive Management of the Upper-Limb Amputee.* New York, NY: Springer-Verlag New York Inc; 1988:227–239.

39 Gibson DA. Child and juvenile amputees. In: Banerjee SN, ed. *Rehabilitation Management of Amputees.* Baltimore, Md: Williams & Wilkins; 1982:391–414.

40 Trefler E. Terminal device activation for infant amputees. *Inter-Clinic Information Bulletin.* 1970;9:11–14.

41 DiCowden M, Ballard A, Robinette H, Ortiz O. Benefit of early fitting and behavior modification training with a voluntary closing terminal device. *J Assoc Child Prosthet Orthot Clin.* 1987;22:47–50.

42 Fishman S, Berger N, Edelstein JE. ISNY flexible sockets for upper-limb amputees. *J Assoc Child Prosthet Orthot Clin.* 1989; 24:8–11.

43 Sauter WF, Dakpa R, Galway R, et al. Development of layered "onionized" silicone sockets for juvenile below-elbow amputees. *J Assoc Child Prosthet Orthot Clin.* 1987;22:57–59.

44 Hodgins J, Sullivan R, Jain S. A modular below elbow prosthesis for children. *Orthot Prosthet.* 1982;36:15–21.

45 D'Onofrio F, Cope PC. Crutches for the quadrimembral amputee. *Inter-Clinic Information Bulletin.* 1972;11:13–15.

46 Friedmann L. Functional skills training in multiple limb anomalies. In: Atkins DJ, Meier RH, eds. *Comprehensive Management of the Upper-Limb Amputee.* New York, NY: Springer-Verlag New York Inc; 1988:150–164.

47 Kostuik JP, ed. *Amputation Surgery and Rehabilitation: The Toronto Experience.* New York, NY: Churchill Livingstone Inc; 1981.

48 Jentschura G, Marquardt E, Rudel EM. *Malformations and Amputations of the Upper Extremity.* New York, NY: Grune & Stratton Inc; 1967:6–21.

49 Molnar GE, ed. *Pediatric Rehabilitation.* Baltimore, Md: Williams & Wilkins; 1985: 342–353.

50 Sanders GT. *Lower Limb Amputations: A Guide to Rehabilitation.* Philadelphia, Pa: FA Davis Co; 1986.

51 Angliss VE. Upper-limb-deficient children. *Am J Occup Ther.* 1974;28:407–414.

52 Patton JG. Developmental approach to pediatric prosthetic evaluation and training. In: Atkins DJ, Meier RH, eds. *Comprehensive Management of the Upper-Limb Amputee.* New York, NY: Springer-Verlag New York Inc; 1988:137–164.

53 Banerjee SN. *Rehabilitation Management of Amputees.* Baltimore, Md: Williams & Wilkins; 1982:137–164.

54 Radford J, Steensma J. The lower extremity toddler amputee: training procedures. *Phys Ther Rev.* 1957;37:32–41.

55 Lamb DW, Law HT. *Upper-Limb Deficiencies in Children: Prosthetic, Orthotic, and Surgical Management.* Boston, Mass: Little, Brown & Co Inc; 1987.

56 Fisher AG. Initial prosthetic fitting of the congenital below-elbow amputee: Are we fitting them early enough? *Inter-Clinic Information Bulletin.* 1976;11-12:7–10.

57 Thornby MA. Pediatric below-elbow amputee bimanual skill development. *Neurology Report.* 1989;13(4):17. Abstract.

58 Ballance R, Wilson BN, Harder JA. Factors affecting myoelectric prosthetic use and wearing patterns in the juvenile unilateral below-elbow amputee. *Canadian Journal of Occupational Therapy.* 1989;56:132–137.

59 Robertson E. *Rehabilitation of Arm Amputees and Limb-Deficient Children.* London, England: Baillière Tindall; 1978.

60 Shepard RB. *Physiotherapy in Paediatrics.* Rockville, Md: Aspen Systems Corp; 1986: 288–306.

61 Lowrey GH. *Growth and Development of Children.* Chicago, Ill: Year Book Medical Publishers Inc; 1986:171–176.

62 Statham L, Murray MP. Early walking patterns of normal children. *Clin Orthop.* 1971;79:8–24.

63 Krebs D, ed. *Prehension Assessment: Prosthetic Therapy for the Upper-Limb Child Amputee.* Thorofare, NJ: Slack Inc; 1987.

Myelodysplasia—the Musculoskeletal Problem: Habilitation from Infancy to Adulthood

The physical therapy and orthopedic management of patients with myelodysplasia from infancy to adulthood are reviewed. The overall goal for the child with myelodysplasia is functional independence. Physical therapy and orthopedic intervention enable the individual to achieve this goal. Associated problems, however, such as Arnold-Chiari malformation, hydrocephalus, and tethered spinal cord, influence functional expectations. Physical therapy management begins in the neonatal period and continues through adolescence. Treatment is modified at the various stages of development. Knowledge of current orthotic and adaptive equipment is necessary to achieve optimal locomotor function. Orthopedic management decisions are based on musculoskeletal and neurologic assessments, to which the physical therapist provides a significant contribution. Controversies exist over the orthopedic management of dislocated hips, scoliosis, and kyphosis. [Ryan KD, Ploski C, Emans JB. Myelodysplasia—the musculoskeletal problem: habilitation from infancy to adulthood. Phys Ther. 1991;71:935–946.]

Kimberly D Ryan
Christine Ploski
John B Emans

Key Words: *Adaptive equipment, Function, Musculoskeletal deformities, Myelodysplasia, Orthotics, Strength.*

Myelodysplasia, or myelomeningocele, is a complex congenital disorder that primarily affects the nervous system and secondarily affects the musculoskeletal and urologic systems (Tab. 1). The myelodysplastic defect involves a failure of the fusion of the caudal end of the neural tube or rupture of the nearly closed neural tube, occurring early in embryonic development before the 28th day of gestation. The etiology is unknown but is believed to be multifactorial and includes genetic and environmental influences.[1]

The incidence of myelodysplasia varies in different parts of the world but is generally 1 per 1,000 births.[2] A slightly higher incidence is found in individuals of northern Europe origin. There is a 1% to 2% greater chance of a child being born with myelodysplasia if a sibling is already affected.[3]

Prenatal screening can lead to early detection of the defect. Elevated levels of alpha-fetoprotein in the maternal serum after the 16th week of gestation may be indicative of a neural tube defect.[4] Ultrasound testing performed between the 16th and 24th

weeks of gestation may decrease the need for a subsequent amniocentesis.[5] Amniocentesis performed at this time detects almost all open myelomeningoceles but not closed (skin-covered) myeloceles.[6] Early detection may present a difficult decision for the parents, because termination of the pregnancy is the only way to prevent the defect. Prior knowledge, however, can prepare parents for the need for a cesarean birth and immediate postnatal care.

Most infants born with myelodysplasia are treated aggressively with immediate closure and shunt insertion to manage hydrocephalus,[7] but this approach has not always been followed. Lorber,[8] in 1971, found that even those children who were treated had considerable problems with self-esteem and the attainment of functional independence. He recommended "selective treatment" based on four criteria identified at birth: the

KD Ryan, BS, PT, is Supervisor and Clinic Consultant, Department of Physical Therapy and Occupational Therapy Services, Children's Hospital, 300 Longwood Ave, Boston, MA 02115 (USA). Address all correspondence to Ms Ryan.

C Ploski, MS, PT, PCS, is Assistant Supervisor and Clinic Consultant, Department of Physical Therapy and Occupational Therapy Services, Children's Hospital.

JB Emans, MD, is Associate in Orthopaedic Surgery, Department of Orthopaedics, and Clinical Director, Myelodysplasia Clinic, Children's Hospital. He is also Assistant Clinical Professor, Department of Orthopedic Surgery, Harvard University, Cambridge, MA 02138.

Table 1. *Basic Myelodysplastic Defect Definitions*

Defect	Definition
Spina bifida occulta	Vertebral defect characterized by failure of closure of the posterior elements of the vertebral arch without a sac containing neural tissue visible on the back. The vertebral defect may or may not be associated with an abnormality of the spinal cord.
Spina bifida cystica	Vertebral defect with cystic protrusion of the meninges or of the spinal cord and meninges.
Meningocele	Protrusion of the meninges and cerebrospinal fluid into a sac that is covered by epithelium. Clinical symptoms vary according to underlying spinal cord anomalies or may not be apparent.
Myelomeningocele	Most common and serious defect, which includes the spinal cord, nerve roots, meninges, and cerebrospinal fluid. Commonly noted in the lumbar area, the level of the lesion is usually reflected in the severity of the clinical deficit, with higher lesions having more pronounced deficits.
Lipomeningocele	Vertebral defect associated with a superficial fatty mass that merges with lower levels of the spinal cord. Neurologic deficits vary. There is no associated hydrocephalus.
Encephalocele	A protrusion of scarred brain, cerebrospinal fluid, and meninges through a bony defect in the skull. This defect is usually occipital, but can be frontal or through the skull base.
Anencephaly	Failure of fusion of the cranial end of the neural tube, resulting in exposure of a malformed brain at birth.

degree of paralysis, the degree of increased head circumference, the presence of kyphosis and other associated congenital anomalies, and birth injuries. Gross and colleagues,[9] using criteria similar to the criteria used by Lorber, as recently as 1983 also suggested that treatment be withheld for some infants. Most authorities today, however, agree that children with myelodysplasia should be treated aggressively to minimize neurologic deficits. In recent years, improved closure techniques and other medical advances and increased societal acceptance of the disability have contributed to a better quality of life for these individuals.[10]

Optimal management of the child with myelodysplasia occurs in a clinical setting with a team of knowledgeable professionals.[11] The treatment team should include a neurosurgeon, orthopedic surgeon, urologist, pediatrician, nurse, physical therapist, occupational therapist, social worker, and orthotist. We believe the availability of a nutritionist, speech and language pathologist, and psychologist is also essential for comprehensive management.

The purpose of this article is to review current physical therapy and orthopedic management of children with myelodysplasia from infancy through adolescence. A philosophy and controversies of care will be addressed.

Associated Problems

Neurologic Deficits

The primary neurologic problems in persons with myelodysplasia are the variable motor and sensory deficits, which will be discussed in detail in the "Physical Therapy and Orthopedic Management" section. Associated central nervous system problems are often present.

Hydrocephalus. Evidence of hydrocephalus is present in 80% or more of infants with myelodysplasia.[12] Clinical symptoms are manifested by bulging fontanel, increasing head circumference, downward deviation of the eyes ("sunset eyes"), irritability, projectile vomiting, and seizures.

Hydrocephalus is managed by the insertion of a shunt, most commonly a ventriculoperitoneal shunt.[13] Shunt insertion may be performed when the defect is closed or later when the symptoms of hydrocephalus are apparent. Revisions are necessary if the shunt tubing becomes occluded, disconnected, or infected.

Some studies[14,15] have shown that children with hydrocephalus may have reduced intelligence and perceptual-motor impairments. More recently, however, Mapsstone and colleagues[16] demonstrated that intellectual function is also affected by complications from shunting and by other central nervous system anomalies. Advances in shunt-placement techniques and infection control have improved the outcome. Perceptual-motor impairment affects school performance. Evaluation for perceptual-motor dysfunction is frequently handled by an occupational therapist.

Arnold-Chiari malformation. In the Arnold-Chiari defect, the lower brain stem and cerebellum, including the fourth ventricle, herniate through the foramen magnum into the spinal canal. The fourth ventricle may become obstructed and the flow of cerebrospinal fluid impeded, resulting in hydrocephalus.[17]

Virtually every child with myelomeningocele has the malformation, and its presence and severity are confirmed by magnetic resonance imaging (MRI), as well as the presence of clinical manifestations.[18] Clinical signs include respiratory symptoms, such as apnea, stridor, vocal cord paralysis, and upper-extremity weakness or spasticity. A shunt insertion or revision is the usual management technique, but severe cases occasionally require cervical laminectomy and posterior decompression.[19]

Syringomyelia and hydromyelia.

Syringomyelia is present if there is a dilatation of the central canal of the spinal cord, resulting in an elongated cavity (syrinx) within the spinal cord filled with cerebrospinal fluid.[20] Hydromyelia or syringohydromyelia are other terms commonly used for this condition. Symptoms such as the development of scoliosis, upper-extremity weakness, or sensory changes may occur if the syndrome progresses. The treatment is complicated and varies according to the etiology of the syrinx.[21,22]

Tethered spinal cord.

Progressive neurologic dysfunction may indicate tethering of the conus medullaris and lower spinal cord roots.[23] Tethering results from scar formation and binding of the spinal cord tissue to the bony column at the site of the initial repair, with subsequent inhibition of normal spinal cord movement with growth or activity. A clinical diagnosis is made based on deterioration of urologic function, progressive orthopedic deformities, changes in motor status, back or leg pain, or deterioration in gait. Usually, the change in motor function entails loss of muscle strength, although muscle activity not previously seen and not under voluntary control may also appear. Surgical untethering is performed to halt the progression of the symptoms, but is not always successful.[24] Existing deformities or problems may persist and require orthopedic intervention.

Musculoskeletal Problems

A variety of bone and joint deformities that affect function are encountered in children with myelodysplasia. Affected extremities usually exhibit muscle atrophy and osteopenia. Together, osteopenia, limited joint proprioception, and resistant contractures make fractures a frequent occurrence.[25,26] Some deformities are congenital, but the majority are acquired through growth and abnormal forces

introduced by muscle imbalances, static positioning and gravity, and weight bearing on joints with insufficient muscular support. The source of the deformity should be determined before intervention, because the success of treatment can be hindered by a changing neurological picture, such as the progressive deformities seen with a tethered spinal cord.

Lower extremities.

Hip subluxation and dislocation are common.[27] They may be present at birth or develop with growth because of the unbalanced action of the hip flexors and adductors. Hip flexion contractures also occur frequently.

Knee flexion contractures occur in children with high neurosegmental levels of involvement,[28] and such contractures may impede the use of braces or a standing frame. Progressive knee flexion deformities may also accompany spasticity (hypertonia) resulting from a tethered spinal cord. Ambulatory individuals with strong ankle dorsiflexors but weak gastrocnemius muscle function may develop knee flexion deformities from a crouched stance. Knee hyperextension deformities and rectus femoris muscle contracture can result from strong quadriceps femoris muscle function unopposed by hamstring muscle activity. Hypertrophy of the sartorius muscle secondary to overuse can be accompanied by a functionally insignificant snapping of the muscle as it glides across the medial knee structures. Patellofemoral overuse syndromes are common in community ambulators with low-lumbar neurosegmental levels of involvement, who rely heavily on their quadriceps femoris muscles, particularly if a knee flexion contracture is present.

Congenital foot deformities (eg, clubfoot, vertical talus) are most common in children with mid-lumbar neurosegmental levels of involvement. Acquired foot deformities such as talipes calcaneus, talipes cavus, and talipes planovalgus, which develop from unbalanced muscle forces and unsupported weight bearing, occur most commonly in children with lower neurosegmental

levels of involvement. As foot sensation is often incomplete, neurotrophic ulceration can become a problem and may interfere with ambulation.

Spinal deformities.

Scoliosis and kyphosis have many etiologies in children with myelodysplasia. In addition to abnormal skin covering and displacement of neural elements, the bony spine is abnormal. The stabilizing effect of the paraspinal muscles is often lost, because the muscles are displaced laterally or may be denervated. In individuals with kyphotic deformities, the muscles may be anterior as well as lateral to the spinal column. Spinal deformities may result from unbalanced growth attributable to congenital abnormalities (congenital scoliosis or kyphosis), from abnormal stresses of pelvic obliquity or hip contracture, or from paralytic collapse. Significant scoliosis in a structurally normal part of the spine or a rapid increase in spinal deformity may result from spinal cord tethering or other neurologic problems.[24]

Bowel and Bladder Problems

The child with myelomeningocele may experience problems with bladder control, which may adversely affect renal function.[29] Clean, intermittent catheterization, in combination with pharmacologic agents, has enabled most children to become continent.[29] Urodynamic studies are performed in the neonatal period and at regular intervals as the child matures. The results provide baseline information that is useful in predicting future function and in detecting changes that may indicate neurological deterioration.[30]

Fecal incontinence affects the child's self-esteem and social acceptance.[31] Management includes a combination of regular toileting, diet, medication, biofeedback, and behavior modification.[32]

Physical Therapy Assessment

A comprehensive evaluation includes testing range of motion (ROM), posture, sensation, muscle strength, de-

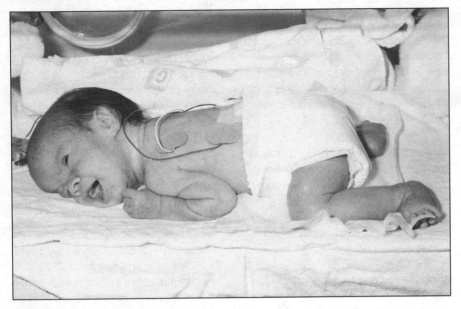

Figure 1. *Newborn infant with myelodysplasia and hydrocephalus after closure. Note abduction; externally rotated position of hips; and dorsiflexed, everted position of the feet.*

velopmental reflexes, motor development, and functional status. Qualitative and quantitative assessments are used to assess motor development, identify strengths and weaknesses, and provide a basis for intervention. Abnormal or immature patterns of movement and any asymmetries should also be documented. Both upper and lower extremities are tested because associated central nervous system problems can affect the upper extremity and affect mobility.[18,20,24,33–36] Assessments are repeated at intervals ranging from 1 month to 1 year, according to the age and needs of the child. Results of sequential examinations allow comparisons to determine the rate of progress, to detect changes that may be indicative of deterioration, and to judge the effectiveness of interventions. The findings within each test area should be interpreted separately as well as jointly when impressions of status, prognosis, and physical therapy intervention are formed.

Range of Motion

Standard test procedures have been established for measurement of joint ROM[37,38] Modifications are necessary in the neonate who may have position restrictions (Fig. 1) or for any child

who is unable to assume test positions because of deformity or discomfort.

The interpretation of the results of the joint ROM measurement should always be based on the individual's age, muscle strength, and potential functional status. For example, in neonates and young infants, limitations of hip and knee extension and hip adduction are normal and do not necessarily indicate a problem.[39] If there is an accompanying muscle imbalance or the limitations persist over time, however, the findings should be considered abnormal.

Posture

Alignment of the trunk and extremities should be assessed through palpation of bony landmarks and observation. Asymmetries and deviations from normal are recorded. Real and apparent leg-length discrepancies may be indicative of a dislocated hip, pelvic obliquity, or scoliosis. Abnormal findings, particularly if new or progressive, warrant orthopedic assessment.

Sensation

The results of sensory testing establish the sensory level and, more impor-

tantly, identify areas that may be at risk for skin breakdown. The presence of any joint or postural deformities further increases the risk for skin breakdown in insensate areas because of unequal weight bearing.

The behavioral state of the infant affects the sensory testing, which should normally be performed when the infant is quiet. The infant's medical status and the effects of any medications must be considered. Reactions to appropriate stimuli that may indicate intact sensation include grimacing, crying, or withdrawal from the stimulus. We believe sensory testing becomes more accurate and precise at later ages. Light touch, position sense, temperature, and two-point discrimination, in addition to pain, can be assessed in the older child.

Strength

The results of the initial and subsequent muscle examinations are used to identify the affected neurosegmental levels and to predict the functional outcome (Tab. 2).[40–43] Realistic interventions are determined based on the upper- and lower-extremity muscle strength in combination with the child's developmental level.

The procedure and grading for muscle testing must be modified in infants and young children according to their age and developmental level, as well as their medical status.[44,45] Grades that have resistance as a criterion, Fair plus or above,[46] may be difficult to assign, because the infant or young child is unable to cooperate or to understand the concept of resistance. If an infant resists passive movement, however, the muscle strength may be graded as at least Fair plus. In a young child, the ability to lift body weight in an activity such as bridging can be used to determine whether the strength of the gluteus maximus muscle is above the Fair level.

The initial muscle examination is usually performed following closure of the defect, once the infant is medically stable. The infant is usually re-

Table 2. *Function in Myelodysplasia*

Neurosegmental Level	Muscles Innervated	Preambulation Orthosis	Ambulation Orthosis[a]	Assistive Device	Functional Prognosis	Musculoskeletal Problem
Thoracic	Abdominal	Standing frame	Reciprocating gait orthoses, swivel walker, parapodium	Parallel bars | Walker | Forearm crutches	Wheelchair	Spinal deformity
Upper lumbar	Abdominal, hip flexors	Standing frame	Reciprocating gait orthoses, parapodium	Parallel bars | Walker | Forearm crutches	Wheelchair Possible household or therapeutic ambulation Standing transfers	Hip flexion contractures Spinal deformity
Mid lumbar	Abdominal, hip flexors, knee extensors, hip adductors	None	HKAFO | KAFO | AFO (depending on quadriceps femoris muscle strength)	Parallel bars | Walker | Forearm crutches	Wheelchair for community mobility or orthoses for household ambulation	Hip dislocation, subluxation
Low lumbar	Abdominal; knee extensors; hip abductors and adductors; knee, hip, and toe flexors; ankle and toe dorsiflexors, evertors, and invertors	None	KAFO | AFO	Parallel bars | Walker | Forearm crutches | None	Household or community ambulators	Foot deformities
Lumbosacral	Abdominal; ankle plantar flexors; foot intrinsic muscles; knee extensors; hip abductors and adductors; knee, hip, and toe flexors; ankle and toe dorsiflexors, evertors, and inventors	None	AFO, UCBL, or none	Walker | None	Community ambulators	

[a]HKAFO=hip-knee-ankle-foot orthosis; KAFO=knee-ankle-foot orthosis; AFO=ankle-foot orthosis; FO=foot orthosis; UCBL=University of California Biomechanics Laboratory shoe insert.

stricted to the prone or side-lying position in order to allow the back to heal. If hydrocephalus is present, there may be further restrictions on upright positioning. Once the positioning restrictions are discontinued, the infant's strength can be assessed in the supine and upright positions.

The infant should be awake and alert, which is often just prior to feeding. Resting posture is observed as well as spontaneous movement. Muscles must be palpated for contraction in order to differentiate between the activity of individual muscles and muscle groups. Tactile stimuli in the area of the deficits as well as at sites innervated by nerves from levels above the spinal defect are used to elicit movement. Positioning a joint or joints in extreme ROM (eg, maximum hip and knee flexion) may stimulate the infant to contract the antagonist. Responses such as the plantar-grasp or equilibrium reactions may also be used to elicit muscle contractions. The presence of muscle activity with reflex stimulation only should be documented, but does not necessarily indicate voluntary control.

Modifications of muscle testing procedures are also necessary for testing the older infant and young child. Developmental activities, such as rolling to elicit hip flexion or pulling to a standing position to determine quadriceps femoris muscle function, may be used. The use of traditional techniques of muscle testing depends on the child's ability to cooperate and follow directions, but, in our experience, these techniques can usually be used by the age of 4 years. Hand-held dynamometers have also been used in pediatric populations to assess muscle strength.[47] Strength assessments should be performed every 6 months in the growing child and yearly in the adolescent to monitor for changes.

Developmental Reflexes and Postural Reactions

Procedures have been established for testing developmental reflexes and postural reactions.[48,49] The presence or absence of certain responses may have a direct influence on gross motor skills[50] and, therefore, treatment decisions. For example, we believe the attainment of independent upright stance cannot be achieved without effective righting and equilibrium reactions or in the presence of certain primitive reflexes. The physical therapy program often includes techniques to facilitate more mature reactions while inhibiting the primitive responses.

Development and Function

The rate of development of motor skills is slower in children with myelodysplasia than in children without myelodysplasia and is related to the neurosegmental level that is affected.[51] Medical problems, such as shunt infections, may result in regression or delay of motor development.[52]

Developmental testing is frequently used for the infant and young child. Developmental tests that are standardized (ie, norm or criterion referenced) provide quantitative, objective information about motor abilities.[53–55] Scores from standardized tests document the degree of developmental delay and may be required in order to justify the need for intervention. Modifications may be necessary when administering and scoring test items, particularly if the child uses adaptive equipment. Statements regarding the influence of factors such as the child's

motor level and associated neurologic or orthopedic problems should be included in the interpretation of the overall scores.

The achievement of specific developmental milestones has implications for decisions regarding orthopedic intervention. For example, if an infant has not achieved adequate sitting balance by the age of 10 months because of trunk instability, a spinal orthosis may be a treatment option. Conversely, if an infant has not developed good head control, surgical intervention to decrease lower-extremity contractures and to allow use of an ambulatory device may not be appropriate.

Functional assessments are used to determine the readiness and need for adaptive equipment such as bracing. These assessments are also used to determine the older child's ability to function in various environments (eg, school, home). Functional assessments include evaluations of gross motor abilities, mobility, and self-care activities. Assessment of motor abilities includes a description of the child's ability to move into, within, and out of various positions and to maintain those positions, as well as a description of the child's ability to function within each position. Assessment of mobility includes an evaluation of gait, wheelchair activities, and transfers. If the child is ambulatory, the type of gait (eg, reciprocal, swing-through), gait deviations, use of assistive devices, and level of ambulation[56] (eg, household, community ambulator) should be described. The ability and ease with which the child ambulates or maneuvers a wheelchair on various terrains and levels and the child's endurance are also assessed. Activities of daily living include hygiene activities (eg, toileting, bathing, skin care), feeding, and dressing. The child's level of independence and need for adaptive equipment should be noted.

Physical Therapy and Orthopedic Management

The overall goal of orthopedic and physical therapy management is the habilitation of the child by maximizing the child's function, independence, and self-esteem while minimizing family stress. Specific goals for each child are formulated, depending on the results of the assessment. Conservative or nonsurgical treatments include physical therapy, casting, bracing, and splinting. We believe that carefully planned surgical interventions may save unnecessary casting or bracing and may help foster independence.

The Neonate

Physical therapy management of the neonate is usually initiated in the period immediately following closure of the back defect. General objectives include increasing ROM and active movement and promoting the achievement of developmental milestones.

Early treatment is limited by the infant's medical status and position restrictions, which are dependent on the type of closure, rate of healing, postoperative complications, the management of hydrocephalus, and the physician's judgment. Prone and side-lying positioning are usually allowed before supine positioning. When the infant can be positioned supine and upright, the developmental program can be expanded.

We believe that appropriate tactile, visual, and auditory stimuli should be introduced to facilitate movement and development. Passive exercises, facilitation of active movement, and positioning techniques are used to oppose any contractures and muscle imbalances.

Parent education is a major focus. The role of and rationale for physical therapy are explained. Parents are instructed in a home program that includes exercises, positioning and handling techniques, and appropriate developmental activities. Skin-care instructions are also given, and standard child care equipment is modified, if needed. Follow-up visits are arranged prior to discharge, and referrals are made to local treatment programs.

The Infant

During infancy, attainment of age-appropriate developmental motor milestones is emphasized. Achievement of upright stance is the overall goal. Activities are incorporated into the program to facilitate head and trunk control in the developmental positions. Prone activities are used to increase upper-extremity strength. Early mobility through rolling, belly crawling, and quadrupedal creeping is encouraged and facilitated, because these achievements provide the foundation for future motor progress. Postural and balance reactions are facilitated, because they are prerequisites for independent standing. Righting and equilibrium reactions will also help strengthen the neck and trunk musculature and promote independent sitting. Modifications in seating may be needed if the child has a severe kyphosis or lacks appropriate head and trunk control.

The Preschool-Aged Child

Physical therapy has an active role at this time, particularly in assisting the child in attaining some form of independent mobility. As the child begins to pull to a standing position, orthopedic intervention may be needed to achieve upright stance. Intervention may include bracing, casting, bony or soft tissue procedures around the hip, and release of contractures that interfere with function. Treatment of foot deformities must be individualized. In our experience, in spite of casting and stretching, most severe foot deformities will require surgery. A plantigrade, supple, braceable foot is the goal.

General principles of surgical treatment include correction of bony deformity and balancing of muscle forces. With the use of internal fixation, postoperative immobilization is kept to a minimum to diminish osteopenia and subsequent fractures.[57]

In our view, as many procedures as possible should be performed during the same hospitalization or same operative session. We attempt to complete all orthopedic surgeries prior to age 5 years, in order to minimize interference with schooling.

Orthopedic management of hip deformities.
Treatment of hip dislocation in children with myelodysplasia is individualized and differs greatly from the management of congenital hip dislocation in children without myelodysplasia or the management of paralytic dislocation in children with spastic cerebral palsy. Hip subluxation in myelodysplasia, unlike that in spastic cerebral palsy is generally not associated with pain. The presence of dislocation or subluxation noted on a radiograph is less important than maintenance of hip joint motion and avoidance of joint contractures. Treatment generally depends on the child's ambulatory potential, which correlates best to the neurosegmental level of involvement.[56,58,59]

Hip subluxation occurs infrequently with lumbosacral neurosegmental levels of involvement, but is usually treated aggressively because of the excellent ambulatory potential of these children. In individuals with thoracic or upper-lumbar neurosegmental levels of involvement, community ambulation is not anticipated beyond childhood. Because little demand will be placed on the hips, contracture releases are performed as needed to maintain ROM. We believe surgical reductions, osteotomies, and muscle transfers are generally not indicated, because the benefits do not outweigh the risks of postoperative stiffness or heterotopic ossification. A severe postoperative hip contracture may prevent the patient from assuming either a sitting or standing position. We also believe a mobile, dislocated hip is preferable to a stiff, reduced hip, particularly in the nonambulatory patient.

There is a relatively high incidence of hip subluxation in children with mid- to low-lumbar neurosegmental levels of involvement.[27] In these individuals,

the presence of quadriceps femoris muscle function makes community ambulation a possibility. Unopposed hip adductors and flexors tend to produce progressive subluxation and eventual dislocation. Management of subluxations in these individuals is an area of considerable controversy. In the infant, abduction splinting and stretching will help maintain ROM and may facilitate acetabular and femoral development. As subluxation and dislocation gradually develop, a decision must be made as to whether to treat the hip dislocation. If the child has little ambulatory potential because of neurologic problems, reduction is not indicated and muscle releases are performed as needed to maintain ROM. If there is good ambulatory potential, as indicated by the presence of a strong quadriceps femoris musculature, and in the absence of other complicating factors, then the child is a potential candidate for surgical treatment of the hip subluxation.

Proponents of hip reduction and muscle transfer argue that optimal ROM is achieved by hip reduction.[60-64] Better posture and gait mechanics may result from keeping the hips reduced and from associated muscle transfers. Opponents of hip reduction believe that operative reduction exposes the child to the risk of hip stiffness without functional benefit and that soft tissue releases alone are sufficient to maintain ROM and ambulatory ability.[65-68]

Studies[56,65-68] have shown no correlation between the level of ambulation and the status of the hips in children with mid-lumbar neurosegmental levels of involvement. Because other factors, such as severe hydrocephalus, Arnold-Chiari malformation, obesity, motivation, and contractures, also influence ambulation, the results of these studies remain somewhat inconclusive.

If the decision is made to relocate the hips, open reduction with capsulorrhaphy is generally required.[60] Pelvic or femoral osteotomy, or both, may also be necessary. Because the iliopsoas and adductor muscle groups are largely unopposed in these children,

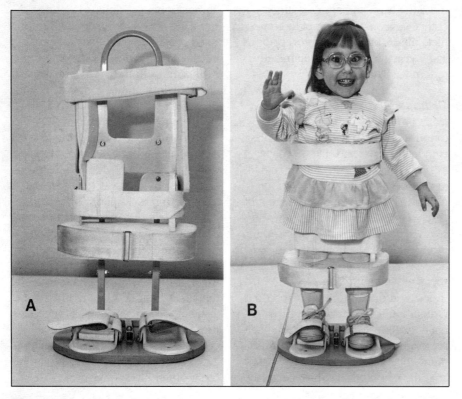

Figure 2. *Standing frame: (A) anterior view; (B) adapted to accommodate child's leg-length discrepancy and tendency to lean to the right.*

some attempt is usually made to balance the musculature, or dislocation will gradually recur. Most procedures include adductor release or posterior transfer of the adductor origin.[69] Lateral transfer of the external oblique muscle to the greater trochanter[70] to provide stabilizing force is now widely used. Another approach consists of lateral transfer of the iliopsoas muscle, through a hole created in the wing of the ilium, to the greater trochanter.[71] This transfer alleviates the deforming force of the iliopsoas muscle and provides a tenodesis or active hip abduction. Both approaches have their advocates. Many feel the external oblique muscle transfer allows better ambulation and does not diminish the patient's ability to flex the hips and climb stairs (RE Lindseth, L Dias; personal communication), although follow-up studies of iliopsoas muscle transfers do not show impairment in climbing stairs.[63] Others feel iliopsoas muscle transfer is more likely to ensure maintenance of reduction. Tailoring treatment to the individual child is crucial and must be based on a realistic assessment of walking potential.

Orthotic management. Some degree of contracture may be accommodated by orthoses. Surgical release, however, is indicated to facilitate orthotic management if hip flexion contractures are greater than 30 degrees, knee flexion contractures are greater than 20 degrees, and plantar-flexion deformities are greater than 10 degrees.

We believe all children, except those with severe central nervous system involvement, should be given the opportunity to be upright, regardless of their functional prognosis. This philosophy is based on the premise that weight bearing increases bone density,[72] helps to maintain urinary tract function, and develops self-esteem.

Either a parapodium or a standing frame (Fig. 2) can be used as the first orthosis for the child with a neurosegmental level of L-3 or above to achieve upright stance and early mobility. The swivel walker, parapodium, and standing frame may also be used for long-term mobility. We have found, however, that few children

learn to release the joints of the parapodium. We therefore prefer the standing frame, which is less expensive and easier to apply.

Time spent in the standing frame depends on the child's tolerance and skin integrity. Once the desire to move in the frame is evident, consideration is given to orthotic devices that allow more functional ambulation. The overall goal is to provide maximum mobility with the minimum amount of bracing.[73]

The reciprocating gait orthosis (RGO) is used for children with thoracic and high-lumbar neurosegmental levels of involvement as young as 18 months of age. Some practitioners prefer to wait until the children are 30 to 36 months of age before prescribing the RGO (see article by Knutson and Clark in this issue). Individuals using the RGO are more likely to achieve household ambulation and remain functional longer than if they used other braces.[74,75]

General guidelines have been established for determining appropriate orthoses for functional mobility (see article by Knutson and Clark in this issue). Hip-knee-ankle-foot orthoses (HKAFOs), knee-ankle-foot orthoses (KAFOs), ankle-foot orthoses (AFOs), and foot orthoses (FOs) are prescribed, depending on the child's neurosegmental level of involvement. The pelvic band of the HKAFO assists in the control of hip abduction, adduction, and rotation during gait. If placement of the lower extremity is not a problem, a KAFO may be used for individuals with little or no quadriceps femoris muscle strength. An AFO or FO is indicated if foot and ankle support are needed.

Functional mobility. Gait training is initiated in the parallel bars. Activities to develop balance and the ability to weight shift are utilized. Progression to either an anterior- or reverse-facing (posterior) walker is made once independent ambulation in the parallel bars is achieved. We prefer the reverse-facing walker whenever possible, as it promotes better postural

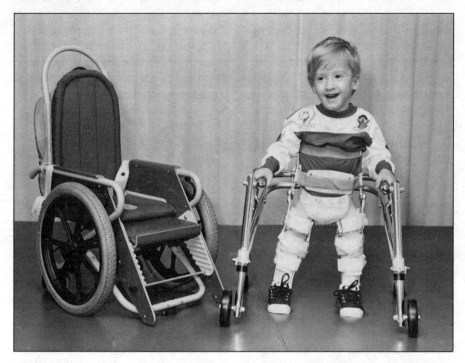

Figure 3. *Two-year-old boy with reciprocating gait orthosis, reverse-facing walker, and wheelchair.*

alignment than does the anterior-facing walker.[76] If a reverse-facing walker is selected for a child, the depth should be sufficient to allow posterior clearance for orthoses that have pelvic components. Once the child is able to maintain standing balance and ambulate confidently with the walker without assistance, forearm crutches may be introduced.

Independent mobility by walking is the goal during early childhood. In our experience, however, many children will require a wheelchair to improve access to the environment, despite optimal bracing and gait training (Fig. 3). Considerable controversy exists surrounding the timing of the introduction of a wheelchair for children who are unlikely to achieve independent community ambulation. The proponents of early wheelchair introduction have argued that early training will maximize eventual wheelchair skills. The opposing view is that early introduction limits the child's ambulatory potential. Mazur and colleagues,[77] in a recent comparative study of two groups of patients, found that the timing of the introduction made no differ-

ence in the ultimate level of wheelchair skill or ambulation.

We introduce the wheelchair as early as 18 months of age if it is apparent that this device will enhance mobility and independence. Early introduction usually enables children to keep up with their peers. In our experience, early wheelchair use has not led to the cessation of ambulation, even in marginal ambulators. Rather, the boost in self-confidence and independence that may accompany wheelchair use seems to increase their activity level and overall mobility. We view the wheelchair as an aid to mobility and do not believe that its use represents a "failure" of management.

Orthopedic management of kyphosis. Seating arrangements and bracing will be complicated by the presence of a kyphotic deformity. Some children, generally those with low-thoracic or high-lumbar level of paralysis, have a severe congenital kyphosis or a collapsing thoracolumbar kyphosis. These deformities normally increase with growth and commonly result in functional and cosmetic difficulties.

Chronic skin breakdown over the kyphotic area may result from pressure against the back of a chair, friction during wheelchair use, or irritation from pelvic bands. Compensatory thoracic lordosis may develop above the thoracolumbar kyphosis and can cause respiratory difficulties. Care of abdominal ileal loops or colostomies becomes difficult when the child is collapsed forward into kyphosis and the contour of the abdomen is distorted. The child's body image may be severely altered by the trunk distortion accompanying severe kyphosis.

Brace or cast treatment of congenital kyphosis or collapsing kyphosis rarely stops progression of the deformity and frequently contributes to skin breakdown. Orthoses, nevertheless, can improve sitting posture and balance, particularly in individuals with flexible collapsing kyphosis.

The most common surgical procedure when kyphosis is present in individuals with paraplegia is excision of the deformed spinal segment (kyphectomy) and the nonfunctional cord at the level of the kyphosis.[78] The remaining relatively straight upper- and lower-spine segments are united by instrumentation and fusion. This procedure effectively removes the kyphosis, but results in a shorter-than-normal trunk. Growth over the fused spinal segment is halted; hence, this procedure is delayed, if possible, until late childhood. Care must be taken when excising the nonfunctional cord to ensure that bladder function will not be adversely affected, because some individuals have a functioning sacral cord in spite of no lower-extremity motor function.

The School-Aged Child

Because most children with myelodysplasia are mainstreamed in public or private schools,[79] physical therapy programs during childhood are based in the school. Services may be direct, indirect, or consultative, but the overall goal of functional independence remains unchanged. Activities of daily living, such as dressing and brace management, as well as continued work on mobility skills, are addressed during the school years.

Orthopedic management of scoliosis. In late childhood and early adolescence, the effects of progressive scoliosis may become apparent. Nonambulatory individuals with severe scoliosis sit with their trunk out of balance in relation to their pelvis. They may require the use of one or both upper extremities to maintain their sitting balance and may need extensive adaptive seating. Pressure from unequal weight bearing during sitting increases the likelihood of ulceration. In our experience, bracing has limited usefulness in preventing progressive scoliosis and the need for eventual surgery. For the child who has difficulty with trunk control, however, bracing may help to improve balance and therefore upper-extremity function.

Surgery for scoliosis is complicated by the presence of rigid bony deformities, deficient skin coverage, soft bone, and lack of posterior bony elements. Combined anterior and posterior fusion and segmental instrumentation has made surgical correction, instrumentation, and fusion more predictable.[80] Infection, loss of correction, neurologic injury, and failure of fusion remain common complications. Stronger segmental instrumentation has improved correction and often allowed the child to be brace or cast free in the postoperative period.

Correction of scoliosis in the individual who is nonambulatory equalizes weight bearing on bony areas for sitting and minimizes the likelihood of ulceration. Care must be taken to maintain lumbar lordosis. Obliteration of the lordosis will cause the individual to sit more posteriorly on the ischii and sacrum and may actually increase seating problems.

Ambulatory individuals may find it difficult to be mobile if they are constantly working to maintain their balance when upright. The complex relationship between the pelvis and the spine should be taken into account when considering spinal fusion. Some individuals are able to stand and walk independently by virtue of a mobile hyperlordotic lumbar spine, which may be compensatory for existing hip flexion contractures. Mobility of the trunk and trunk musculature may be used to assist lower-extremity movement in gait, such as with the RGO. Fusion resulting in the loss of lumbar lordosis will accentuate existing hip flexion contractures and make upright stance more difficult. In turn, increased weight bearing on the upper extremities may be required. A retrospective study by Mazur et al,[81] indicated that nearly one third of ambulatory individuals who underwent spinal fusion lost a functional level of ambulatory ability.

The Adolescent

The energy cost of ambulation is high in adolescents with thoracic and high- to mid-lumbar neurosegmental levels.[82] Body weight, which usually increases at this time, contributes to the difficulties.[83] Ambulation becomes less efficient in adolescence, and it becomes more difficult for the adolescent to keep up with peers. The adolescent, therefore, may choose the wheelchair for full-time functional mobility. Ambulation is usually done for therapeutic reasons only, with standing used for the purpose of transfers.

Adolescents with lower neurosegmental levels of involvement may request a wheelchair for community mobility and for participation in sports. We believe participation in sports should be encouraged, not only for the beneficial effects on coordination and trunk and upper-extremity strength, but also for the benefit of self-esteem. Many adolescents enjoy athletic activities such as basketball, tennis, weight lifting, swimming, and wheelchair racing.

Because wheelchair use may increase in adolescence, daily skin inspection and frequent push-ups to unweight the buttocks are imperative. Special wheelchair cushions are used to promote equal weight distribution and provide a firm base of support for the pelvis; however, they do not take the place of pressure-relief maneuvers. Skin ulceration has a major effect on the adolescent's function, because treatment may require surgical intervention, lengthy hospitalizations with restricted positioning, and major financial and personal costs, such as decreased peer and family interaction.[84]

Preparation for transition to adulthood takes place during late adolescence. The adult with myelodysplasia faces problems with separation from family, locating independent living arrangements, developing vocational skills, and finding appropriate medical care.[85,86] The more prepared the adolescent, the easier the transition. The therapist may help by visiting the proposed living and vocational environments and making suggestions for accessibility. If medical care is to be assumed under adult services, communication by the treatment team who has monitored the individual will ensure an easier transition.

Summary

The physical therapist and orthopedist have a significant role in the assessment and treatment of the child with myelodysplasia. Care of the individual with myelodysplasia is a complex process and continues throughout life. Because the neurologic deficit may change over time in some individuals, treatment programs must be individualized and flexible. The nature and timing of various interventions may vary. The needs and status of the individual, the level of function, and stage of life should be considered.

Acknowledgments

We thank Alice Shea, ScD, PT, R Michael Scott, MD, Director of the Section of Pediatric Neurosurgery, and James Koepfler, medical photographer, all of Children's Hospital, Boston, Mass, for their assistance in preparing the manuscript.

References

1 Carter CO. Spina bifida and anencephaly: a problem in genetic-environmental interaction. *J Biosoc Sci.* 1969;1:71–83.

2 Shurtleff DB, Lemir RJ, Warkany J. Embryology, etiology, and epidemiology. In: Shurtleff DB, ed. *Myelodysplasias and Extrophies: Significance, Prevention, and Treatment*. New York, NY: Grune & Stratton Inc; 1986:39–64.

3 Lipman-Hand A, Fraser FC, Cushman Biddle CJ. Indications for prenatal diagnosis in relatives of patients with neural tube defects. *Obstet Gynecol*. 1978;51:72–76.

4 Alan LD, Donald I, Gibson AA, et al. Amniotic fluid alpha-fetoprotein in the antenatal diagnosis of spina bifida. *Lancet*. 1973;2:522–525.

5 Nadel AS, Green JK, Holmes LB, et al. Absence of need for amniocentesis in patients with elevated levels of maternal serum alphafetoprotein and normal ultrasonographic examinations. *N Engl J Med*. 1990;323:557–561.

6 Milinsky A. The prenatal diagnosis of neural tube and other congenital defects. In: Milinsky A, ed. *Genetic Disorders and the Fetus: Diagnosis, Prevention, and Treatment*. New York, NY: Plenum Publishing Corp; 1986:453–519.

7 McLone DG. Treatment of myelomeningocele: arguments against selection. *Clin Neurosurg*. 1986;3:359–370.

8 Lorber J. Results of treatment of myelomeningocele. *Dev Med Child Neurol*. 1971;13:279–303.

9 Gross RH, Cox A, Tatyrek R, et al. Early management and decision making for the treatment of myelomeningocele. *Pediatrics*. 1983;72:450–458.

10 McLaughlin JF, Shurtleff DB, Lamers JY, et al. Influence of prognosis on decisions regarding the care of newborns with myelodysplasia. *N Engl J Med*. 1985;312:1589–1594.

11 Banta JV, Lin R, Peterson M, Dagenais T. The team approach in the care of the child with myelomeningocele. *Journal of Prosthetics and Orthotics*. 1989;2:263–273.

12 Chauvel P. Spina bifida and hydrocephalus. In: Capute AJ, Accardo PJ, eds. *Developmental Disabilities in Infancy and Childhood*. Baltimore, Md: Paul H Brookes Publishing Co; 1991:383–393.

13 Stark GD, Drummond MB, Poneprasert S, Robarts FH. Primary ventriculoperitoneal shunts in treatment of hydrocephalus associated with myelomeningocele. *Arch Dis Child*. 1974;9:112–117.

14 Soare PL, Raimondi AJ. Intellectual and perceptual-motor characteristics of treated myelomeningocele children. *Am J Dis Child*. 1977;131:199–204.

15 Miller E, Sethi L. The effect of hydrocephalus on perception. *Dev Med Child Neurol*. 1971;13(suppl 25):77–81.

16 Mapsstone TB, Rekate HL, Nulsen FE, et al. Relationship of CNS shunting and IQ in children with myelomeningocele. *Child's Brain*. 1984;11:112–118.

17 Schut L, Bruce DA. The Arnold-Chiari malformation. *Orthop Clin North Am*. 1978; 9:913–923.

18 Raynor RB. The Arnold-Chiari malformation. *Spine*. 1986;11:343–344.

19 Park TS, Hoffman HJ, Hendrick EB, Humphreys RP. Experience with surgical decompression of the Arnold-Chiari malformation in young infants with myelomeningocele. *Neurosurgery*. 1983;13:147–152.

20 Hall PV, Campbell RN. Myelomeningocele and progressive hydromyelia. *J Neurosurg*. 1975;43:457–463.

21 Barnett HJM, Foster JB, Hudgson P. *Syringomyelia: Major Problems in Neurosurgery*. Philadelphia, Pa: WB Saunders Co; 1973:vol 1.

22 Barbaro NM, Wilson CB, Gutin PH, Edwards MS. Surgical treatment of syringomyelia: favorable results with syringoperitoneal shunting. *J Neurosurg*. 1984;61:531–538.

23 James CCM, Lassman LP. Spinal dysraphism: the diagnosis and treatment of progressive lesions in spina bifida occulta. *J Bone Joint Surg [Br]*. 1962;44:828–840.

24 Schmidt D, Robinson B, Jones D. The tethered spinal cord: etiology and clinical manifestations. *Orthopedic Review*. 1990;19:870–876.

25 Katz JF. Spontaneous fractures in paraplegic children. *J Bone Joint Surg [Am]*. 1953; 35:220–226.

26 Lock TR, Aronson DD. Fractures in patients who have myelomeningocele. *J Bone Joint Surg [Am]*. 1989;71:1153–1157.

27 Samuelsson L, Eklof O. Hip instability in myelomeningocele: 158 patients followed for 15 years. *Acta Orthop Scand*. 1990;61:3–6.

28 Abraham E, Verinder DG, Sharrad WJ. The treatment of flexion contracture of the knee in myelomeningocele. *J Bone Joint Surg [Br]*. 1977;59:433–438.

29 Bauer SB. Urologic management of the myelodysplastic child. *Problems in Urology*. 1989;3:86–101.

30 Bauer SB, Hallet M, Khoshbin S, et al. Predictive value of urodynamic evaluation in newborns with myelodysplasia. *JAMA*. 1984; 252:650–652.

31 Evans K, Hickman V, Carter CO. Handicap and social status of adults with spina bifida cystica. *Br J Prev Soc Med*. 1974;28:85–92.

32 Whitehead WE, Parker LH, Bosmajian L, et al. Treatment of fecal incontinence in children with spinal bifida: comparison of biofeedback and behavior modification. *Arch Phys Med Rehabil*. 1986;17:218–224.

33 Mazur JM, Aylward GP, Colliver J, et al. Impaired mental capabilities and hand function in myelomeningocele patients. *Z Kinderchir*. 1988;43(suppl 2):24–27.

34 Mazur JM, Menelaus MB, Hudson I, Stillwell A. Hand function in patients with spina bifida cystica. *J Pediatr Orthop*. 1986;6:442–447.

35 Strecker WB, Riordan MT, Daily L. Hand grasp measurements in myelomeningocele patients. Presented at the annual meeting of the American Academy of Orthopedic Surgeons; February 8–15, 1990; New Orleans, La.

36 Wallace SJ. The effect of upper-limb function on mobility of children with myelomeningocele. *Dev Med Child Neurol*. 1973;15(suppl 29):84–91.

37 *Joint Motion: Method of Measuring and Recording*. Park Ridge, Ill: American Academy of Orthopedic Surgeons; 1965.

38 Moore ML. The measurement of joint motion, part II: the technic of goniometry. *Phys Ther Rev*. 1949;29:256–264.

39 Forero N, Okamura L, Larson M. Normal ranges of hip motion in neonates. *J Pediatr Orthop*. 1989;9:391–395.

40 McDonald C, Jaffe K, Shurtleff DB. Assessment of muscle strength in children with meningomyelocele: accuracy and stability of measurements over time. *Arch Phys Med Rehabil*. 1986;67:855–861.

41 Asher M, Olson J. Factors affecting the ambulatory status of patients with spina bifida cystica. *J Bone Joint Surg [Am]*. 1983; 65:350–356.

42 DeSouza L, Carroll N. Ambulation of the braced myelomeningocele patient. *J Bone Joint Surg [Am]*. 1976;58:1112–1118.

43 Mazur JM, Menelaus MB. Neurologic status of spina bifida patients and the orthopedic surgeon. *Clin Orthop*. 1991;264:54–64.

44 Kendall FP, McCreary EK. *Muscles: Testing and Function*. 3rd ed. Baltimore, Md: Williams & Wilkins; 1983.

45 Zausmer E. Evaluation of strength and motor development in infants: parts I and II. *Phys Ther Rev*. 1953;33:575–581, 621–629.

46 Daniels L, Worthingham C. *Muscle Testing: Techniques of Manual Examination*. 4th ed. Philadelphia, Pa: WB Saunders Co; 1980.

47 Stuberg WA, Metcalf WK. Reliability of quantitative muscle testing in healthy children and in children with Duchenne muscular dystrophy using a hand-held dynamometer. *Phys Ther*. 1988;68:977–982.

48 Fiorentino MR. *Reflex Testing Methods for Evaluating Central Nervous System Development*. 2nd ed. Springfield, Ill: Charles C Thomas, Publisher; 1981.

49 Barnes MR, Crutchfield CA, Heriza CB, Herdman SJ. *Reflex and Vestibular Aspsects of Motor Control, Motor Development, and Motor Learning*. Morgantown, WV: Stokesville Publishing Co; 1990.

50 Wolf LS, McLaughlin JFJ. Early motor development of children with myelomeningocele. Presented at the annual meeting of the American Academy of Cerebral Palsy and Developmental Medicine; October 1984; Washington, DC.

51 Sousa JC, Telzrow RW, Holm RA, et al. Developmental guidelines for children with myelodysplasia. *Phys Ther*. 1983;63:21–29.

52 Shurtleff DB. Myelodysplasia: management and treatment. *Curr Probl Pediatr*. 1980; 10:7–98.

53 Folio MR, Fewell RR. *Peabody Developmental Motor Scales and Activity Cards Manual*. Hingham, Mass: DLM Teaching Resources; 1983.

54 Bayley N. *Bayley Scales of Infant Development*. New York, NY: The Psychological Corp; 1969.

55 Knobloch H, Stevens F, Malone A. *A Manual of Developmental Diagnosis: The Administration and Interpretation of the Revised Gesell and Amatruda Developmental and Neurological Examination*. New York, NY: Harper & Row, Publishers Inc; 1980.

56 Hoffer MM, Feiwell E, Perry R, et al. Functional ambulation in patients with myelomeningocele. *J Bone Joint Surg [Am]*. 1973; 55:137–148.

57 Drummond DS, Moreau M, Cruess RL. Post-operative neuropathic fractures in patients with myelomeningocele. *Dev Med Child Neurol*. 1981;23:147–150.

58 Samuelsson L, Skoog M. Ambulation in patients with myelomeningocele: a multivariate statistical analysis. *Pediatric Orthopedics*. 1988;8:569–575.

59 Dudgeon BJ, Jaffe KM, Shurtleff DB. Variations in midlumbar myelomeningocele: impli-

cations for ambulation. *Pediatric Physical Therapy.* 1991;3:57–62.

60 Carroll NC. Assessment and management of the lower extremity in myelodysplasia. *Orthop Clin North Am.* 1987;18:709–724.

61 Lee EH, Carroll NC. Hip stability and ambulatory status in myelomeningocele. *J Pediatr Orthop.* 1985;5:522–527.

62 Molloy MK. The unstable paralytic hip: treatment by combined pelvic and femoral osteotomy and transiliac psoas transfer. *J Pediatr Orthop.* 1986;6:533–538.

63 Stillwell A, Menelaus MB. Walking ability after transplantation of the iliopsoas: a long-term follow-up. *J Bone Joint Surg [Br].* 1984;66:656–659.

64 Bunch WH, Hakala MW. Iliopsoas transfers in children with myelomeningocele. *J Bone Joint Surg [Am].* 1984;66:224–227.

65 Crandall RC, Birkebak RC, Winter RB. The role of hip location and dislocation in the functional status of the myelodysplastic patient: a review of 100 patients. *Orthopedics.* 1989;12:675–684.

66 Sherk HH, Melchionne J, Smith R. The natural history of hip dislocations in ambulatory myelomeningoceles. *Z Kinderchir.* 1987;42(suppl 1):48–49.

67 Riggins RS, Kraus J, Fontanetta P. Hip dislocations in myelodysplasia: a functional assessment. *South Med J.* 1983;76:736–739.

68 Bazih J, Gross RH. Hip surgery in the lumbar level myelomeningocele patient. *J Pediatr Orthop.* 1981;1:405–411.

69 Gugenheim JJ, Rosenthal RK, Dabrowski S, Hall JE. Adductor transfer in the high-risk hip in myelodysplasia. *Clin Orthop.* 1978;132:108–114.

70 Thomas LI, Thompson TC, Strub LR. Transplantation of the external oblique muscle for abductor paralysis. *J Bone Joint Surg [Am].* 1950;32:207–217.

71 Sharrard WJW. Posterior iliopsoas transplantation in the treatment of paralytic dislocation of the hip. *J Bone Joint Surg [Br].* 1964;46:426–444.

72 Rosenstein BD, Greene WB, Herrington RT, Blum AS. Bone density in myelomeningocele: the effects of ambulatory status and other factors. *Dev Med Child Neurol.* 1987;29:486–494.

73 Lindseth RE, Glancy J. Polypropylene lower extremity braces for paraplegia due to myelomeningocele. *J Bone Joint Surg [Am].* 1974;56:556–563.

74 McCall RE, Schmidt WT. Clinical experience with the reciprocal gait orthosis in myelodysplasia. *J Pediatr Orthop.* 1986;6:157–161.

75 Flandry F, Burke S, Roberts J, et al. Functional ambulation in myelodysplasia: the effect of orthotic selection on physical and physiologic performance. *J Pediatr Orthop.* 1986;6:661–665.

76 Logan L, Byers-Hinkley K, Ciccone CD. Anterior vs posterior walkers: a gait analysis study. *Dev Med Child Neurol.* 1990;32:1044–1048.

77 Mazur JM, Shurtleff DB, Menelaus MB, Colliver J. Orthopaedic management of high-level spina bifida: early walking compared with early use of a wheelchair. *J Bone Joint Surg [Br].* 1989;71:56–61.

78 McMaster M. The long-term results of kyphectomy and spinal stabilization in children with myelomeningocele. *Spine.* 1988;13:417–424.

79 Lord J, Varzos N, Behrman B, et al. Implication of mainstream classrooms for adolescents with spina bifida. *Dev Med Child Neurol.* 1990;32:20–29.

80 Ward WT, Wenger DR, Roach JW. Surgical correction of myelomeningocele scoliosis: a critical appraisal of various spinal instrumentation systems. *J Pediatr Orthop.* 1989;9:262–268.

81 Mazur JM, Menelaus MB, Dickens DR, Doig WG. Efficacy of surgical management for scoliosis in myelomeningocele: correction of deformity and alteration of functional status. *J Pediatr Orthop.* 1986;6:568–575.

82 Findley TW, Agre JC, Birkebak RC, et al. Ambulation in adolescent with myelomeningocele, I: early childhood predictors. *Arch Phys Med Rehabil.* 1987;68:518–522.

83 Agre JC, Findley TW, McNally MC, et al. Physical activity in children with myelomeningocele. *Arch Phys Med Rehabil.* 1987;68:372–377.

84 Harris M, Banta J. Cost of skin care in the myelomeningocele population. *J Pediatr Orthop.* 1990;10:355–361.

85 Castree B, Walker TH. The young adult with spina bifida. *Br Med J.* 1981;283:1040–1042.

86 McLone DG. Spina bifida today: problems adults face. *Semin Neurol.* 1989;9:169–175.

Orthotic Devices for Ambulation in Children with Cerebral Palsy and Myelomeningocele

Children with cerebral palsy and children with myelomeningocele frequently require orthotic devices for standing and walking. The purpose of this article is to review the literature on orthotic devices for walking, present principles of lower-extremity orthoses, discuss designs of orthoses, and consider criteria for selecting orthotic devices. Although discussion of the devices is specific to children with myelomeningocele and to children with cerebral palsy, the orthoses can be used with children having other disabilities. The information presented should be of value to clinicians, educators, and researchers interested in reviewing orthotic applications for children with disabilities. [Knutson LM, Clark DE. Orthotic devices for ambulation in children with cerebral palsy and myelomeningocele. Phys Ther. 1991;71:947–960.]

Loretta M Knutson
Dennis E Clark

Key Words: *Cerebral palsy, Children, Meningomyelocele, Orthoses, Orthotic devices, Physical therapy.*

The prevalence of cerebral palsy (CP) at school entry is 2.0 per 1,000 live births.[1–3] The school-entry prevalence for myelomeningocele (MMC) may be slightly less than the MMC birth incidence of 1.0 per 1,000.[4] Collectively, approximately 3.0 children per 1,000 have one of these disabilities. Projecting from the statistics that 4,021,000 children were born in the United States in 1989,[5] over 12,000 children in a given year can be expected to be affected by one of these neurological disabilities. A majority of these children will have orthotic needs for which the attention of a physical therapist will be required. In a public health survey on payment for services, 54% of the 380 children with mixed diagnoses studied used braces.[6] Because so many children will use orthoses, physical therapists should be knowledgeable about orthotic programming.

The purpose of this article is to review contemporary practice in orthotic management, focusing on devices used for ambulation in children with CP and children with MMC. These two patient populations were chosen for four reasons. First, these children commonly need orthoses to walk. Second, their needs extend through and change during their lifetime. Third, their orthotic and gait training programs frequently fall under the direction of a physical therapist. Fourth, the orthotic management of these children can often be generalized to the care of children with other disabilities. This article is divided into sections organized to review the literature on orthotic devices for walking, present principles of lower-extremity orthoses, discuss orthotic design, and consider criteria for selecting orthotic devices according to patient needs.

Review of Literature

Although numerous references to and discussions of orthotic devices can be found in the literature, there are fewer reports of an investigative nature. Only recently have reports of studies been published on the effects of orthotic devices for children with disabilities. Table 1 summarizes key studies of pediatric orthotic use.

Cerebral Palsy

The use of orthoses in the management of children with CP has varied from the discussion by Little of "mechanical apparatus" in the mid-1800s and advocacy by Phelps and Deaver between 1930 and 1950 to avoidance

LM Knutson, PhD, PT, PCS, is Lecturer, Physical Therapy Graduate Program, and Senior Physical Therapist, Division of Developmental Disabilities, The University of Iowa, 2600 Steindler Bldg, Iowa City, IA 52242 (USA). Address correspondence to Dr Knutson.

DE Clark, BA, CPO, is Prosthetist/Orthotist and Owner of Dale Clark Prosthetics in Waterloo, Coralville, and Dubuque, Iowa. He is also on the Board of Directors of the American Board for Certification in Orthotics and Prosthetics.

Table 1. *Original Investigative Studies in Pediatric Orthotics*

| Orthosis | Investigator(s) | Subject Population | | | Variables Studied[b] |
		Diagnosis[a]	N	Age (y)	
Foot orthoses	Wenger et al,[54] 1989	Flatfeet	129	1–6	Radiographs
	Penneau et al,[55] 1982	Pes planus	10	1.5–4.5	Radiographs
	Bordelon,[56] 1983	Flatfeet	50	3–9	Radiographs
	Bleck and Berzins,[57] 1977	Pes planus	71	1–12	Radiographs
	Mereday et al,[58] 1972	Pes planus	10	3.5–12.5	Radiographs
Supramalleolar orthoses	Embrey et al,[24] 1990	CP	1	2.7	Knee kinematics
Inhibitive casts and splints	Hinderer et al,[22] 1988	CP	1	. . .	Stride characteristics
	Bertoti,[25] 1986	CP	16	0.8–9	Stride characteristics
	Watt et al,[26] 1986	CP	28	1.5–5	Tone, motor skills, PROM, observational kinematics
	Mills,[27] 1984	HI (7), aneurysm (1)	8	10–22	EMG
Ankle-foot orthoses	Lough,[28] 1990	CP	15	3–12	EMG, walking velocity, foot radiographs, kinematics
	Mossberg et al,[10] 1990	CP	18	3–14	HR, walking velocity
	Thomas et al,[42] 1989	MMC	. . .	. . .	EMG, kinematics
	Brodke et al,[11] 1989	Nondisabled child	5	6–12	EMG, kinematics, kinetics, walking velocity
	Middleton et al,[21] 1988	CP	1	4.5	Kinematics, kinetics, walking velocity
	Harris and Riffle,[23] 1986	CP	1	4.5	Standing balance time
Knee-ankle-foot orthoses	Krebs et al,[43] 1988	MMC (12), upper motoneuron pathology (2), myopathy (1)	15	5–21	Gait kinematics, ADL, child and parent opinion
Reciprocating gait orthosis	Mazur et al,[37] 1989	MMC	3	. . .	Walking velocity, stride characteristics, EMG, kinematics
	Flandry et al,[41] 1986	MMC	8	4–19	HR, EE, walking velocity
	McCall and Schmidt,[49] 1986	MMC	37	1.3–1.6	Pulse rate, walking velocity
	Yngve et al,[48] 1984	MMC	3	3–16	Walking velocity
Hip guidance orthosis	Rose et al,[46] 1981	MMC	27	5.7–12.6	HR, walking velocity, ambulation status
Swivel walker	Stallard et al,[45] 1978	MMC	1	. . .	HR, walking velocity
	Davies,[44] 1977	MMC	. . .	. . .	HR
Parapodium	Lough and Nielsen,[47] 1986	MMC (9), SCI (1)	10	4–8	EE, HR, walking velocity

[a]CP=cerebral palsy, HI=head injury, MMC=myelomeningocele, SCI=spinal cord injury.

[b]PROM=passive range of motion, EMG=electromyographic activity, HR=heart rate, ADL=activities of daily living, EE=energy expenditure.

of orthotic devices, particularly full-control orthoses, during the peak of the neurodevelopmental treatment (NDT) era.[7,8] Today, a new enthusiasm for the use of orthoses has surfaced, specifically for below-knee devices used by children who are ambulatory.[9]

A 1985 report on a group of English children with CP born between 1970 and 1974 states that 50% to 75% of the children were ambulatory.[2] Because a majority of children with CP will use orthoses to assist walking, research that complements orthotic selection or adds to an understanding of orthoses is helpful. In one such recent study, Mossberg and colleagues[10] evaluated walking velocity and heart rate in 18 children with spastic diplegia walking with and without plastic ankle-foot orthoses (AFOs). Use of orthoses increased walking velocity and reduced the heart rate compared with walking without AFOs; however, the differences were not statistically significant.

Fifteen years ago, steel or aluminum braces with adjustable ankle joints were common. Although today metal braces are rarely used for children with CP, the purported advantages of polypropylene orthotic designs have not been well studied. Brodke and co-workers[11] evaluated five nondisabled children walking barefoot and using both traditional metal AFOs and fixed polypropylene AFOs. Walking speed and cadence were observed to decrease with either AFO compared with the barefoot condition; however, the decrease was more pronounced with the metal AFOs. The duration of quadriceps femoris muscle electromyographic (EMG) activity was greater with molded plastic AFOs than with metal AFOs and was greater for both braces than for barefoot walking. Changes in lower-extremity (ie, hip and knee), motion were not significantly different, but maximum knee extension during stance tended to be greater with polypropylene AFOs than with metal AFOs or barefoot walking. Both types of orthoses effectively limited ankle motion. The researchers concluded that metal AFOs impaired

normal gait more than did polypropylene AFOs.

Polypropylene orthoses were first introduced in the 1960s.[12] Their use in children with CP did not become established until the mid- to late-1970s when clinical experience and satisfaction gradually dispelled views that plastic orthoses would increase spasticity (excessive contraction of the muscle and stiffness that prevents or opposes normal muscle lengthening) or would not be sufficiently strong to support the spastic (affected by spasticity) limb. The first designs of polypropylene orthoses, as described by Hoffer et al[13] in 1974, were strictly of the fixed design.

By the early 1980s, fixed polypropylene AFOs were being molded with features designed to hold the subtalar joint in neutral and inhibit spasticity.[14] The "subtalar-neutral" AFO was intended to oppose foot valgus or pronation during weight bearing, a problem that occurs frequently in children with spastic diplegia or quadriplegia.[15,16] The concept of subtalar-neutral alignment and "tone reduction," or reduction of the state of muscle contraction, was first introduced in inhibitive casts[17,18] and was later applied to orthoses.[14,19] Descriptive reports have been supplemented by case reports[20,21] and single-subject design research.[22–24] Hinderer and co-workers[22] found tone-reducing casts yielded a longer stride length than standard casts in two children under 6 years of age with CP.[22] Harris and Riffle[23] found inhibitive AFOs (right supramalleolar orthosis and left AFO) increased standing balance time in a 4½-year-old child with quadriplegia. Embrey and colleagues[24] demonstrated knee flexion could be reduced during gait in a 2½-year-old child who had hypotonia by the use of NDT and "ankle-height orthoses."

Early contoured AFO designs did not allow ankle motion. Recently, however, hinged polypropylene AFOs have been introduced and have received positive responses by physical therapy clinicians. Middleton and colleagues[21] reported the first compari-

son of fixed AFOs with hinged AFOs by studying a 4½-year-old child with spastic diplegia. The child's pattern of ankle dorsiflexion was more normal and the knee muscle moments were lower during the stance phase of gait with the hinged AFOs than with the fixed AFOs. The investigators concluded that hinged AFOs appear to be more effective than fixed AFOs for treating children who have spastic CP.

Without replication, the results of the case reports and single-subject studies cannot be generalized to other children. Some investigators, however, have studied groups of patients using inhibitive short leg casts,[25,26] splints,[27] and AFOs.[28] In studying two groups of children before and after 10 weeks of NDT, Bertoti[25] found the group of eight children wearing short leg casts had a 27% increase in stride compared with a 13% decrease in stride for the group of eight children who were uncasted. Watt and colleagues[26] examined the long-term effects of a 3-week treatment course involving inhibitive casting and NDT. Whereas improvements in passive ankle dorsiflexion and foot-floor contact when walking were seen 2 weeks after treatment, these changes were less evident after 5 months. Specifically, right ankle dorsiflexion showed an increase of 8.8 degrees 2 weeks after cast removal but only 3.6 degrees after 5 months. Right foot-floor contact was seen in 64% of the patients 2 weeks after casting and in 39% of the patients 5 months after casting. Mills[27] studied the EMG and range-of-motion (ROM) effects of inhibitive splints on eight adolescent and young adult subjects who had neurological insults. Compared with the presplint condition, no effects on integrated EMG activity during splint use were noted, but the ROM into extension increased. In a study by Lough,[28] the effects of no orthoses, fixed AFOs, and hinged AFOs were contrasted in 15 children with CP. Mean walking velocity increased by 5.6 cm/s, and ankle dorsiflexion increased during mid-stance of gait by 4.9 degrees for hinged orthoses compared with no orthoses. The EMG amplitudes were examined at 5% intervals across an ensemble average created for each of four muscles. Of 80 possible intervals of significant difference, only 3 were different—2 for the vastus lateralis muscle and 1 for the tibialis anterior muscle. No differences were found among the treatments for the medial hamstring or gastrocnemius muscles. The reduction in foot pronation, as determined from standing dorsoplantar radiographic measurements of the talonavicular angle, was significant for fixed AFOs (4.5° less) and approached significance for hinged AFOs (3.6° less) compared with no orthoses.

Myelomeningocele

The prognosis for ambulation by children with MMC is related to level of motor function. The effect of the spinal cord dysfunction level on energy expenditure was well documented in adults with paraplegia by Clinkingbeard and associates[29] and is in accord with reports of function for children with MMC.[30–38] Children with higher levels of spinal defect (eg, at and above L-2) require more extensive orthotic support and can be expected to expend more energy than children with defects below L-2. Table 2 summarizes reports on the status of and prognosis for ambulation in children with MMC. Consensus generally exists that the higher the level of defect, the smaller will be the percentage of the group who are ambulatory. Other factors influencing ambulation include mental retardation, muscle power within the level of defect, orthopedic deformities, hydrocephalus, and walking status at age 7 years.[30–39]

Whether children with high lumbar- and thoracic-level defects are provided early instruction for walking appears to be influenced by practice patterns of the geographic area. Although reports agree the majority of children with thoracic MMC who walk will later become nonambulatory, the study by Mazur and colleagues[37] supports the value of bracing and walking. Subjects who walked as children had fewer fractures and pressure sores, were more independent, and were better able to transfer than were

patients who used a wheelchair from early in life. Sankarankutty et al[41] stressed the importance of effective bracing and suggested that modern orthoses can prolong ambulation in patients who otherwise may discard their devices. This notion was reinforced by Flandry et al[41] in their study, which demonstrated that the energy cost values for walking with the reciprocating gait orthosis (RGO) approximated those for wheelchair use.

Limited research has addressed the effects of orthotic designs on ambulation in children with MMC. In most practices, clinical experiences of the prescriber serve as guideposts in orthotic selection. A recent quantitative study by Thomas et al[42] revealed that children with MMC who wore AFOs showed reduced hip, knee, and ankle flexion; decreased muscle activation time; and decreased muscle coactivation during gait. Krebs and colleagues[43] found specific differences for children with MMC using metal versus polypropylene knee-ankle-foot orthoses (KAFOs); children preferred the polypropylene KAFOs and appeared to have better control of hip, knee, and ankle motion.

Studies in the 1970s and early 1980s at the Orthotic Research and Locomotor Assessment Unit (ORLAU) in Oswestry, England, measured velocity, heart rate, and ambulatory status with different orthoses used primarily for children with high-level spinal defects.[44–46] Descriptive results suggested improvements in all variables when children switched from previous bracing (ie, conventional hip-knee-ankle-foot orthosis [HKAFO] or swivel walker) to a hip guidance orthosis. In 1986, Lough and Nielsen[47] reported that children with MMC walked faster, but had higher energy expenditure and were less efficient, with their use of parapodiums than with their use of parapodiums adapted with a swivel-walker base.

Comparing the RGO used with different hip joint and cable configurations (normal reciprocal action, locked, or free motion), Yngve and colleagues[48]

and McCall and Schmidt[49] favored the normal reciprocal mode based on patients achieving a faster walking velocity. Patients in both studies also reported preferring the reciprocal to the swing-through pattern of gait.

Principles of Lower-Extremity Orthoses

Several textbooks are available that provide a more comprehensive coverage of orthoses; each of these textbooks presents a list of principles, purposes, and goals of bracing.[50–53] Following are guiding principles that should be applied with the pediatric client.

1. Prevent deformity. Orthoses may be prescribed to prevent a deformity that is anticipated to occur or that might increase without treatment. Orthoses can also be used following surgery or serial casting to maintain correction of a deformity. Occasionally, orthoses are used to correct a deformity.

2. Support normal joint alignment and mechanics. Molded orthoses often have a greater chance of achieving this goal than do conventional metal devices because they provide total contact. Options in molded AFOs (solid, variable range, or free motion) can all support joint alignment. Even foot orthoses (FOs) can facilitate this goal as long as alignment includes the ankle joint, the subtalar joint, and other midfoot and forefoot structures. This principle is inherent in what some clinicians refer to as "tone reduction." Good alignment may be more important than the addition of extra pressure at selected sites in reducing tone.

3. Provide variable range of motion when appropriate. For ambulatory patients, restriction of some ROM is often necessary to assist weak muscles, oppose spastic muscles, enhance balance, protect certain soft tissues postsurgically, or improve the appearance of gait for the patient who lacks selective control to achieve a normal pattern. At the ankle, this may require restricting plantar flexion while allowing free dorsiflexion or allowing plan-

Table 2. *Studies Addressing the Status and/or Prognosis for Ambulation in Children with Myelomeningocele*

Investigator(s)	No. of Subjects[a]	Mobility Status	Factors Influencing Prognosis
Taylor and McNamara,[38] 1990	32—thoracic 32—lumbar 16—lumbosacral 1—sacral 6—unknown	58 wheelchair users; 23 community ambulators; 6 household ambulators	Level of neurological deficit and type of orthoses used
Mazur et al,[37,b] 1989	22—T10-12 14—L1-2	17 (47%) no longer walked; 12 (33%) were community ambulators; 7 (20%) were household ambulators	Those who had discontinued walking specified reasons including energy expenditure and ease
Samuelsson and Skoog,[39] 1988	163—total	0% of thoracic and L1-2, 54% of L-3, 67% of L-4, 80% of L-5, and 100% of sacral patients ambulate	Level of defect and associated neurological findings influence walking
Findley et al,[36] 1987	14—thoracic 4—L1-2 16—L3-4 19—L5-S1 24—sacral	20 not walking; 56 community ambulators, 26 of 56 occasionally used a wheelchair; 1 therapeutic ambulator	Walking outdoors independently and using a wheelchair by age 7 y was more predictive of adolescent ambulation than was neurologic level
Schopler and Menelaus,[35] 1987	109—total (sites of lesion not specified)	88% with grade 0–2 quadriceps femoris muscle strength exclusively used wheelchairs; 82% with grade 4–5 muscle strength were community ambulators; 89% with grade 3–5 muscle strength were at least household ambulators	Strong quadriceps femoris muscles predict good ambulation
Sankarankutty et al,[40] 1979	102—total 52—thoracic	5.7% were wheelchair users; 3 subjects over 15 y old (1 wheelchair user, 1 household ambulator, 1 therapeutic ambulator)	Level of defect important, but thoracic lesions do not prevent independence; improved orthotic design is needed
DeSouza and Carroll,[33] 1976	4—thoracic 19—upper lumbar 13—lower lumbar 32—sacral	1 of 4 with thoracic defects was a wheelchair user, 1 was a household ambulator, and 1 was a therapeutic ambulator	Level of defect, motor power, and orthopedic deformity influenced progress
Barden et al,[34] 1975	9—thoracolumbar 20—lumbar	2 of 9 with T12-L2 defects and 19 of 20 with L-3 defects still walked	Final hip position did not correlate with walking status
Hoffer et al,[13] 1974	10—thoracic 40—lumbar 6—sacral	52% were wheelchair users; all 10 with thoracic defects were nonambulators; all 6 with sacral defects were community ambulators	Factors other than level of spinal defect were age; presence of hydrocephalus, spasticity, and skeletal deformities; intelligence; and societal factors
Lorber,[31] 1971	134—total (sites of defects not specified)	1/3 limited to wheelchair use; 1/3 used calipers at least part time; 1/3 walked independently	. . .
Richings and Eckstein,[30,c] 1970	4—encephalocele 8—cervical 15—thoracic 5—thoracolumbar 51—lumbar 27—lumbosacral 15—sacral	7 (6%) used wheelchairs; 105 (94%) had some degree of mobility; 16 of 23 with complete paralysis of lower extremities achieved some mobility with braces	Improved orthotic design is needed

[a]When indicated, the total number of subjects was reduced according to the number of subjects for whom locomotor behavior was reported.

[b]Comparison study of early walking group (n=36) to matched early use of wheelchair group (n=36).

[c]Number at each level of defect was estimated from a figure.

tar flexion while restricting dorsiflexion. The plantar-flexion stop, for example, might be used for a child with CP who has an equinus deformity, whereas the dorsiflexion stop might be used to eliminate a crouched gait by stopping anterior motion of the tibia in the presence of an overlengthened heelcord. The dorsiflexion stop could also be used for the child with an MMC at L-5 who heel walks or has excessive ankle dorsiflexion. Various combinations of motion and restriction are possible.

4. Facilitate function. The orthotic device should not restrict the child, but should encourage function. The physical therapist is particularly important for assessing the fit and function of an orthosis. Changes in the orthosis may be needed as the patient's ability or muscle function changes, thus ensuring the device facilitates and does not restrain the patient's progress.

Orthotic Design

Foot Orthoses

With FOs (Fig. 1), attention must be given to achieving a close-contact fit that does not impinge on the medial or lateral malleoli. The distal trimline should extend just proximal to the metatarsal heads. The high medial and lateral walls should extend to the dorsum of the foot. Studies on FOs are reported in Table 1.[54-58]

Supramalleolar Orthoses

Supramalleolar orthoses (SMOs) (Fig. 2) have proximal trimlines that extend 30 to 50 mm above the malleoli. Although the malleoli are covered by the orthotic walls, the orthoses are trimmed anteriorly and posteriorly to allow plantar flexion and dorsiflexion.

Ankle-Foot Orthoses

Ankle-foot orthoses (Fig. 3) should be designed to extend 10 to 15 mm distal to the head of the fibula on the pediatric patient. All below-knee supports, whether AFOs (fixed or hinged AFOs), SMOs, or FOs, should incorpo-

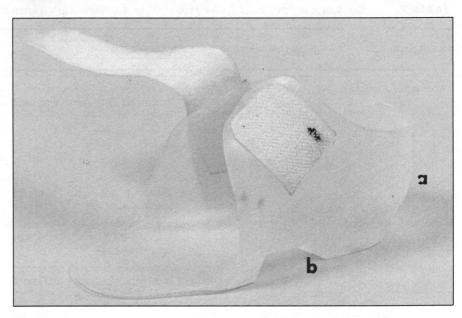

Figure 1. *Foot orthosis designed to oppose pronation by molding the heel cup to grasp the calcaneus firmly (a) and wedging, or posting, the heel medially (b).*

rate supportive features to align the foot in a subtalar-neutral position. An anterior floor-reaction AFO is a variation on the design of an AFO used for children with excessive flexible knee flexion posture. This design has particularly been recommended for children with L-4 myelomeningocele and for children with CP who stand with knee flexion attributable to overlengthened heelcords. The polypropylene mold includes an anterior rather than a posterior shell only. An illustration of the floor-reaction AFO is shown in the article by Rose and colleagues in this issue. If the FO is cut low or supports only beneath the foot, it will not contain all key components of ankle and foot support.

Five Key Components of Ankle and Foot Support

Control of the subtalar joint. The AFO, SMO, and some FOs should grasp the calcaneus firmly (Fig. 1) to prevent medial and lateral motion with subsequent collapse of the heel into valgus and the subtalar joint into pronation. A medial heel post with slight wedging of the plantar surface will also oppose pronation and encourage normal alignment (Fig. 1).

Control of the midtarsal joint. The AFO, SMO, and FO must resist forefoot abduction or adduction. This can be accomplished by ensuring well-molded medial and lateral walls and borders of the orthosis (Fig. 2). At times, the medial or lateral trimlines may extend distal to the metatarsal heads (eg, in a child with MMC following treatment of clubfoot deformity). In this case, consideration should be given to the effect this extension will have on restricting toe extension late in the stance phase.

High (flexible) medial and lateral walls. If the walls of the AFO, SMO, or FO wrap over the dorsum of the foot, the force exerted by the walls will help restrain the heel for maximum control (Fig. 2). Additional benefits of the high walls are (1) control of forefoot abduction or adduction, (2) distribution of pressures over the foot for reducing unwanted stimulation, and, (3) assurance of constant contact with the orthosis during the entire gait cycle. A potential disadvantage is the lack of ease with which the child can don the orthosis. Some parents have reported their children have difficulty keeping the orthosis walls spread while sliding the foot into the device.

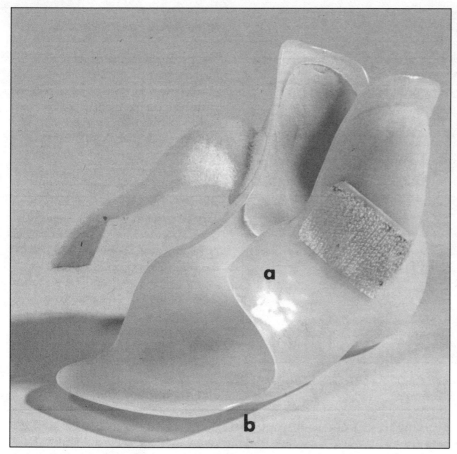

Figure 2. *Supramalleolar orthosis extending proximally to the malleoli. Well-molded medial and lateral walls that wrap over the dorsum of the foot (a) help control the midtarsal joint and keep the heel seated. Dorsal flaps also disperse pressure and may reduce sensitivity of the foot. Intrinsic toe elevation (b) can prevent stimulating the plantar grasp reflex.*

Toe elevation. Toe elevations may be intrinsic (ie, built into the plastic) (Fig. 2) or extrinsic (ie, removable and repositionable) (Fig. 3). Intrinsic toe elevations may shorten the life of the orthosis because the child's growth cannot be readily accommodated. By contrast, extrinsic elevations can be repositioned as the child grows. Additionally, the height of the elevations can be more easily increased or decreased.

Transmetatarsal arch. As with toe elevations, the transmetatarsal arch can be intrinsic or extrinsic. Caution must be taken to ensure appropriate placement of this feature so the child does not feel inappropriately posi-

tioned pressure. This feature has particularly been used with toe elevation for tone reduction.

Variable-Motion Ankle Joints

Until the past 5 years, the solid, molded, fixed orthosis was standard. Recently, however, hinged ankle joints have been introduced, in part, to encourage a more normal gait pattern. Hinged or variable-motion ankle joints can be used in KAFOs and AFOs. The following variable-motion ankle joints represent commonly used designs at the present time.

Overlap articulation. This joint is constructed from polypropylene or

copolymer (Fig. 4). The overlap articulation design is the most widely used hinged ankle joint. When used alone, the joint allows free dorsiflexion or plantar flexion. When used in combination with other features of the brace, several possibilities for controlling motion emerge. Typically, the orthosis will be molded with a plantar-flexion stop at neutral. Modifications to the polypropylene, however, can place the stop in dorsiflexion or in plantar flexion. A plantar-flexion stop set in dorsiflexion is commonly used to restrict knee hyperextension. If the goal is to stop dorsiflexion, a posterior strap can be added. A further adaptation involves the addition of screws to restrict motion. A screw placed horizontally through the posterior overlap can stop all motion until the therapist is ready to allow dorsiflexion. A posteriorly placed vertical screw will allow variable ROM. Turning the screw adjusts the plantar flexion.

Gillette joint. The Gillette joint* is made of rubber vacuformed into polypropylene (Fig. 5). This hinge is normally used to provide a

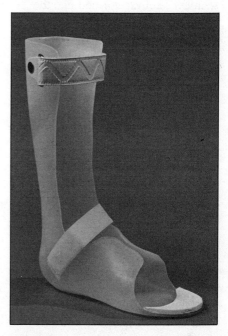

Figure 3. *Fixed molded ankle-foot orthosis with an ankle strap to restrain the heel. Extrinsic toe elevation to unload the metatarsal heads is optional.*

---

*Becker Orthopedic Appliance, 635 Executive Dr, Troy, MI 48083-4576.

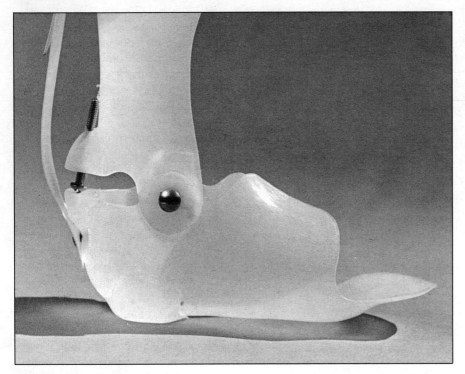

Figure 4. *Overlap articulation joint used in a hinged, variable-motion ankle-foot orthosis showing the posterior strap and the vertical screw.*

hinge joint allows all the flexibility of the plastic overlap joint.

Knee-Ankle-Foot Orthoses

The proximal medial aspect of the thigh portion of a KAFO (Fig. 9) should extend to within 45 mm of the perineum on the medial side and to within 75 mm of the greater trochanter on the lateral side. Various knee joints can be used, and the reader is referred to other references for coverage of the options available.[50–53] The knee joint must be aligned in all three planes—sagittal, coronal, and transverse. In the sagittal plane, the joint should be one half the distance between the posterior aspect of the patella and the posterior aspect of the leg. From the coronal plane, the joint should be at the midpoint of the patella. In the transverse plane, the joints must be aligned with the line of gait progression.

Hip-Knee-Ankle-Foot Orthosis

Conventional metal HKAFOs are rarely used today by children with CP or children with MMC. If these devices are prescribed, however, their fit must be examined in the sitting and standing positions. If the patient is being fitted bilaterally, the critical fitting is done in a sitting position. Ideally, the hip joint should be positioned 10 mm superior to the greater trochanter.

Special designs of HKAFOs (parapodium, swivel walker, and RGO) are described in the next section. Only the Rochester HKAFO, which is not used for walking, is mentioned here. This orthosis is mainly used by the very young child with MMC as a nighttime sleeping brace. The orthosis can also be helpful to encourage early weight bearing in the child under 15 months of age who has a high lumbar- or thoracic-level MMC. Parents are instructed to support and supervise their child in standing with this device. A belt across the chest, and thigh and calf straps, help restrain body position for standing.

plantar-flexion stop and free dorsiflexion. By grinding the plastic posteriorly, some increased plantar-flexion ROM is possible.

Gaffney joint. This joint[†] is made of stainless steel vacuformed into the polypropylene (Fig. 6). Seven sizes of hinges are available. This design of hinged ankle joint is normally used to provide a plantar-flexion stop and unrestricted dorsiflexion.

Select joint. These joints[‡] are made of color-coded aluminum disks vacuformed into plastic (Fig. 7). Two sizes of disks are available. Within each size, five variations in disks allow the therapist to insert different disks and change selectively the ROM allowed at the ankle. Because each color-coded disk has its ROM stamped on it, the changes are easy to document. One drawback is the joint's lack of durability. Both the inserts and the plastic forms housing them are subject to

wear. The anterior stops seem particularly susceptible to the forces imposed on them during active, forceful walking and may yield to increased ROM. A second drawback is that the metal hinges must be mechanically aligned and thus are not anatomically aligned. Generally, anatomic alignment is used for joint placement, because cosmesis and function are assumed to be better when the brace's joint overlies the true (ie, human or anatomic) joint. A third disadvantage is the bulk of the brace. The bulk of the brace makes it difficult to place a shoe over the hinge and reduces the cosmesis of the device. Some difficulty may also be encountered by the child clicking his or her ankles together.

Oklahoma ankle joint. This joint* is made from polypropylene vacuformed in plastic (Fig. 8). Five sizes, pediatric to adult, are scheduled to be available commercially in 1991. This

---

[†]Gaffney Technology, 2575 NE Kathryn St, #26, Hillsboro, OR 97124.

[‡]United States Manufacturing Co, 180 N San Gabriel Blvd, Pasadena, CA 91107-3488.

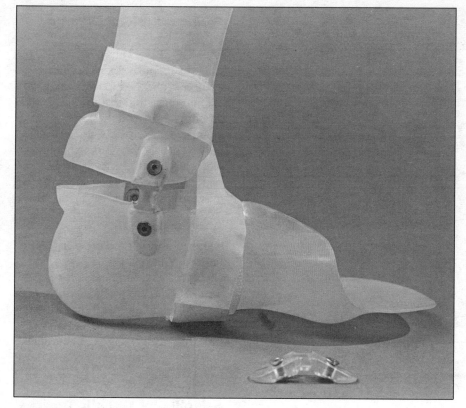

Figure 5. *Ankle-foot orthosis (AFO) with Gillette joint vacuformed in polypropylene. Joint shown in foreground is freestanding. Self-adhesive fastener adhered to the AFO is configured for a figure-eight ankle strap.*

Parapodium

The Toronto parapodium (Fig. 10) has one lock for both hip and knee joints, whereas the Rochester parapodium has separate hip and knee joint locks.[59,60] With the child standing, the parapodium should fit such that the center of the chest pad is at the xiphoid, the knee pad is across the patellae, and the metal portion of the trunk support clears the axillae by one to two fingers. If the metal expends too proximally, the brace may restrict arm use. If too low, the child may outgrow the appliance quickly. From the side, alignment of the trunk, hips, knees, and ankle joints should be checked. Cutouts on the knee pad should neither be so minimal they cause knee hyperextension nor so extreme they allow excessive knee flexion. The foot mold should align the malleoli slightly posterior to the knee. The final step of a parapodium fit check involves determining whether the child's pelvis rotates ex-

cessively to one side of the pelvic support when the child moves. This check can be performed after the child has been rolling, pushing to a standing position, or walking in the brace. If excessive rotation occurs, increasing the anterior-posterior depth and the tightness of the pelvic support across the greater trochanters may help prevent the shifting.

Swivel Walker

The first swivel walker (Fig. 11) was designed at ORLAU in the 1970s as a modification of an earlier prosthetic device used for children affected by the thalidomide crisis in the 1960s.[61] The fit considerations of the swivel walker parallel those of the parapodium, except for the unique point of spacing for the swivel-walker footplates. Based on a case report, recommendation has been made for the spacing to be one-fifth of body height.[62] The crutchless mode of walking is characteristic of this brace. A modification merging the parapodium with the base and footplate assembly of the swivel walker was used

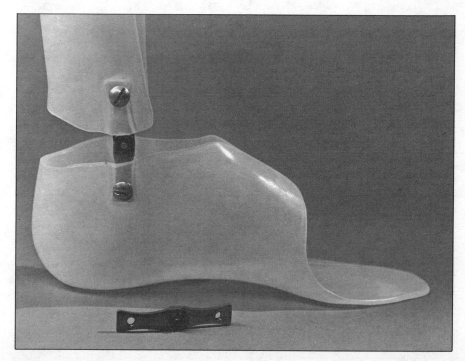

Figure 6. *Lateral view of the ankle region of a hinged ankle-foot orthosis displaying the Gaffney joint. The joint is shown freestanding in the foreground.*

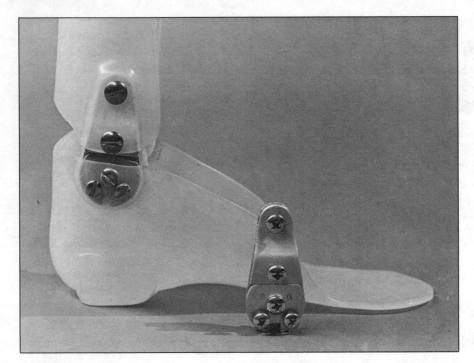

Figure 7. *Medial view of the lower portion of an ankle-foot orthosis with a Select joint inserted at the ankle. Another disk is freestanding in the foreground. Numbers impressed into the metal designate the degrees of motion possible; for example, the disk shown prevents motion.*

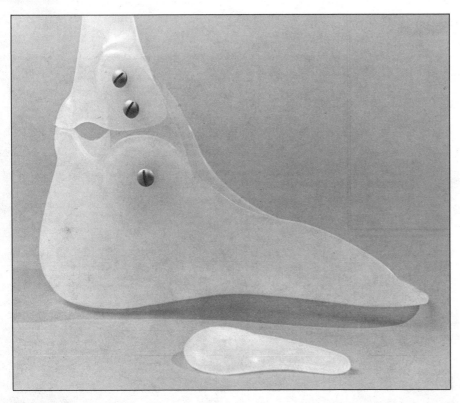

Figure 8. *Medial view of the lower portion of a hinged ankle-foot orthosis designed with an Oklahoma joint. The joint is shown freestanding in the foreground.*

by Lough and Nielsen[47] to contrast swing-to walking with swivel walking.

Reciprocating Gait Orthosis

The RGO (Fig. 12) has extensions that extend superiorly above the hip joints to the level of the xiphoid with a circumferential strap that extends around the torso at the level of the xiphoid. A wide pad is also placed at the level of the hip joints to hold the pelvis into the control of the butterfly-shaped pelvic band and thus maximize the reciprocal action created by the cable system. The cable system couples flexion of one hip with extension of the opposite hip. Release of the cables on both sides allows bilateral hip flexion for sitting. A modification to the RGO that includes muscle electrical stimulation and a new hip joint release mechanism has been designed, but evaluation has only been reported in adults with paraplegia.[63]

Selection of Orthotic Devices

Although generalizations can be made regarding the best orthosis to use according to the child's age, disability type, and degree of motor impairment, unique features about the child and his or her family and community should be considered. The following information provides general guidelines only and assumes good clinical judgment will be used when making orthotic choices for specific patients.

Cerebral Palsy

Children with hemiplegia, diplegia, or mild to moderate spastic quadriplegia can all benefit from the orthotic devices discussed in this article. Although children with severe quadriplegia are not likely to ambulate, a number of the orthoses mentioned may be appropriate for preventing deformity and assisting postural support in sitting.

In the United States today, neither HKAFOs nor KAFOs are commonly prescribed for children with CP. As mentioned earlier, this may have stemmed from a shift in the 1950s and 1960s to an NDT philosophy and a departure from the previous orthopedic approach described by Deaver and Phelps in which extensive bracing was common.[7,8] Because new orthotic materials have been introduced, reconsideration of the present philosophy may be warranted.

The use of AFOs has remained a standard treatment because of their usefulness in preventing equinus contractures. Some clinicians have recommended a progression from casts before the child walks to AFOs once walking begins. Although debate continues over the relative advantages of hinged versus fixed AFOs, studies by Middleton et al[21] and Lough[28] have favored hinged AFOs. Because specific guidelines for selecting the style of hinged ankle joint do not exist, the choice should be made jointly by members of the treatment team consisting of physician, physical therapist, and orthotist.

Issues related to orthotic prescription for children with hypotonia or athetoid (dyskinetic) CP have not been well addressed in the literature. Many clinicians believe children with hypotonia are more stable with molded FOs, SMOs, or AFOs. By contrast, children with dyskinesia frequently have difficulty with molded orthoses because of friction irritation created by writhing movement. Partial or full lining of the orthosis may reduce the irritation.

The selection of an AFO for a child with CP will change depending on age, nature of the disability, associated findings, and surgical history. The following recommendations are based on reports in the literature, as well as personal clinical and research experience.

1. The preambulatory child under 30 months of age who appears to be at risk for plantar-flexion contracture should begin with a fixed AFO or an "inhibitive cast." Hinged AFOs are more complex and should be postponed until the second fitting. Ankle straps or high medial-lateral walls will help secure the heel.

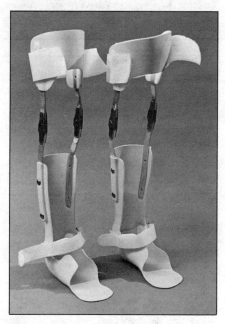

Figure 9. *Oblique view of knee-ankle-foot orthoses with an anterior thigh cuff.*

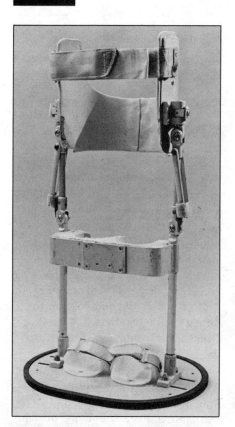

Figure 10. *Front view of the Toronto parapodium.*

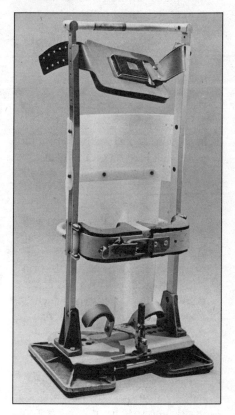

Figure 11. *Front view of the Orthotic Research and Locomotor Assessment Unit (ORLAU) swivel walker.*

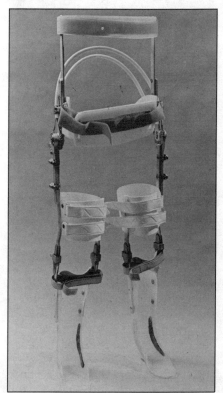

Figure 12. *Front view of a reciprocating gait orthosis (RGO).*

2. The child who walks in equinus will likely require restriction of plantar flexion to neutral. This can be accomplished with a hinged AFO or a fixed AFO. The hinged AFO will facilitate a more normal gait pattern.

3. When genu recurvatum is present, an AFO that blocks plantar flexion at 5 degrees of dorsiflexion should create a knee flexion moment at the onset of stance phase that will counter the hyperextension.

4. If the child with CP responds well to a hinged AFO that restricts plantar flexion, gradual reintroduction of a small range of plantar flexion may be possible. When this is anticipated, the Select joint, which allows several joint settings, may be the best choice.

5. The child who is heavy or large, is extremely active, or does not reside near an orthotist may not be a good candidate for the Select joint because of the potential for earlier wear with this type of hinge.

6. For a child with very mild hypertonia and medial-lateral instability, but not equinus, a free-motion hinged AFO or SMO may suffice. Caution is needed to identify increasing plantar-flexor tightness, which would indicate the need for an AFO that restricts plantar flexion.

7. A child with weak plantar flexors because of surgical lengthening or selective posterior rhizotomy should have an AFO that restricts dorsiflexion.

Myelomeningocele

The type of orthosis prescribed for a child with MMC is influenced by the child's level of motor function. The physical therapist should assume a key role in clarifying muscle function before an orthosis is prescribed. If a child demonstrates muscle activity in the lower extremities that is not willful or strong, or is reflective, a judgment about "functional motor level"

Table 3. *Factors Limiting Ambulation Progress in Young Children with Myelomeningocele*

Limitations to Progress	Guidelines/Suggestions
1. Developmental delay (in mental, language, social, or fine motor areas)	Begin experiences according to the child's developmental readiness unless structural benefits warrant attention earlier; 18 months is usually the upper limit of chronological age for beginning upright experiences
2. Upper-extremity dysfunction	Children having dysfunction of one or both hands may have difficulty learning to use a walker or crutches; an orthosis that does not require use of a walking aid (eg, a swivel walker) may be the best choice for children with high lesion levels
3. Structural limitations such as congenitally dislocated hips, clubfoot deformity, extremity contractures, or gibbus (convex spine)	Casting or surgical correction may be needed first; persisting deviances, such as a leg-length discrepancy, may restrict use of some orthoses (eg, a reciprocating gait orthosis)
4. Health issues necessitating focus in other areas or resulting in hospitalization, surgery, casting, and so forth	Once issues are managed, the work on ambulation can be resumed; the timetable for sequencing changes in braces may be slower than for other children
5. Visual status (acuity and perception)	Progress beyond standing in an orthosis may come slowly or not at all if visual acuity is very impaired
6. Social-environmental restraints	Time spent learning to use a brace may be longer and rate of progress slower than expected

should be made. We believe that the functional motor level reflects the child's ability to use muscles for skilled activities rather than the muscles innervated. When a discrepancy exists between the functional motor level and the motor level represented by the muscle activity present, the functional motor level should guide selection of the orthosis.

An early consideration in selecting an orthosis for a child with MMC is the timing for the first device. Whereas Drennan[64] recommended bracing at the neurodevelopmental age when children normally learn to stand and walk, Carroll[65] advocated beginning standing when the child begins to demonstrate interest in being upright. Based on Drennan's recommendation,

an orthosis would be prescribed when a child is 9 to 12 months old. Carroll's recommendation appears preferable, because it encourages adjustment for individual differences in social or cognitive developmental readiness. If the developmental readiness guideline is used, however, an exception becomes necessary for orthopedic benefits when the child reaches 20 to 24 months of age but remains below the 9-month level developmentally. In such cases, an orthosis should be ordered and the parapodium may be the best choice for a first device, even if the child has a low lumbar MMC.

A further consideration related to orthotic selection is that the types of orthoses used by children with MMC

90

typically change with age. Changes are particularly common during the first 6 years of life, and families should be assisted in planning for these changes. Before changing from the current orthosis to a more sophisticated design, a child should be able to walk with the current device. Table 3 presents guidelines for responding to factors that may impede walking progress in young children learning to use their first orthosis. Minor changes may be indicated within 6 months of initiating orthotic use. Such changes could include addition or removal of a swivel base to the bottom of a parapodium or addition of an above-knee component of AFOs.

Based on clinical reports, personal experience, and research, the following guidelines for initial to later orthotic devices are provided.

1. A child with an S-2 motor level may begin standing and walking without an orthosis but may later benefit from FOs.

2. A child with an L4-5 motor level may ambulate throughout life with AFOs or SMOs. Rarely would a parapodium be needed as a first device.

3. A child with an L3-4 motor level will benefit from the postural support and stability provided by a parapodium used as a first standing and walking orthosis. Although some reports[48,49] have cited the use of an RGO at this motor level, the child should eventually ambulate with AFOS, AFOs attached to twister cables or a single lateral upright and pelvic band, or standard KAFOs.

4. A child with a motor level above L-2 will likely require an HKAFO as a first and later device. The child may begin with a parapodium on a swivel walker, then switch to an RGO. Transition from a parapodium to an RGO is not recommended before 30 to 36 months' developmental age. The likelihood of a child with high spinal-level MMC using only a wheelchair after

age 15 years is great; however, factors including the orthosis used, the philosophy of the program, and personal characteristics of the child and family can influence outcome.

5. A child with discrepant motor and "functional motor" levels, should be fitted with an orthosis according to the functional motor level. For example, a child having some muscle activity through the L-5 level, who belly crawls rather than creeps, does not pull to stand or support body weight in vertical, and uses mainly hip flexors, should be considered to have a functional motor level of L-2. A parapodium or standing frame would be more appropriate than AFOS for a first device. Changes can be made as indicated with age.

Summary

This article has provided a summary of research on orthoses used for children with CP and children with MMC. Principles of orthotic application and guidelines for orthotic selection have been presented. Each child needs to be assessed individually, with consideration given to functional ability, management goals, and orthotic options. Although progress has been made in the development of orthoses and in the understanding of how the orthoses affect gait variables, further research will be needed as advances in material properties and designs are made available. Additionally, physical therapists should give further consideration to such matters as critical timing for introducing or progressing gait and methods for gait and other functional skill training with orthoses. The issue of using a total-mobility approach, which represents a combined program of seated mobility and ambulation versus either mobility mode used exclusively, also warrants attention from clinical researchers.

References

1 Paneth N, Kiely N. The frequency of cerebral palsy: a review of population studies in industrialized nations since 1950. In: Stanley F, Alberman E, eds. *The Epidemiology of the Cerebral Palsies*. Philadelphia, Pa: JB Lippincott Co; 1984:46–56.

2 Evans P, Elliott M, Alberman E, Evans S. Prevalence and disabilities in 4 to 8 year olds with cerebral palsy. *Arch Dis Child*. 1985; 60:940–945.

3 Kudrjavcev T, Schoenberg BS, Kurland KT, Groover RV. Cerebral palsy: survival rates, associated handicaps, and distribution by clinical subtype (Rochester, MN, 1950–1976). *Neurology*. 1985;35:900–903.

4 Shurtleff DB, Lemir RJ, Warkany J. Embryology, etiology, and epidemiology. In: Shurtleff DB, ed. *Myelodysplasias and Extrophies: Significance, Prevention, and Treatment*. New York, NY: Grune & Stratton Inc; 1986:39–64.

5 Wegman ME. Special article: annual summary of vital statistics—1989. *Pediatrics*. 1990; 86:835–847.

6 Walker DK, Palfrey JS, Butler JA, Singer J. Use and sources of payment for health and community services for children with impaired mobility. *Public Health Rep*. 1988;103:411–415.

7 Wolf JM, ed. *The Results of Treatment in Cerebral Palsy*. Springfield, Ill: Charles C Thomas, Publisher; 1969:18–26.

8 Bleck EE. *Orthopaedic Management in Cerebral Palsy*. London, England: MacKeith Press; 1987:142–183.

9 Cusick BD. *Progressive Casting and Splinting for Lower Extremity Deformities in Children with Neuromotor Dysfunction*. Tucson, Ariz: Therapy Skill Builders; 1990.

10 Mossberg KA, Linton KA, Friske K. Ankle-foot orthoses: effect on energy expenditure of gait in spastic diplegic children. *Arch Phys Med Rehabil*. 1990;71:490–494.

11 Brodke DS, Skinner SR, Lamoreux LW, et al. Effects of ankle-foot orthoses on the gait of children. *J Pediatr Orthop*. 1989;9:702–708.

12 Yates G. Molded plastics in bracing. *Clin Orthop*. 1974;102:46–57.

13 Hoffer MM, Garrett A, Koffman M, et al. New concepts in orthotics for cerebral palsy. *Clin Orthop*. 1974;102:100–107.

14 Rosenthal RK. The use of orthotics in foot and ankle problems in cerebral palsy. *Foot Ankle*. 1984;4:195–200.

15 Banks HH. The management of spastic deformities of the foot and ankle. *Clin Orthop*. 1977;122:70–76.

16 Bennet GC, Rang M, Jones D. Varus and valgus deformities of the foot in cerebral palsy. *Dev Med Child Neurol*. 1982;24:499–503.

17 Cusick BD, Sussman MD. Short leg casts: their role in the management of cerebral palsy. *Physical and Occupational Therapy in Pediatrics*. Binghamton, NY: The Haworth Press Inc; 1982;2:93–110.

18 Duncan WR, Mott DH. Foot reflexes and the use of the "inhibitive cast." *Foot Ankle*. 1983;4:145–148.

19 Jordan RP. Therapeutic considerations of the feet and lower extremities in the cerebral palsied child. *Clin Podiatr Med Surg*. 1984;1:547–561.

20 Selby L. Remediation of toe-walking behavior with neutral-position, serial-inhibitory casts: a case report. *Phys Ther*. 1988;68: 1921–1923.

21 Middleton EA, Hurley GRB, McIlwain JS. The role of rigid and hinged polypropylene ankle-foot-orthoses in the management of

cerebral palsy: a case study. *Prosthet Orthot Int*. 1988;12:129–135.

22 Hinderer KA, Harris SR, Purdy AH, et al. Effects of "tone-reducing" vs standard plaster-casts on gait improvement of children with cerebral palsy. *Dev Med Child Neurol*. 1988;30:370–377.

23 Harris SR, Riffle K. Effects of inhibitive ankle-foot orthoses on standing balance in a child with cerebral palsy: a single-subject design. *Phys Ther*. 1986;66:663–667.

24 Embrey DG, Yates L, Mott DH. Effects of neuro-developmental treatment and orthoses on knee flexion during gait: a single-subject design. *Phys Ther*. 1990;70:626–636.

25 Bertoti DB. Effect of short leg casting on ambulation in children with cerebral palsy. *Phys Ther*. 1986;66:1522–1529.

26 Watt J, Sims D, Harckham F, et al. A prospective study of inhibitive casting as an adjunct to physiotherapy for cerebral-palsied children. *Dev Med Child Neurol*. 1986;28:480–488.

27 Mills VM. Electromyographic results of inhibitory splinting. *Phys Ther*. 1984;64:190–193.

28 Lough LK (Knutson LM). *The Effects of Fixed and Hinged Ankle-Foot Orthoses on Gait Myoelectric Activity and Standing Joint Alignment in Children with Cerebral Palsy*. Iowa City, Iowa: The University of Iowa; 1990. Doctoral dissertation.

29 Clinkingbeard JR, Gersten MW, Hoehn D. Energy cost of ambulation in the traumatic paraplegic. *Am J Phys Med*. 1964;43:157–165.

30 Richings JC, Eckstein HB. Locomotor and educational achievements of children with myelomeningocele. *Ann Phys Med*. 1970;10:291–298.

31 Lorber J. Results of treatment of myelomeningocele: an analysis of 524 unselected cases, with special reference to possible selection for treatment. *Dev Med Child Neurol*. 1971;13:279–303.

32 Hoffer MM, Feiwell E, Perry R, et al. Functional ambulation in patients with myelomeningocele. *J Bone Joint Surg [Am]*. 1973;55:137–148.

33 DeSouza LJ, Carroll N. Ambulation of the braced myelomeningocele patient. *J Bone Joint Surg [Am]*. 1976;58:1112–1118.

34 Barden GA, Meyer LC, Stelling FH. Myelodysplastics: fate of those followed for twenty years or more. *J Bone Joint Surg [Am]*. 1975;57:643–647.

35 Schopler SA, Menelaus MB. Significance of the strength of the quadriceps muscles in children with myelomeningocele. *J Pediatr Orthop*. 1987;7:507–512.

36 Findley TW, Agre JC, Habeck RV, et al. Ambulation in the adolescent with myelomeningocele, I: early childhood predictors. *Arch Phys Med Rehabil*. 1987;68:518–522.

37 Mazur JM, Shurtleff DB, Menelaus MB, Colliver J. Orthopaedic management of high-level spina bifida: early walking compared with early use of a wheelchair. *J Bone Joint Surg [Am]*. 1989;71:56–61.

38 Taylor A, McNamara A. Ambulation status of adults with myelomeningocele. *Z Kinderchir*. 1990;45:32–33.

39 Samuelsson L, Skoog M. Ambulation in patients with myelomeningocele: a multivariate statistical analysis. *J Pediatr Orthop*. 1988;8:569–575.

40 Sankarankutty M, Rose GK, Stallard J. The effect of orthotic treatment on spina bifida patients. *Spina Bifida Therapy*. 1979;1:187–196.

41 Flandry F, Burke S, Roberts JM, et al. Functional ambulation in myelodysplasia: the effect of orthotic selection on physical and physiologic performance. *J Pediatr Orthop*. 1986;6:661–665.

42 Thomas SE, Mazur JM, Child ME, Supan TJ. Quantitative evaluation of AFO use with myelomeningocele children. *Z Kinderchir*. 1989;44:38–40.

43 Krebs DE, Edelstein JE, Fishman S. Comparison of plastic/metal and leather/metal knee-ankle-foot orthoses. *Am J Phys Med*. 1988;67:175–185.

44 Davies JB. Use of heart rate in assessment of orthoses. *Physiotherapy*. 1977;63:112–115.

45 Stallard J, Rose GK, Farmer IR. The ORLAU swivel walker. *Prosthet Orthot Int*. 1978;2:35–42.

46 Rose GK, Stallard J, Sankarankutty M. Clinical evaluation of spina bifida patients using hip guidance orthosis. *Dev Med Child Neurol*. 1981;23:30–40.

47 Lough LK (Knutson LM), Nielsen DH. Ambulation in myelomeningocele: parapodium versus parapodium with ORLAU swivel modification. *Dev Med Child Neurol*. 1986;28:489–497.

48 Yngve DA, Douglas R, Roberts JM. The reciprocating gait orthosis in myelomeningocele. *J Pediatr Orthop*. 1984;4:304–310.

49 McCall RE, Schmidt WT. Clinical experience with the reciprocal gait orthosis in myelodysplasia. *J Pediatr Orthop*. 1986;6:157–161.

50 Bunch WH, Keagy RD. *Principles of Orthotic Treatment*. St Louis, Mo: CV Mosby Co; 1976.

51 Rose GK. *Orthotics: Principles and Practice*. London, England: William Heinemann Medical Books Ltd; 1986.

52 Redford JB, ed. *Orthotics Etcetera*. 3rd ed. Baltimore, Md: Williams & Wilkins; 1986.

53 Shurr D, Cook T. *Prosthetics and Orthotics*. East Norwalk, Conn: Appleton & Lange; 1990.

54 Wenger DR, Mauldin D, Speck G, et al. Corrective shoes and inserts as treatment for flexible flatfoot in infants and children. *J Bone Joint Surg [Am]*. 1989;71:800–810.

55 Penneau K, Lutter LD, Winter RD. Pes planus: radiographic changes with foot orthoses and shoes. *Foot Ankle*. 1982;2:299–303.

56 Bordelon RL. Hypermobile flatfoot in children: comprehension, evaluation, and treatment. *Clin Orthop*. 1983;181:7–14.

57 Bleck EE, Berzins UJ. Conservative management of pes valgus with plantar flexed talus, flexible. *Clin Orthop*. 1977;122:85–94.

58 Mereday C, Dolan CME, Lusskin R. Evaluation of the University of California biomechanics laboratory shoe insert in "flexible" pes planus. *Clin Orthop*. 1972;82:45–58.

59 Motloch WM. The parapodium: an orthotic device for neuromuscular disorders. *Artificial Limbs*. 1971;15:36–47.

60 Kinnen E, Gram M, Jackman KV, et al. Rochester parapodium. *Clin Prosthet Orthot*. 1984;8(4):24–25.

61 Rose GK, Henshaw JT. Swivel walkers for paraplegics: considerations and problems in their design and application. *Bull Prosthet Res*. 1973;10-20:62–74.

62 Stallard J, Rose GK, Tait JH, Davies JB. Assessment of orthoses by means of speed and heart rate. *J Med Eng Technol*. 1978;2:22–24.

63 Solomonow M, Baratta R, Hirokawa S, et al. The RGO Generation II: muscle stimulation powered orthosis as a practical walking system for thoracic paraplegics. *Orthopedics*. 1989;12:1309–1315.

64 Drennan JC. Orthotic management of the myelomeningocele spine. *Dev Med Child Neurol*. 1976;18(suppl 37):97–103.

65 Carroll N. The orthotic management of the spina bifida child. *Clin Orthop*. 1974;102:108–114.

Strategies for the Assessment of Pediatric Gait in the Clinical Setting

Clinical gait analysis is a term that can be applied to numerous methods of evaluating a subject's walking pattern. These methods may include observation, videotaping, electromyography, kinematics, kinetics, and energetics. Modern gait analysis is based on the integration of these component methods of measurement to derive a complete analysis of gait. The data may then be used to help determine the treatment course of a patient with ambulatory problems or to document the effects of treatment. The purpose of this article is to provide an overview of the individual components of gait analysis. Emphasis will be placed on the type of information that can be derived from each component and how the information may be used clinically. Normal pediatric kinematics and kinetics are provided with literature references for phasic electromyography and temporal and stride variables. Two case examples illustrate the clinical utility of gait analysis information applied to cerebral palsy in surgical decision making and orthotic assessment. Guidelines are also provided for the referral of patients to a gait analysis laboratory. [Rose SA, Õunpuu S, DeLuca PA. Strategies for the assessment of pediatric gait in the clinical setting. Phys Ther. 1991;71:961–980.]

Key Words: *Electromyography, Gait analysis, Kinematics, Kinetics, Orthotic decision making, Surgical decision making.*

Sally A Rose
Sylvia Õunpuu
Peter A DeLuca

The value of objective gait analysis in clinical decision making has been demonstrated through applications for surgical, orthotic, and therapeutic treatment planning.[1–10] Normal gait is complex, but pathological gait is even more complex. For example, children with cerebral palsy (CP) have complex gait deviations occurring in three planes of motion, primary deviations are often confounded with compensations, and findings can be missed by observational gait analysis.[11] The gait of children with CP may best be analyzed using a three-dimensional (3D) computerized motion measurement system that can aid the clinician in delineating primary problems and secondary compensations. Coupled with information from other measures of gait assessment, the clinician is then able to make more scientific decisions regarding surgical treatment and objectively evaluate the outcome.[3–7]

The purpose of this article is to review the various components of computerized gait analysis with an emphasis on the type of information that can, and cannot, be derived from each component. A review of normal kinematics and kinetics with references for phasic electromyographic (EMG) activity and time–distance variables for the pediatric population is provided. Two case examples of children with CP are provided to demonstrate the value of objective computerized gait assessment in neuromuscular disorders, one in which gait analysis information was applied to surgical treatment planning and outcome and one demonstrating the evaluation of orthoses. Finally, guidelines for referral of patients to a gait analysis laboratory will be reviewed.

SA Rose, BS, PT, is Senior Physical Therapist, Rehabilitation Services and Gait Analysis Laboratory, Newington Children's Hospital, 181 E Cedar St, Newington, CT 06111 (USA). Address all correspondence to Ms Rose.

S Õunpuu, MS, is Kinesiologist, Gait Analysis Laboratory, Newington Children's Hospital, and Instructor, Department of Orthopaedic Surgery, School of Medicine, University of Connecticut Health Center, 10 Talcott Notch Rd, Farmington, CT 06032.

PA DeLuca, MD, is Co-Director, Gait Analysis Laboratory, Director, Cerebral Palsy Service, and Director, Hip and Foot Service, Newington Children's Hospital; Assistant Professor of Orthopaedic Surgery, School of Medicine, University of Connecticut Health Center; and Assistant Clinical Professor, Department of Orthopaedic Surgery and Rehabilitation, Yale New Haven Hospital, 333 Cedar St, New Haven, CT 06510.

Gait Analysis Measures: the Pros and Cons of Individual Components

Gait analysis is a broad term that can refer to many different methods of evaluating a subject's walking pattern. The most comprehensive gait analysis today is one that provides an assessment of videotaped recordings, clinical measures, EMG activity, 3D joint kinematics and kinetics, and energy expenditure. Each mode of evaluation provides important information, yet none, we believe, is complete in and of itself. Each component has limitations that should be recognized and understood. Proper interpretation of gait analysis information is possible only with a knowledge of how the information is collected, processed, and calculated. For example, on clinical evaluation, if one were to report the degree of tibial torsion, it would be important to know how it was measured. Measurement by bisecting the malleolar axes may produce different results than evaluating the foot/thigh angle in the prone position with the knee flexed to 90 degrees. Likewise, the angle definitions on the kinematic plots are based on the marker set used and how it is aligned. In both circumstances, it is critical to understand exactly what information a particular measurement provides in order to make appropriate recommendations based on the information.

Observational and Video Gait Analysis

Observational gait analysis appears to be the technique most often used in clinical settings.[12] Qualitative descriptions of ambulation can be made by observing stability and balance, velocity and control, symmetry and movements of the upper and lower extremities and trunk, weight transfer, foot placement, deformities such as hindfoot varus, and the influence of assistive devices. Such descriptions provide the clinician with general information about the child's overall walking pattern. It is only through observation that we can assess the "functional" ambulation of a child. *Function*, during gait, may be defined as the ability to

ambulate during activities of daily living. Factors influencing functional ambulation include uneven terrain, curbs and hills, and obstacles in the school and home settings. One of the assumptions made with computerized analysis is that the type of walking pattern demonstrated in a laboratory setting is typical of the patients' community ambulation. This is an assumption that may have the greatest impact on the more severely impaired patient who is able to ambulate over smooth, level surfaces, yet is greatly challenged by the least of environmental constraints. We believe these differences in functional gait can be noted by observational gait analysis.

To aid the clinician in describing gait, documentation forms have been designed to help organize the clinician's observations and facilitate a more comprehensive evaluation of gait.[13,14] After practice, these forms are relatively easy to use, and they can be used across different environments. Many aspects of gait cannot be observed at normal speed. *Video analysis* is an excellent tool that can be used to supplement observational gait analysis. This analysis allows the clinician more time to observe gait by reviewing the information repeatedly without the effect of patient fatigue. When used in combination with a preset documentation process, video analysis can be helpful in recognizing deviations. A video machine with stop-framing and slow-motion capabilities allows multiple joint-level comparisons during a particular portion of the gait cycle. Sagittal- and coronal-plane motion can be viewed simultaneously when the output of two video cameras are displayed on one screen. One major advantage of observational and video analyses is that encumbering measurement devices or invasive electrodes are not required. These analyses, therefore, may provide the best representation of a patient's typical walking pattern. There is some evidence that equipment may affect gait patterns. Young et al[15] found that temporal and stride variables changed as a result of surface electrode application and

changed even further when fine-wire electrodes were used.

It has been shown that two-dimensional (2D) cinematography and the measurement of joint angles using a goniometer on a video screen yield similar results when evaluating sagittal-plane motion of the hip, knee, and ankle in mid-stance in patients with and without pathology.[16] The meaningfulness of a 2D analysis of a 3D activity, however, must be considered. Specifically, neither video nor 2D cinematography account for out-of-plane motion (ie, the combination of eversion that occurs with ankle dorsiflexion during the swing phase of gait). As a result, a sagittal-plane view alone will give misleading results if there are significant coronal- or transverse-plane motions. The error associated with out-of-plane movement in normal gait has been demonstrated and is greatly magnified as the degree of out-of-plane movement increases, as may be seen in children with CP.[17] One major limitation of observational or video analysis is the lack of objective measurement of specific gait descriptors, such as joint angles. The error associated with attempting to measure angles directly from a screen that is a 2D representation of a 3D activity is also a major limitation. Interrater reliability of observational gait analysis is limited even in highly trained clinicians using stop-motion video recording.[12]

Time-Distance Variables

Time-distance variables in gait that can be measured include step length, stride length, cadence, cycle time, and walking velocity. Fairly simple techniques can be used to measure these variables, such as using a stopwatch with a marked walkway and powder on the feet. *Step length* is the distance from initial contact of one extremity to initial contact of the opposite extremity. *Cadence* is the number of steps taken per unit of time, and *walking velocity* is the distance traveled per unit of time. These measures provide information about symmetry in the lower extremities by comparing step lengths and stance-phase/

swing–phase ratios, about stability by examining the time spent in the stance phase versus the swing phase, and about function by examining walking velocity in reference to cadence. That is, a high cadence may indicate instability and decreased function, especially if step lengths are less than normal. Although time–distance measures may be good indicators of overall function, they are descriptors of an end product and do not provide information about the component segments that interact to produce these measures. In this way, these measures do not aid the clinician in determining the origin of the pathology requiring treatment. It is also important to note that variables such as stride length, step length, and walking velocity are related to stature.[18] Therefore, conclusions regarding an increase in function over time based on these measures may be a function of an increase in growth and not the treatment itself. In these cases, the contribution of growth must be factored out.

Sutherland et al[18] evaluated the walking patterns of 309 children ranging in age from 1 to 7 years. They concluded that, whereas a mature gait pattern is established by 7 years of age, time–distance variables vary with age and stature. These variables were reported for each age group from 1 to 7 years and are available for comparison with similar patient populations. Caution should be taken, however, when comparing similar–aged subjects with and without pathologies that may affect leg length.

Electromyography

The EMG is the electrical signal associated with a muscular contraction.[19] Electromyographic analysis can provide information about the timing and intensity of a muscle contraction. Use of EMGs for the purpose of obtaining timing or phasic information is popular. Phasic data allow us to determine whether a certain muscle's EMG activity is normal, out of phase, continuous, or clonic. This application can prove useful in evaluating the cause of a movement abnormality and aid in

planning for tendon transfers.[3,4] For example, if an inversion posturing of the foot is noted during the stance or swing phase, the EMG of the anterior and posterior tibialis muscles may provide information on which muscle is contributing to the deformity. The interpretation, however, may be more difficult if EMG data are analyzed alone, without consideration of whether the muscle's activity is abnormal or in response to the demands placed on the joint. For example, if a nondisabled person walks in a crouched position, the activity of the quadriceps femoris muscle will be noted throughout the stance phase (JR Gage, Newington Children's Hospital [NCH]; personal communication; 1990). If a patient with CP walks with a crouched gait and demonstrates continuous activity of the quadriceps femoris muscle in stance, the conclusion may be incorrectly drawn that this activity is an abnormal spastic response, when the contraction is required to prevent falling.[2]

Because EMG amplitude, under some conditions, has been shown to be correlated with force (ie, higher amplitudes are seen with greater force production), the study of EMG activity during gait has also taken an amplitude focus. In this way, activity level can be related to work.[19] Caution is needed with this interpretation, however, because the nature of the relationship (ie, linear or curvilinear) between EMG activity and force has not been well established. Additionally, studies of this relationship have mainly been limited to measurements taken under isometric test conditions.[20,21] Interpretation of the EMG signal in terms of amplitude across different muscles is difficult. The amplitude of an EMG signal is affected by many factors including electrode location with respect to the muscle of interest, interelectrode distance, subcutaneous fat, and skin/electrode gel temperature.[22] Therefore, to compare EMG amplitudes across muscles, within or between subjects, the data should be normalized to a reference.[23-25]

The clinical utility of EMG data, therefore, may not lie in the assessment of

amplitudes, but rather in identifying the phase activity of muscles. Recognition of the limitations should lead to cautious interpretation of EMG data. Nonetheless, when abnormal activity is noted, conclusions regarding the causes of the abnormality are best drawn after coupling the EMG data to the kinematic, kinetic, and clinical data.

In order to interpret EMG data from patients with pathologies, a reference to normal EMG activity is usually made. Normal EMG patterns for adults[26,27] and children[18,28] are well documented. The inherent variability of EMG patterns within and between subjects should always be taken into account when interpreting EMG data.[26] One should also be aware of the changes in EMG patterns that occur with age in children without pathology before interpreting EMG patterns in patient populations.[18,29]

Electromyographic data can be collected by using surface or indwelling electrodes. Detailed reviews on the advantages and disadvantages of each have been published.[22,30] Indwelling electrodes are more definitive than surface electrodes in terms of sampling activity from a particular muscle, and they are necessary for the evaluation of deep muscles, such as the posterior tibialis muscle. Indwelling electrodes are less reliable than surface electrodes,[30] and the location of the wire may migrate as a result of tissue contracting along the length of the wire.[22] When isolated movements are not possible, the only way to be sure of appropriate placement in a particular muscle is through electrical stimulation. Indwelling electrodes are also invasive and may promote local muscle cramping and ultimately modify the gait pattern.[15] Surface electrodes are noninvasive and less variable than indwelling electrodes and can provide general information about the activity of large surface muscle groups.[19,23,30,31] The major limitation of surface electrodes is that they are not as selective as indwelling electrodes.[32] The use of surface electrodes, therefore, increases the risk of cross talk, or picking up activity from muscles other than the specific muscle of interest. The larger the muscle of interest, the less the likelihood will be that cross talk from other muscles will be recorded.

Kinematics

Kinematics is a term used to describe movement such as angular displacements of joints and angular velocities and accelerations of limb segments. Kinematic data do not give information about the cause of movement. The analysis of joint angular displacements using computerized motion measurement systems provides measurements of joint motions.

Common to all computerized motion analysis is some type of reference system such as the use of markers that are placed and aligned with respect to specific anatomical landmarks. This reference system is used to estimate the segment orientations, which in turn are used to calculate the joint angles (Fig. 1). These markers are either active markers, emitting light for camera detection, or passive reflective markers illuminated for the camera by a separate light source. One of the major advantages of passive reflective markers is that they do not require direct connection with a power source and therefore tend to be less encumbering to the subject. The marker alignment illustrated in Figure 1 may differ among gait laboratories. Therefore, the direct comparison of joint kinematic data among institutions must be approached cautiously.

This advantage is of particular importance in the assessment of children. Examples of commercially available systems that use active markers are those marketed by Northern Digital

Incorporated[*] and Selspot Systems Limited.[†] Some examples of commercially available systems that use reflective markers are those marketed by Ariel Performance Analysis System Incorporated,[‡] Motion Analysis Corporation,[§] Oxford Metrics Incorporated,[||] and Peak Performance Technologies Incorporated.[#] The major advantages and disadvantages of these systems have been described by Whittle.[33] Computer automated tracking, which is available to various extents in all of these systems, has significantly decreased the time required for processing the motion data for routine clinical use. Cinematography, using manual digitization of film frame by frame, was the precursor to the more recent optico-electronic motion measurement systems described. Cinematography, however, has never been a clinically viable tool because of the excessive time required for data processing.

Joint kinematic data may be collected in either two or three dimensions. There are very important differences in the two methods with respect to the way in which the joint angles are calculated and the final data output. In brief, 2D motion systems provide joint angles that are a direct measure of the angles created by the marker set placed on the skin. Normally, 2D data are collected with respect to the sagittal plane. The majority of the data on gait until recently have been calculated in two dimensions.[2,9,19] In a 2D analysis, out-of-plane motion is not accounted for and, if significant, may introduce substantial error in the sagittal-plane measurements.[17] A similar problem occurs when extracting angles off a video image. The limitations of a 2D analysis are of particular concern in patients with CP who have abnormal motion in the coronal and

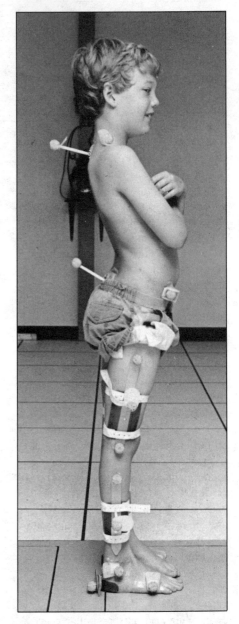

Figure 1. *Passive retroreflective marker set used at Newington Children's Hospital (Newington, Conn) for three-dimensional evaluation of the foot, shank, thigh, pelvis, and shoulder segments.*

transverse planes. Sagittal-plane data, however, may be collected in three dimensions and thus account for motion in the other two planes.

When motion data are presented in three dimensions, that is, motion of each joint in the coronal, sagittal, and transverse planes is represented, calculation of the joint angles may incorporate some type of joint centering. Joint centering requires the use of a

---

[*]Northern Digital Inc, 403 Albert St, Waterloo, Ontario, Canada N2L 3V2.

[†]Selspot Systems Ltd, 21654 Melrose St, Southfield, MI 48075.

[‡]Ariel Performance Analysis System Inc, 6 Alicante St, Trabuco Canyon, CA 92679.

[§]Motion Analysis Corp, 3650 N Laughlin Rd, Santa Rosa, CA 95403.

[||]Oxford Metrics Inc, Unit 8, 7 West Way, Oxford, England OX2 OJB.

[#]Peak Performance Technologies Inc, 7388 S Revere Pkwy, Ste 801, Englewood, CO 80112.

mathematical estimation of the location of the actual joint centers based on the markers and other anatomical relationships that may be measured directly from the patient. Essentially, the marker set that is placed on the outside of the body is "translated" mathematically to the inside so that the final joint angles are a better representation of the actual joint motion. Joint angles are determined for every frame of data and plotted as points across the gait cycle. These points are then connected to produce a curve representing the joint motion through the gait cycle.

Many assumptions and estimations are involved in the calculation of joint kinematics. System users should be aware of these assumptions and estimations and interpret the data accordingly. These assumptions will vary depending on the motion system and the modeling used to provide the joint kinematics. There is also measurement error associated with each system that must be recognized. System error itself is usually believed to be small, because the camera resolution is so high.[28] The major source of error stems from the marker set that is placed externally on the body and thus does not directly represent skeletal motion. The use of bone pins is the best way to measure skeletal movement during gait; however, bone pins are not practical for clinical use. The error attributable to skin movement under the markers is difficult to quantify, yet can be insignificant if skin movement is minimal. In general, interpretation of joint kinematics to the nearest degree in any motion system is not appropriate.

The value of kinematic analysis of gait in children with pathology lies in the ability to document joint ranges during function. Kinematic data can be compared with values collected from a population of children without pathology as well as with values obtained before and after a prescribed treatment.[18,28] Interpretation of kinematic curves should be approached with knowledge of the following: (1) the angle definitions based on the particular marker set and marker set

alignment, (2) whether the measurements and data reduction are 2D or 3D, (3) the measurement error of the system used, and (4) the trial-to-trial variability of the subject being tested. When comparing a subject's data with the normal curve, it is important to make this comparison to the mean, plus or minus one standard deviation from the mean. The variability of the normal curve is then demonstrated, which helps to avoid overinterpretation of deviations from normal.[34]

The joint kinematic data collected on 124 children without pathology between 5 and 16 years of age at the NCH Gait Analysis Laboratory are presented in Figure 2. A detailed description of the motion measurement system used to collect these data has been published previously.[35] A description of how the joint angles are measured is included in the figure legend.

Kinetics

Kinetics, used in the context of gait analysis, refers to those factors that cause or control movement. The joint kinetic patterns, which refer more specifically to joint moments and powers, are more complex to understand than joint kinematic patterns, because they are not as "visual" and require more complex procedures to be determined. The complexity increases if the calculations are made as part of a 3D analysis. Some appreciation for the methods of calculation for joint kinetic data is necessary to be able to understand and interpret joint kinetic patterns. The following is a brief description of the method used for calculation of joint kinetics. For details of these computations, the reader is referred to other published work.[19] When comparing the magnitudes of the moments and powers in all three planes of motion, the sagittal-plane moments and powers are the greatest. In the coronal plane, the moments and powers are greatest in magnitude at the hip followed by the knee and the ankle. It is not yet clear whether there is any clinical significance in the transverse-plane kinetics.[19] Because the majority of

power for forward progression appears to occur in the sagittal plane, we will focus on the sagittal-plane moments and powers. The sagittal-plane joint kinematic and kinetic patterns calculated on 31 children without gait abnormalities between 5 and 16 years of age at the NCH Gait Analysis Laboratory are presented in Figure 3. It is important to note that the sagittal-plane kinetic data presented in this article were calculated as part of a 3D analysis.

A joint moment represents the body's internal response to an external load. The net joint moment (what is plotted) represents the sum of all internal joint moments in a particular plane of motion at a specific joint. During normal gait, the influence of soft tissues other than muscles on joint rotations is minimal.[19] Therefore, the moments that are described refer primarily to muscular forces that are acting to control segmental rotation (ie, the algebraic sum of agonist, antagonist, and synergistic muscle groups). As a result, the net joint moment indicates which muscle group is dominant without indicating the contribution of the muscle groups on either side of the joint. In pathological gait, the influence of other soft tissues on joint moments may occur more frequently and more dramatically. For example, a hyperextended knee may be stabilized in stance by the posterior capsule and ligaments. In this case, difficulty arises in determining whether the internal flexor moment is being produced by ligamentous structures or muscular contractions of the hamstring and gastrocnemius muscles. Only if EMG activity is absent in these muscles can one conclude that the forces being produced are of ligamentous origin. Otherwise, the contribution of ligamentous and muscular structures individually cannot be readily determined.

There are two basic methods for calculating joint moments. The first is the ground reaction force (GRF) method. In this method, the resultant GRF is multiplied by its perpendicular distance from the axis of rotation. This method is simple and easy to

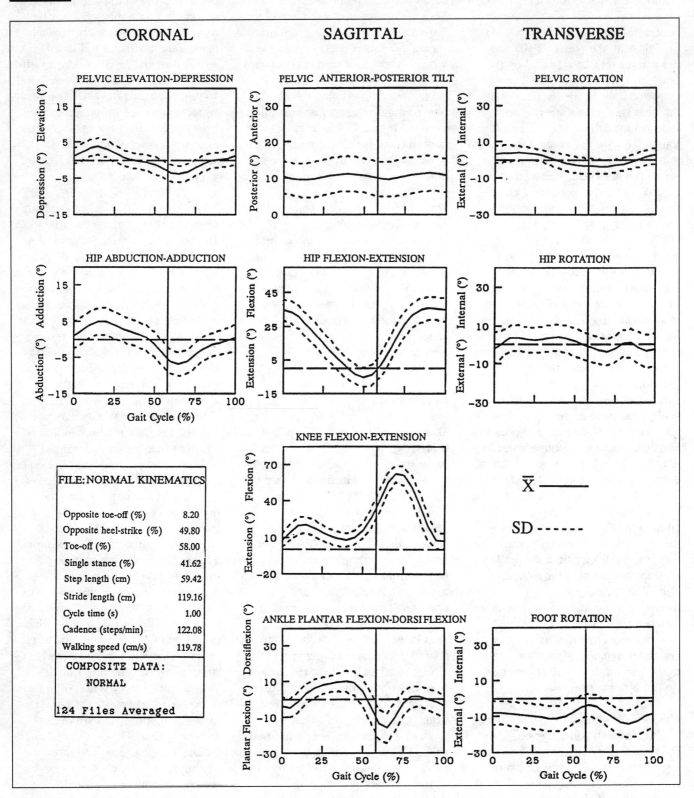

Figure 2. *Normal kinematics of the pelvis, hip, knee, and ankle in the coronal, sagittal, and transverse planes collected at 30 frames/s and plotted every 5% of the gait cycle. One gait cycle is depicted and is normalized to 100% of stride. Stance phase (left) is separated from swing phase (right) at toe-off, indicated by the vertical line at approximately 60% of stride. The pelvis is measured with respect to laboratory coordinates. The hip angles are the angles between the pelvic and thigh segments. The knee angle is the angle between the thigh and shank segments, and the ankle angle in the sagittal plane is the angle between the shank and foot segments. The ankle in the transverse plane (ie, foot rotation) is measured with respect to the line of forward progression. The mean (±1 standard deviation) is plotted.*

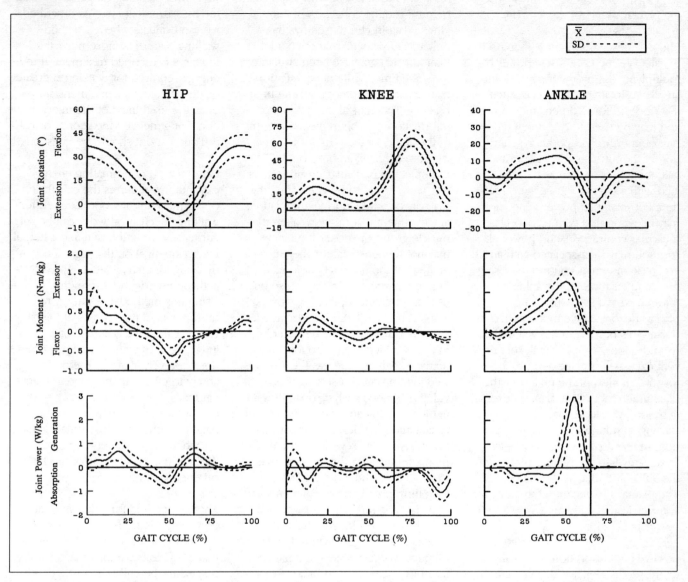

$$\overline{X} \quad \text{————}$$
$$SD \quad \text{- - - -}$$

Figure 3. *Normal sagittal-plane kinematics and kinetics of the hip, knee, and ankle. The motion (top), moment (middle), and power curves (bottom) are displayed. One gait cycle is depicted and is normalized to 100% of stride. The vertical line designates toe-off. A complete description of the power curves is provided in Ōunpuu et al.[28] The mean (±1 standard deviation) is plotted.*

apply, yet has numerous limitations.[19] With the GRF method, the error associated with the moment calculations greatly increases at the more proximal joints (ie, the hip). The calculations do not incorporate the influence of gravitational and inertial forces on the segments and do not account for out-of-plane motion. Calculations of moments and powers in the swing phase are not possible. In the second method for calculating joint moments, inverse dynamics based on a link-segment model approach are used.[19] This method also utilizes knowledge of the magnitude and direction of the GRF and its point of application (obtained from force-plate data), as well as the location of the joint centers. This 3D method requires additional information associated with each segment (ie, the location and linear acceleration of the center of mass, the angular acceleration [obtained from the motion data], and the inertial characteristics [estimated from anthropometric relationships]).[36] The collection of valid force-plate data is not always possible, because insufficient step length may allow only one foot to have contact with a particular plate. Therefore, in small children or patients with pathology severe enough to significantly limit step length, the calculation of joint kinetics is not always possible.

To help explain the net joint moment, an example of the ankle during stance may be used. In mid-stance, the ankle dorsiflexes as the tibia rotates over the plantigrade foot. The line of action of the resultant GRF passes in front of the ankle joint center, which will tend to dorsiflex the ankle. The body's response is a net plantar-flexor moment produced by the ankle plantar flexors that counteracts the external force producing dorsiflexion. The net plantar-flexor moment increases as the center of pressure (ie, point of application of the resultant GRF on the foot) moves more distally along the plantar aspect of the foot (Fig. 3).

The net muscle moment is then used to calculate the net muscle power by multiplying the moment by the joint angular velocity.[19] *Power* is defined as the work performed per unit of time and may be used to document the net rate of energy absorption or generation of the muscles. During normal gait, the joint power may be associated with a type of muscular contraction. For example, power generation may be associated with a concentric muscular contraction, and power absorption may be associated with an eccentric muscular contraction. Using the same example of the ankle in mid-stance, we know that a net plantar-flexor muscle moment occurs during this portion of the gait cycle. In mid-stance, the plantar flexors prevent excessive dorsiflexion (ie, the forward motion of the tibia over the plantigrade foot). The plantar flexors, therefore, would be eccentrically contracting, resulting in power absorption. In terminal stance, the plantar flexors reverse the relative motion of the ankle and plantar flexion occurs. The plantar flexors, therefore, are concentrically contracting, resulting in power generation. On a plot, power generation is typically expressed as positive and absorption is typically expressed as negative. A complete explanation of normal 3D joint kinematics and kinetics has been published previously.[28]

In order for forward progression to occur during gait, power must be generated that is consistent with the direction of forward progression. These power generators are the hip extensors during loading response, the plantar flexors in terminal stance, and the hip flexors in terminal stance/initial swing.[37] Kinetic analysis has revealed those muscle groups that are the primary contributors to forward progression during gait. Identification of these power bursts has provided useful information that can be applied to treatment planning for patients with pathology.[9]

The clinical value of joint kinetic assessment has yet to be fully explored, because routine collection of joint kinetic data in clinical settings has only recently begun. Although adult joint kinetic data have been available[38] for some time, pediatric kinetic normative data[28] were not available until recently. The clinical utility of kinetic information may be in the assessment of the ability of the muscles to generate power during ambulation. For example, if a particular group of muscles were found to be generating the majority of power during ambulation, any treatment that might weaken the muscle group or render it inefficient may not be beneficial for the patient. Analysis of the moments of force acting on a particular joint may also be useful in treatment planning. For example, an extended or hyperextended knee in stance can only be described in terms of degrees of motion by kinematic analysis, whereas the associated joint-moment assessment provided by kinetic analysis quantifies the net force acting about the joint (ie, an exaggerated net flexor moment may be present). The severity of the flexor moment may alert the clinician that treatment may be indicated for long-term protection of ligaments and capsular structure. In the assessment of orthoses, joint kinetics have also provided useful information for determining the effectiveness of a particular brace (see case 2 in "The Use of Gait Analysis in Clinical Decision Making" section). Further application of kinetic analysis in the evaluation of surgical intervention is needed before the utility of these measures in preoperative decision making is known. It is possible that only through the evaluation of joint kinetics postoperatively will we better understand the inconsistencies in treatment outcome in children with CP.

Energy Expenditure

The determination of energy expenditure in gait has been undertaken since the 1950s. Ralston[39] first studied adult subjects without gait pathologies. Later, the energy cost of gait in adult disabled populations was studied.[40–43] The necessary analyses have been used much less often in children with pathological gaits.[44–47] With the measurement systems described, we can evaluate whether a child's walking pattern is more normal following a prescribed treatment. If the energy required for walking is greater or unchanged after treatment, however, the usefulness of the intervention that generated the more normal walking pattern should be questioned.

One method of estimating energy expenditure requires the calculation of the mechanical work required for walking. Mechanical work can be calculated by using internal and external loads (kinetics) on the segments or by using kinematic data coupled with anthropometric measurements.[9,19] Using this method, the energy requirements of the individual joints can be calculated. The use of loads to judge work in pathological gait does not, however, measure the body's ability to efficiently respond to external loads. For example, the co-contraction frequently noted in patients with spasticity is unaccounted for when evaluating energy costs through the calculations of mechanical energy alone.

Another method for calculating energy expenditure is through oxygen consumption measures. This method may provide more information with respect to the child's neurologic involvement, as the total end product of the metabolic costs are estimated. Previous studies[44,47] have shown an increase in oxygen uptake in subjects with pathology as compared with subjects without pathology.

The Use of Gait Analysis in Clinical Decision Making

The following are examples of how gait analysis information can be used in clinical decision making. All of the analyses were performed in the Gait Analysis Laboratory at NCH and included the following: videotaping; clinical assessment; surface electromyography; 3D kinematic analysis; and, in case 2, 3D kinetic analysis.

Case 1: Orthopedic Surgery

Subject 1 was an 11-year–5-month-old girl with spastic quadriplegia secondary to CP when she was evaluated prior to orthopedic surgery. She was born prematurely at 6 1/2 months gestation, weighing 1.13 kg (2.5 lb). She began walking with a walker after 2 years of age. Previous lower-extremity surgery included bilateral subtalar arthrodeses at 5 years of age. At the time of the preoperative gait analysis, she ambulated with the use of an anterior rolling walker and bilateral hinged ankle-foot orthoses (AFOs) with free dorsiflexion and a 0-degree plantar-flexion stop. Her endurance was limited, requiring the use of a stroller for long distances. The kinematic information was collected using hand-held assistance, because her walker interfered with marker identification. This was accomplished by

two clinicians on either side of the subject providing upper-extremity support in the same manner as an assistive device. Care was taken during hand-held assistance not to influence her walking velocity or facilitate changes in posture by guiding her or providing additional input through the upper extremities other than weight bearing.

Preoperative gait analysis. Pertinent clinical information is presented in Table 1. Moderate spasticity (grade 2 on a modified Ashworth scale[48]) was noted in the quadriceps femoris, adductor, hamstring, and triceps surae muscles. The subject's barefoot ambulation, as observed, consisted of a crouched pattern at the hips and knees, with apparent bilateral lower-extremity internal rotation, limited sagittal-plane motion of the hips and knees, a foot-flat pattern of initial

contact on the left, and a toe-to-toe pattern on the right. When the orthoses were worn, she had increased difficulty clearing her feet in the swing phase.

Her EMGs showed continuous activity of the quadriceps femoris muscles throughout the gait cycle, prolonged activity of the hamstring muscles in stance and premature activity in mid-swing, and inappropriate activity of the gastrocnemius/soleus muscle complex in initial stance and terminal swing (Fig. 4).

Figure 5 is a graphic representation of the joint angles over one gait cycle. The right and left sides are plotted for comparison of symmetry between sides. This graph can also be compared with the normal curve shown in Figure 2. Subject 1's major gait deviations were:

Table 1. *Preoperative and Postoperative Summary of Pertinent Clinical Measurements—Subject 1*

	Preoperative				Postoperative			
	ROM[a]		MMT[b] Grade		ROM		MMT Grade	
	Right	Left	Right	Left	Right	Left	Right	Left
Hip extension[c] (0°–30°)	−20	−15	2−	2−	0	0	3−	3
Hip abduction (0°–45°)	10	30	3+	3+	25	30	3+	3+
Hip internal rotation (prone) (0°–35°)	75	50			70	40		
Hip external rotation (prone) (0°–45°)	10	40			15	50		
Femoral anteversion[d] (15°)	70	30			5	30		
Popliteal angle[e] (90°–0°)	60	60	4+	4+	30	25	3−	3−
Knee flexion contracture	10	10						
Ankle dorsiflexion								
With knee at 90° (0°–20°)	30	30			20	15		
With knee at 0° (0°–20°)	15	15	2+	3−	20	15	U[f]	3+
Ankle clonus[g]	+	+			+	+		
Leg Length (cm)	69.0	68.0			72.0	71.5		

[a]ROM=range of motion (in degrees) with normal ranges in parentheses.

[b]MMT=manual muscle test (0=Zero, 1−=Trace minus, 1=Trace, 1+=Trace plus, 2−=Poor minus, 2=Poor, 2+=Poor plus, 3−=Fair minus, 3=Fair, 3+=Fair plus, 4−=Good minus, 4=Good, 4+=Good plus, 5=Normal). (Source: Daniels L, Worthingham C. *Muscle Testing: Techniques of Manual Examination*. Philadelphia, Pa: WB Saunders Co; 1986.)

[c]Hip extension measured by the Thomas Test.

[d]Femoral anteversion estimated by measuring the degree of hip internal rotation in the prone position with the knee flexed to 90° when the greater trochanter is palpated to be most lateral or parallel to the supporting surface.

[e]Popliteal angle measured by flexing the hip to 90° and then extending the knee.

[f]U=unable to isolate.

[g]Plus sign (+) indicates presence.

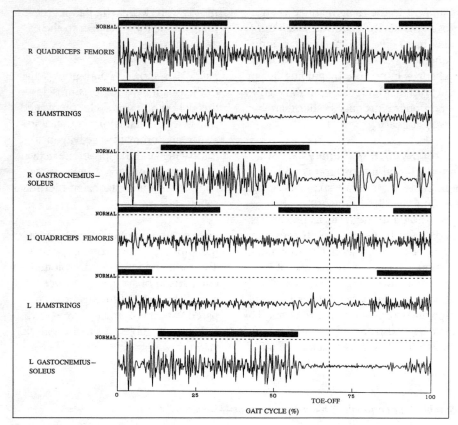

Figure 4. *Subject 1's surface electromyographic data displayed in raw form and normalized to 100% of stride. The vertical dashed line indicates toe-off and separates the stance phase (left) from the swing phase (right). The horizontal bars located above the signals indicate the normal phasic activity of the muscle sampled. The right (R) and left (L) sides are shown. The amplitude of the signal is approximately 500 μV from baseline to peak, or 1,000 μV from peak to peak.*

1. ***Asymmetrical pelvic obliquity.*** In the coronal plane, the right side of the pelvis was in exaggerated depression in terminal stance. This result may have been due to a functionally shorter right lower extremity that lacks extension at the hip and knee during this portion of the gait cycle.

2. ***Excessive anterior pelvic tilt.*** Hip flexor tightness and spasticity, along with hip extensor and abdominal weakness, may have been primary contributors to the increased anterior pelvic tilt.

3. ***Retracted right hemipelvis.*** In the transverse plane, a large asymmetrical pelvic rotation was evident, with the right pelvis retracted throughout the gait cycle. This result may have been due to the subject's decreased ability to protract the pelvis

in terminal swing, or it may have been a compensation for the excessive hip internal rotation on the right. (If the pelvis were to remain in a neutrally rotated position, given the degree of right hip internal rotation, the corresponding foot progression would have been severely internal.) External rotation of the pelvis to align the foot in the direction of forward progression is a common compensation.

4. ***Adducted right hip.*** In the coronal plane, persistent adduction of the right hip was noted and may have been due to adductor tightness or abductor weakness, or it may have been caused by the internally rotated hip in a crouched position.

5. ***Excessive hip flexion.*** In the sagittal plane, the thigh failed to extend fully in relation to the pelvis in

terminal stance. Absence of full extension may have been associated with the excessive anterior pelvic tilt. When the pelvis is tipped anteriorly in stance, the relative motion of the hip is anatomical flexion. Full hip extension, therefore, is not required in terminal stance in order to orient the femur posterior to an absolute vertical position.

6. ***Right hip internal rotation.*** In the transverse plane, excessive right hip internal rotation was evident and was likely due to the excessive femoral anteversion on that side.

7. ***Decreased overall knee motion.*** In stance, greater-than-normal flexion was noted from initial contact to mid-stance. The greater knee flexion may have been due to hamstring muscle tightness and spasticity, gastrocnemius muscle activity pulling at the proximal end, and 10-degree knee flexion contractures. During the swing phase, the decreased knee flexion may have resulted from the abnormal continuous activity of the quadriceps femoris muscle, as is suggested by the EMG recordings (Fig. 5).

8. ***Limited dorsiflexion.*** Less-than-normal dorsiflexion was noted in stance bilaterally (greater on the right side than on the left side) and in swing on the right side. Inadequate dorsiflexion in stance or swing may have been due to gastrocnemius muscle spasticity and decreased anterior tibialis muscle control.

9. ***Internal left-foot progression.*** Because foot rotation was relative to the direction of forward progression, this rotation could have originated from any segment above the foot or from the foot itself. It appeared that the subject's internal left-foot progression originated from the internal or protracted left side of the pelvis.

Recommendations/surgery. Based on clinical and gait analysis information, the following recommendations

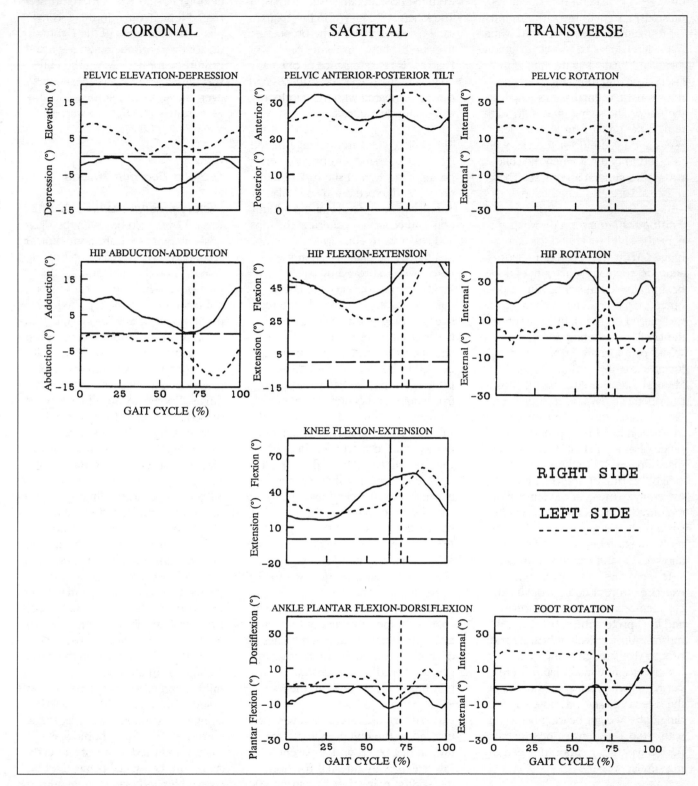

CORONAL SAGITTAL TRANSVERSE

Figure 5. *Subject 1's right and left preoperative kinematic patterns during barefoot ambulation.*

were made: right femoral derotational osteotomy to correct for excessive femoral anteversion and hip internal rotation during gait; right psoas major muscle intramuscular tenotomy to decrease anterior pelvic tilt and im-

prove hip extension in terminal stance; a right adductor tenotomy to improve abduction in stance and swing; bilateral semimembranosus and gracilis muscle lengthenings to improve knee extension at initial con-

tact, mid-stance, and terminal swing; bilateral distal semitendinosus muscle transfers to the distal femur to decrease flexion while trying to preserve hip extension and thus decrease the anterior pelvic tilt (preliminary results, however, do not substantiate this theory); bilateral rectus femoris muscle transfers to the sartorius muscle to maintain knee flexion in swing following hamstring muscle lengthenings[7]; and finally lengthening of the fascia overlying the right gastrocnemius muscle to increase its length in the stance and swing phases. In addition, at the time of surgery, the left psoas and left adductor muscles were assessed to be tight when the child was under general anesthesia. These muscles were also lengthened.

Postoperative care. Following surgery, the child was fitted for new hinged AFOs with posterior check straps to control the amount of dorsiflexion allowed in stance during postoperative gait training. A short leg cast was placed on the right leg to protect the fascial lengthening for 3 to 4 weeks postoperatively. No other lower-extremity casting was used. Physical therapy began on the second postoperative day and included gentle passive-range-of-motion exercises and instruction in a home program of range-of-motion (ROM) and positioning exercises. Precautions included no weight bearing on the right lower extremity because of the femoral osteotomy. To protect the semitendinosus muscle transfer for 3 to 4 weeks, no hip flexion beyond 45 degrees was allowed. Careful handling during assisted transfers and slow, gentle ROM exercises were used to avoid quadriceps femoris muscle reflex activity and thus protect the rectus femoris muscle transfer. Weight bearing and progressive strengthening of the lower-extremity musculature were permitted when adequate healing of the osteotomy site was noted by radiographs. Weight bearing began within the 4- to 6-week postoperative period typical for children undergoing similar surgery.

Postoperative gait analysis. One year following surgery, the subject returned to the Gait Analysis Laboratory for a routine postoperative evaluation. The preoperative and postoperative clinical measurements are presented for comparison in Table 1. Figure 6 is representative of one gait

cycle during barefoot ambulation from the postoperative gait analysis. The kinematic patterns in this figure can be compared with the preoperative curves shown in Figure 5. Figure 7 is representative of one gait cycle with the use of the orthoses and can be compared with the barefoot ambulation in Figure 6.

The subject's posture was determined by visual assessment to be more erect postoperatively, and she reported improved endurance during ambulation. The pelvic obliquity, right hip adduction, and crouched pattern at the hips and knees were eliminated. More normal transverse-plane rotation was noted, with improved overall sagittal-plane motion of the knees. For pelvic stability, she still required strengthening of the lower extremities, especially for the hip extensors and abductors, and hip flexor strength needed to be increased for clearance in swing. Improved hamstring, gastrocnemius, and quadriceps femoris muscle control may help decrease the subject's genu recurvatum. Improved hip external rotation is needed for gait, and improved knee flexion is needed for mobility skills such as transfers and stair climbing. Finally, a heel shim or resetting the plantar-flexion stop of the hinged AFO to stop in 3 to 5 degrees of dorsiflexion may be helpful in controlling the residual genu recurvatum.

Summary. In this example, the gait analysis helped to identify the primary problems in all three planes of motion. Although visual observation appeared to demonstrate bilateral hip internal rotation, the subject's primary problem was excessive right femoral anteversion that led to the compensatory rotation in her pelvis and apparent left lower-extremity internal rotation. In the sagittal plane, her hamstring and quadriceps femoris muscles were limiting the sagittal-plane motion of her knees along with her plantar flexors, which were abnormally active in the swing phase and during loading response. Although the range of dorsiflexion was the same for both ankles, only the right side demon-

strated shortness (ie, limited dorsiflexion) in stance and therefore warranted lengthening. In the coronal plane, the tightness of the right adductors was producing an adducted posture at the hip. When the child was under general anesthesia, however, the surgeon felt the adductors were sufficiently tight to warrant lengthening bilaterally.

Case 2:
Orthotic Decision Making

History/present status. Subject 2 was a 17-year-old boy with the diagnosis of asymmetrical spastic diplegia secondary to CP (greater on the left side than on the right side) at the time of his gait analysis. He was born full-term without any reported complications, weighing 2.7 kg (6 lb). Developmental milestones were delayed, and he did not begin walking until 6 years of age. Approximately 1 year previous to this analysis, rear-entry hinged floor-reaction orthoses were prescribed (Fig. 8) to decrease the flexion of his knees in stance and allow plantar flexion to occur during loading response and terminal stance.

Subject 2's pertinent clinical measurements are summarized in Table 2. The pelvis in the coronal plane was within normal limits (Fig. 9). In the sagittal plane, the baseline degree of pelvic tilt was within normal limits, yet modulated in an abnormal pattern with two phases of exaggerated anterior pelvic tilt. This pattern is typical in patients with spasticity who have poor dissociation between the pelvis and femur. In the transverse plane, a mild asymmetrical pelvic rotation was noted, with the left side retracted compared with the right side. In the coronal plane, the right hip was slightly abducted in swing and early stance. In the sagittal plane, the hips showed limited overall ROM and lacked full extension in terminal stance. At the knees, the subject had difficulty with extension at initial contact, mid-stance, and terminal swing. At the ankles in the sagittal plane, he demonstrated excessive dorsiflexion in the stance and swing phases on the right side. On both sides, he lacked

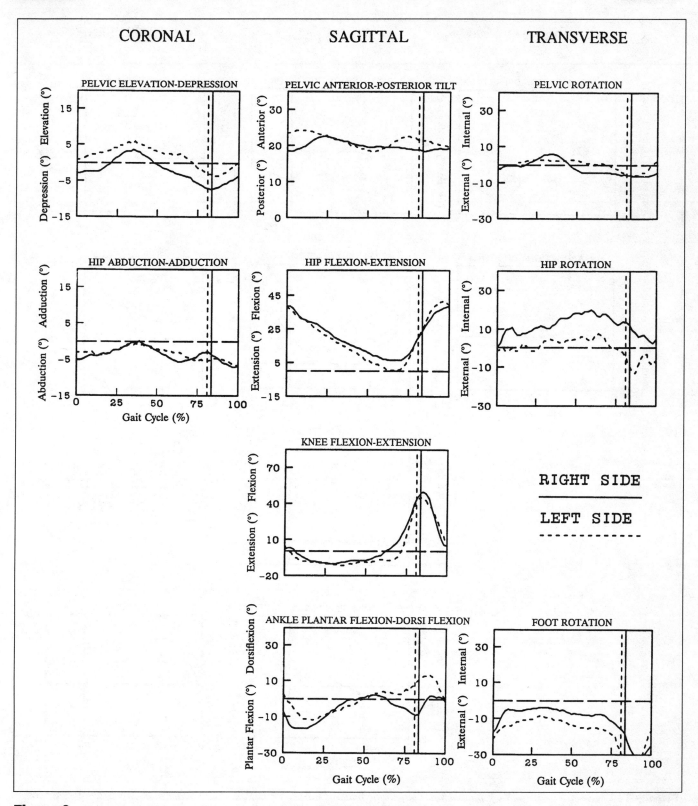

Figure 6. *Subject 1's right and left postoperative kinematic patterns during barefoot ambulation.*

the normal plantar flexion that occurs during loading response as the forefoot is lowered to the floor. In the transverse plane, the left foot rotation was slightly more external than normal. When the orthoses were worn (Fig. 10), there was little change in the kinematic curves at the pelvis, hip, and knee. Both ankles were held in 0 to 10 degrees of dorsiflexion through the gait cycle, and the foot rotations were in a more neutral position.

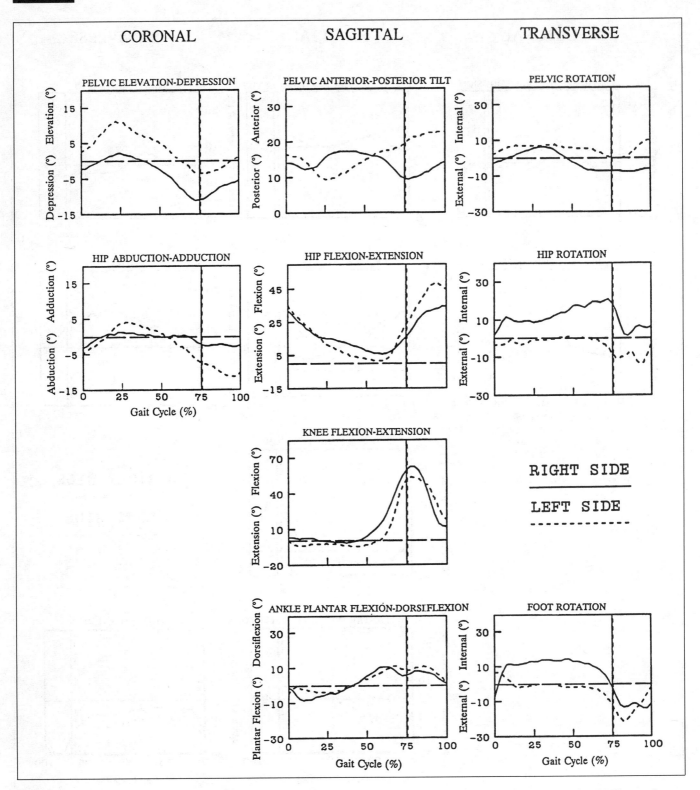

CORONAL　　　　　SAGITTAL　　　　　TRANSVERSE

Figure 7. *Subject 1's right and left postoperative kinematic patterns during ambulation with bilateral hinged ankle-foot orthoses.*

Temporal and stride variables. Step lengths were 104% of normal (56 cm) on the right and 90% of normal on the left. Stride length was 96% of normal (113 cm). Cadence was 79% of normal (128 steps/min), and walking velocity was 76% of normal (120 cm/s).[18] When the orthoses were worn, these values remained relatively unchanged except for cadence and walking velocity, which were both reduced to 59% of normal.

Kinetics. During barefoot ambulation, the hip moments and powers were essentially within normal limits and therefore are not reported. At the knees, a prolonged extensor moment was evident in stance as a result of the persistent flexion of the knees (Fig. 11). With the orthoses, there were no changes in the knee kinetic patterns (Fig. 12). That is, there was a minimal reduction in the excessive extensor moment throughout stance. The minimal reduction in extensor moment may be due to the residual knee flexion contractures that interfered with the use of the GRF transmitted through the brace to the knee.

At the left ankle during barefoot ambulation, no dorsiflexor moment was present during loading response, indi-

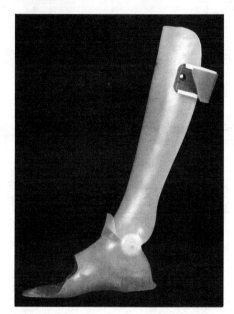

Figure 8. *Rear-entry hinged floor-reaction orthosis. Note the solid anterior shell, articulated ankle, and solid wraparound foot piece that is open at the toes, the heel, and the posterior aspect of the lower leg for donning. The articulated ankle allows for free plantar flexion while limiting ankle dorsiflexion. This orthosis was designed for patients who demonstrate excessive flexion of the knees and dorsiflexion of the ankles in stance. Normally, the gastrocnemius muscle helps to control the forward rotation of the tibia in stance and provides power for push-off in terminal stance.[39] Most brace designs inhibit further development of this muscle because of the plantar-flexion stops. Patients with excessive crouch and ankle dorsiflexion typically do not have a problem with foot drop in swing, but they do have a problem with stance-phase plantar flexion. The rear-entry hinged floor-reaction orthosis inhibits dorsiflexion, allows plantar flexion, and stimulates a plantar-flexion/ knee-extension couple during stance.*

Table 2. *Summary of Pertinent Clinical Measurements—Subject 2*

	ROM[a]		MMT[b] Grade	
	Right	**Left**	**Right**	**Left**
Hip extension[c] (0°–30°)	−10	−10	2	2
Hip abduction (0°–45°)	30	20	3+	3
Hip internal rotation (prone) (0°–35°)	45	40		
Hip external rotation (prone) (0°–45°)	30	35		
Femoral anteversion[d] (15°)	40	30		
Popliteal angle[e] (90°–0°)	55	55	4+	4
Knee flexion contracture	10	15		
Ankle dorsiflexion				
With knee at 90° (0°–20°)	35	25		
With knee at 0° (0°–20°)	25	15	2+	3−
Ankle plantar flexion (0°–50°)	F[f]	F	2	1
Ankle clonus[g]	+	+		
Leg length (cm)	90.0	90.0		

[a]ROM=range of motion (in degrees) with normal ranges in parentheses.

[b]MMT=manual muscle test (see Tab. 1 footnote for description of grades).

[c]Hip extension measured by the Thomas Test.

[d]Femoral anteversion estimated by measuring the degree of hip internal rotation in the prone position with the knee flexed to 90° when the greater trochanter is palpated to be most lateral or parallel to the supporting surface.

[e]Popliteal angle measured by flexing the hip to 90° and then extending the knee.

[f]F=full ROM.

[g]Plus sign (+) indicates presence.

cating a lack of heel contact at initial contact. Even though the magnitude of the ankle power generation in terminal stance was less than normal, a distinct power generation was evident bilaterally. When the braces were worn, however, this power generation was absent. It is possible that the braces may not have allowed power to be generated at the ankle because of the position of the ankles in the braces. The subject may have had more difficulty generating power from 0 degrees of dorsiflexion into plantar flexion, as opposed to from approximately 10 to 15 degrees of dorsiflexion into plantar flexion. During gait, the ankle is normally in a position of dorsiflexion at the end of mid-stance just prior to the initiation of this power burst. Plantar-flexor activity may be triggered by this stretch. With the ankle held at 0 degrees, the plantar flexors may be at a relative disadvantage to generate power for

push-off. The 0-degree dorsiflexion stop, however, is needed in order to provide a plantar-flexion/knee extension couple at the knee in stance. It is also possible that the relative decrease in walking velocity when wearing the orthoses was a result of the decreased power generation at both ankles, as power amplitude is related to walking velocity.[38]

Summary. The orthoses did not provide adequate control of the subject's knee flexion in stance. The hinged ankle joint did not provide any additional benefits for which it was designed (ie, plantar flexion during loading response and plantar flexion in terminal stance for push-off). One might argue that a solid-ankle floor-reaction orthosis would provide the same results during gait, yet with decreased bulk at the ankle joint and reduced possibility for mechanical failure.

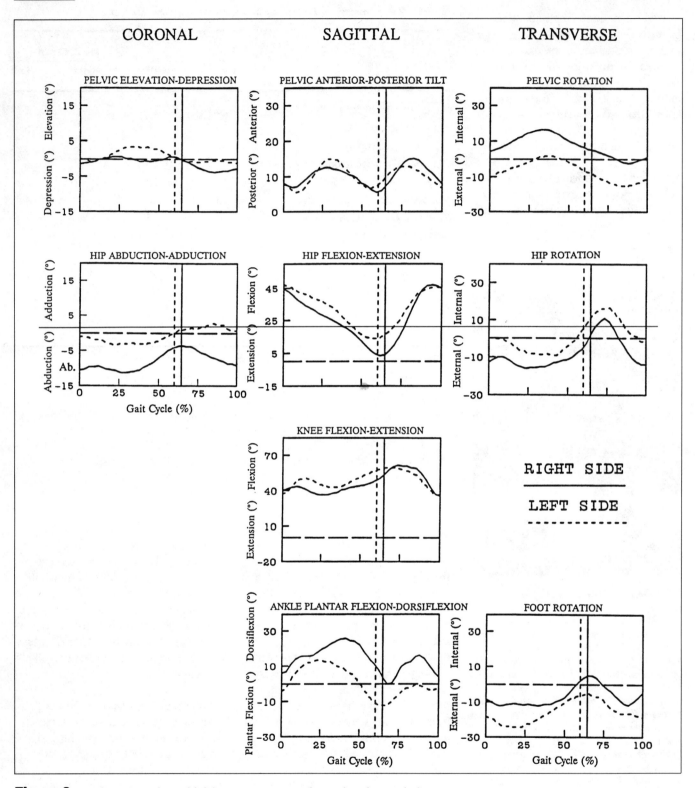

| CORONAL | SAGITTAL | TRANSVERSE |

Figure 9. *Subject 2's right and left kinematic patterns during barefoot ambulation.*

The evaluation of the effectiveness of this orthosis could only be accomplished through computerized gait analysis. Specifically, the kinetic analysis showed that the brace was not functioning at the ankle in the manner for which it was designed.

Criteria for Referral to a Gait Analysis Laboratory

The most common use of gait analysis is in the treatment decision-making process for children with neuromuscu-

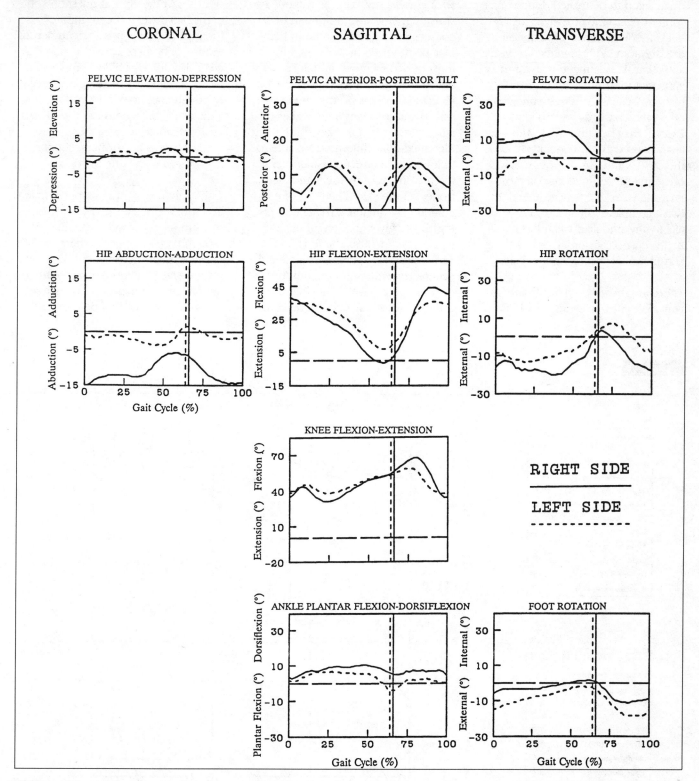

CORONAL

PELVIC ELEVATION-DEPRESSION

HIP ABDUCTION-ADDUCTION

Gait Cycle (%)

SAGITTAL

PELVIC ANTERIOR-POSTERIOR TILT

HIP FLEXION-EXTENSION

KNEE FLEXION-EXTENSION

ANKLE PLANTAR FLEXION-DORSIFLEXION

Gait Cycle (%)

TRANSVERSE

PELVIC ROTATION

HIP ROTATION

RIGHT SIDE
———————
LEFT SIDE
- - - - - - -

FOOT ROTATION

Gait Cycle (%)

Figure 10. *Subject 2's right and left kinematic patterns during ambulation with the rear-entry hinged floor-reaction orthoses.*

lar disorders such as CP.[3–7] As mentioned previously, walking patterns in these children are complex and usually consist of a combination of primary problems and adaptations. Gait analysis will provide objective documentation of the patients' gait pattern and provide more insight into the causes of gait abnormalities. Usually, a referral for gait analysis is made when all methods of conservative treatment have been tried and surgical options are being considered. This typically occurs after the child has reached a plateau in terms of improvement in ambulation or when orthopedic concerns (eg, hip subluxation) necessitate treatment. Multilevel surgical procedures now allow all possible areas of dysfunction to be treated during one surgical session. Gait analysis greatly helps to identify areas of dysfunction that are not readily identified by visual and clinical assessment. With this new approach to treatment, it is possible that the "staging" of single surgeries on a yearly basis, as described by Bleck,[27] may be eliminated. With gait analysis used as a preoperative tool, the child with CP may require only one surgical treatment during the growing years. We believe, therefore, that a complete gait analysis is beneficial to any ambulatory child with a neuromuscular disorder who is being considered for orthopedic surgery.

There are, however, other factors to consider when referring a child for gait analysis. The child must be somewhat ambulatory, with or without assistive devices, for a minimum of 10 consecutive steps. A minimum height may be required (at NCH, children must be 101.6 cm [40 in] tall) in order to position sufficient markers for kinematic analysis on the child and still have a sufficient intermarker distance so that each marker can be identified. The child must be able to follow simple directions and tolerate the placement of markers and electrodes on the skin. The level of cooperation may influence the child's testing ability, given the length of a typical gait analysis. The length of a gait analysis may vary from patient to patient, depending on the number of measurements taken. If a child uses orthoses, tests may need to be completed both barefoot and with the orthoses, if the clinical question concerns brace wear. If collection of force-plate data is possible, numerous trials may be necessary to obtain sufficient data for variability comparisons, which would also increase test length. Although cooperation is typically not a major problem with the use of toys as distractions, in some cases of severe cognitive impairment, cooperation may be an issue of concern.

Gait analysis may not be appropriate as a tool for obtaining "baseline" measurements of walking ability. Although baseline measurements would provide useful information for some progressive conditions, the benefit to the patient is not clear. Gait analysis as a research tool may be more ap-

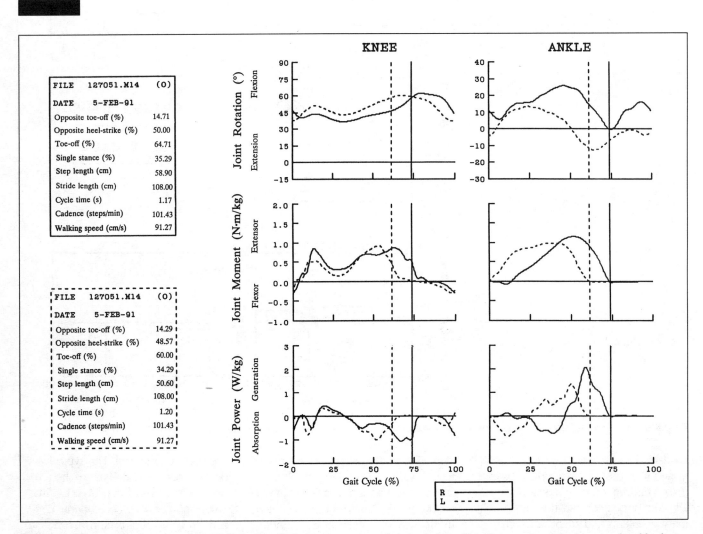

Figure 11. *Subject 2's right and left time-distance measurements and sagittal-plane kinetic patterns of the knee and ankle during barefoot ambulation.*

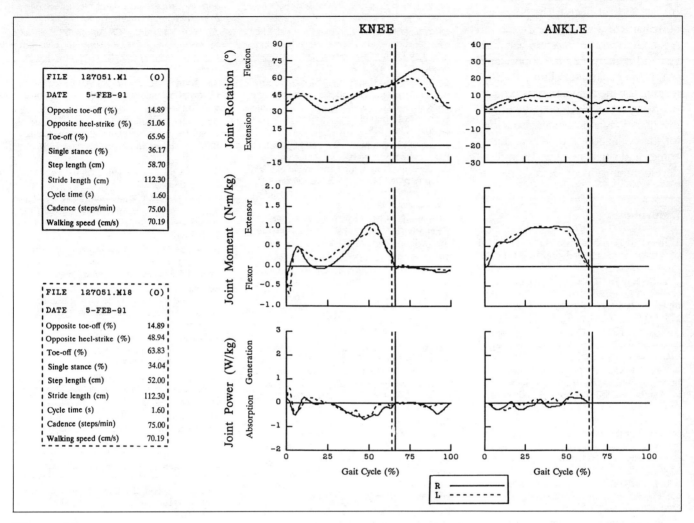

Figure 12. *Subject 2's right and left time-distance measurements and sagittal-plane kinetic patterns of the knee and ankle during ambulation with bilateral rear-entry hinged floor-reaction orthoses.*

propriate in these situations.[49] Another valuable function of gait analysis is in the assessment of surgical intervention.[7] Routine analyses of postoperative status provide the clinician with more objective information to evaluate the effect of the treatment. In general, a gait analysis may be appropriate for any patient who has a gait abnormality for which the cause is unclear or treatment decisions are complex.

Because of the limited number of clinical gait laboratories, most facilities allow referral of patients. At NCH, where gait analysis is a part of the surgical decision-making process, referral is made typically by an orthopedist. Referrals from other physicians are also accepted. A therapist may

initiate a referral process, but the final referral must be made by the patient's physician. Patients who do not have an orthopedist may be initially referred to the appropriate outpatient clinic based on diagnosis, after which a referral to the gait laboratory would be made, if appropriate. Once a patient is scheduled for a gait analysis, input from the referring physician and physical therapist regarding the patient's present status and any other information that may influence the surgical decision-making process is requested.

Summary

Computerized gait analysis provides the tools necessary to evaluate both normal and pathological gait. Through

the study of normal gait, we are better able to understand pathological gait and to prescribe more effective treatments. Recent advances in technology have allowed us to measure gait variables more precisely and in a timely manner. There is no single method of measurement, however, that provides a complete analysis of gait. We believe a complete analysis should include videotaping, clinical evaluation, EMG, 3D joint kinematics, 3D joint kinetics, and the evaluation of energy expenditure. Sophisticated clinical gait analysis requires the integration of many methods of analysis to arrive at a more complete assessment of a child's gait pattern. Proper interpretation and integration of the information obtained from sophisticated gait analysis measures is possible with a basic knowledge of how the information is collected, processed, and calculated. The purpose of this article was to review these various components of modern gait analysis and demonstrate the applications of this information in clinical decision making for the ambulatory child with neurological involvement. The objective documentation of gait also allows for the evaluation of treatment outcomes and subsequently aids in the development of new ideas.

References

1 Simon SR, Deutsh SD, Nuzzo RM, et al. Genu recurvatum in spastic cerebral palsy. *J Bone Joint Surg [Am]*. 1978;60:882–894.

2 Sutherland DH, Cooper L. The pathomechanics of progressive crouch gait in spastic diplegia. *Orthop Clin North Am*. 1978;9:143–154.

3 Perry J, Hoffer MM, Goeovan P, et al. Gait analysis of the triceps surae in cerebral palsy. *J Bone Joint Surg [Am]*. 1974;56:511–520.

4 Perry J, Hoffer MM. Preoperative and postoperative dynamic electromyography as an aid in planning tendon transfers in children with cerebral palsy. *J Bone Joint Surg [Am]*. 1977;56:531–537.

5 Gage JR, Fabian D, Hicks R, Tashman S. Pre- and postoperative gait analysis in patients with spastic diplegia: a preliminary report. *J Pediatr Orthop*. 1984;4:715–725.

6 DeLuca PA. Gait analysis in the treatment of the ambulatory child with cerebral palsy. *Clin Orthop*. 1991;264:65–75.

7 Gage JR. Surgical treatment of knee dysfunction in cerebral palsy. *Clin Orthop*. 1990;253:45–54.

8 Hicks R, Durinick N, Gage JR. Differentiation of idiopathic toe-walking and cerebral palsy. *J Pediatric Orthop*. 1988;8:160–163.

9 Olney SJ, MacPhail HEA, Hedden DM, Boyce WF. Work and power in hemiplegic cerebral palsy gait. *Phys Ther*. 1990;70:431–438.

10 Sutherland DH, Wyatt MP, Biden EN. Use of the motion analysis laboratory. In: *Goldsmith's Practice of Surgery*. Philadelphia, Pa: Harper & Row, Publishers Inc; 1985: chap 8.

11 Gage JR, Õunpuu S. Surgical intervention in the correction of primary and secondary gait abnormalities. In: *Adaptability of Human Gait: Implications for the Control of Locomotion*. Amsterdam, the Netherlands: Elsevier Science Publishers BV; 1991:359–385.

12 Krebs DE, Edelstein JE, Fishman S. Reliability of observational kinematic gait analysis. *Phys Ther*. 1985;65:1027–1033.

13 Pathokinesiology Department and Physical Therapy Department. *Observational Gait Analysis Handbook*. Downey, Calif: The Professional Staff Association, Rancho Los Amigos Medical Center; 1989.

14 Winter DA. Concerning the scientific basis for the diagnosis of pathological gait and for rehabilitation protocols. *Physiotherapy Canada*. 1985;37:245–252.

15 Young CC, Rose SE, Biden EN, et al. The effect of surface and internal electrodes on the gait of children with cerebral palsy spastic diplegic type. *J Orthop Res*. 1989;7:732–737.

16 Stuberg WA, Colerick VL, Blanke DJ, Bruce W. Comparison of clinical gait analysis method using videography and temporal-distance measures with 16-mm cinematography. *Phys Ther*. 1988;68:1211–1225.

17 Davis RB, Õunpuu S, Tyburski DJ, DeLuca PA. A comparison of 2D and 3D techniques for the determination of joint rotation angles. *Proceedings of the Internal Symposium on 3-D Analysis of Human Movement*. Montreal, Quebec, Canada, 1991.

18 Sutherland DH, Olshen RA, Biden EN, Wyatt MP. *The Development of Mature Walking*. London, England: MacKeith Press; 1988.

19 Winter DA. *Biomechanics and Motor Control of Normal Human Movement*. 2nd ed. New York, NY: John Wiley & Sons Inc; 1990.

20 Lippold OCJ. The relationship between integrated action potentials in a human muscle and its isometric tension. *J Physiol* (Lond). 1952;177:492–499.

21 Vredenbregt J, Rau G. Surface electromyography in relation to force, muscle length and endurance. In: Desmedt JE. *Developments in Electromyography and Clinical Neurophysiology*. Basel, Switzerland: S Karger AG, Medical and Scientific Publishers; 1973;1:607–622.

22 Basmajian JV, DeLuca CJ. *Muscles Alive: Their Functions Revealed by Electromyography*. Baltimore, Md: Williams & Wilkins; 1985.

23 Yang JF, Winter DA. Electromyographic normalization methods: improving their sensitivity as a diagnostic tool. *Arch Phys Med Rehabil*. 1984;65:517–521.

24 Õunpuu S, Winter DA. Bilateral electromyographical analysis of the lower limbs during walking in normal adults. *Electroencephalogr Clin Neurophysiol*. 1989;72:429–438.

25 Yang JF, Winter DA. Electromyographic reliability in maximal and submaximal isometric contractions. *Arch Phys Med Rehabil*. 1983;64:417–420.

26 Winter DA, Yack HJ. EMG profiles during normal human walking: stride-to-stride and intersubject variability. *Electroencephalogr Clin Neurophysiol*. 1987;67:402–411.

27 Bleck EE. *Orthopaedic Management in Cerebral Palsy*. Philadelphia, Pa: MacKeith Press; 1987.

28 Õunpuu S, Gage JR, Davis RB. Three-dimensional lower extremity joint kinetics in normal pediatric gait. *J Pediatr Orthop*. 1991;11:341–349.

29 Tata JA, Peat M. Electromyographic characteristics of locomotion in normal children. *Physiotherapy Canada*. 1987;39:167–175.

30 Kadaba MP, Wooten ME, Gainey J, et al. Repeatability of phasic muscle activity: performance of surface and intramuscular wire electrodes in gait analysis. *J Orthop Res*. 1985;3:350–359.

31 Komi PV, Buskirk ER. Reproducibility of electromyographic measures with inserted wire electrodes and surface electrodes. *Electromyography*. 1970;10:357–367.

32 Perry J, Easterday CS, Antonelli DJ. Surface versus intramuscular electrodes for electromyography of superficial and deep muscles. *Phys Ther*. 1981;61:7–15.

33 Whittle M. *Gait Analysis: An Introduction*. Oxford, England: Butterworth & Co (Publishers) Ltd; 1991.

34 Winter DA. Kinematic and kinetic patterns in human gait: variability and compensating factors. *Human Movement Science*. 1984;3:51–76.

35 Davis RB. Clinical gait analysis. *Eng Med Biol*. 1988;17:35–40.

36 Dempster WT, Grabel WC, Felts WJL. The anthropometry of manual work space for the seated subject. *Am J Phys Anthropol*. 1959;17:289–317.

37 Winter DA. *The Biomechanics and Motor Control of Human Gait*: Waterloo, Ontario, Canada: University of Waterloo Press; 1987.

38 Winter DA. Energy generation and absorption at the ankle and knee during fast, natural and slow cadences. *Clin Orthop*. 1983;174:147–154.

39 Ralston HJ. Energy-speed relation and optimal speed during level walking. *Int Z Agnew Physiol*. 1958;17:277–283.

40 Bard G. Energy expenditure of hemiplegic subjects during walking. *Arch Phys Med Rehabil*. 1963;44:368–370.

41 Bard G, Ralston HJ. Measurement of energy expenditure during ambulation with special reference to evaluation of assistive devices. *Arch Phys Med Rehabil*. 1959;40:415–420.

42 Corcoran PJ, Brengelmann GL. Oxygen uptake in normal and handicapped subjects in relation to speed of walking beside velocity-controlled cart. *Arch Phys Med Rehabil*. 1970;51:78–87.

43 Gordon EE, Vanderwalde H. Energy requirements in paraplegic ambulation. *Arch Phys Med Rehabil*. 1956;37:276–285.

44 Campbell J, Ball J. Energetics of walking in cerebral palsy. *Orthop Clin North Am*. 1978;9:358–360.

45 Dahlbäck GO, Norlin R. The effect of corrective surgery on energy expenditure during ambulation in children with cerebral palsy. *Eur J Appl Physiol*. 1985;54:67–70.

46 Lough LK, Nielsen DH. Ambulation of children with myelomeningocele: parapodium versus parapodium with ORLAU swivel modification. *Dev Med Child Neurol*. 1986;28:489–497.

47 Rose JR, Gamble JG, Medeiros J, et al. Energy cost of walking in normal children and those with cerebral palsy: comparison of heart rate and oxygen uptake. *J Pediatr Orthop*. 1989;9:276–279.

48 Bohannon RW, Smith MB. Interrater reliability of a modified Ashworth scale of muscle spasticity. *Phys Ther*. 1987;67:206–207.

49 Winters TF, Hicks R, Gage JR. Gait patterns in spastic hemiplegia in children and young adults. *J Bone Joint Surg [Am]*. 1987;69:4337–4411.

Development of a Clinical Measure of Postural Control for Assessment of Adaptive Seating in Children with Neuromotor Disabilities

The primary purposes of this article are to review the literature on seating assessment and to describe the development of a clinical evaluation scale, the Seated Postural Control Measure (SPCM), for use with children requiring adaptive seating systems. The SPCM is an observational scale of 22 seated postural alignment items and 12 functional movement items, each scored on a four-point, criterion-referenced scale. A secondary purpose of this article is to report the reliability of the seven-point Level of Sitting Scale (LSS). Interrater and test-retest reliability of the SPCM items and the one-item LSS were evaluated on a sample of 40 children with developmental disabilities who sat with and without their seating systems. Kappa values of .75 or higher were considered excellent, .40 to .74 as fair to good, and less than .40 as poor. The interrater reliability tests for the two seated conditions and the two test sessions conducted 3 weeks apart yielded overall item Kappa coefficient means of .45 for the alignment section and .85 for the function section. Test-retest results for the SPCM items were less satisfactory, with item Kappa coefficient means for the two seating conditions and raters of .35 and .29 for alignment and function, respectively. Reliability results did not appear to be consistently better among seating conditions, raters, or test sessions. Kappa coefficients for the LSS were fair to good for both interrater and test-retest reliability. Plans for future development of the SPCM and LSS are discussed. [Fife SE, Roxborough LA, Armstrong RW, et al. Development of a clinical measure of postural control for assessment of adaptive seating in children with neuromotor disabilities. Phys Ther. 1991;71:981–993.]

Key Words: *Adaptive seating, Neuromotor disabilities, Postural control.*

Susan E Fife
Lori A Roxborough
Robert W Armstrong
Susan R Harris
Janice L Gregson
Debbie Field

SF Fife, MSc, PT, is Research Therapist, Therapy Department, Sunny Hill Hospital for Children, 3644 Slocan St, Vancouver, British Columbia, Canada V5M 3E8. Address all correspondence to Miss Fife.

LA Roxborough, BSR, OT/PT, is Director, Therapy Department, Sunny Hill Hospital for Children.

RW Armstrong, MD, Phd, FRCPC, is Coordinator of Research and Medical Director of the Neuromotor Program, Sunny Hill Hospital for Children, and Assistant Professor, Department of Pediatrics, and Associate Member, School of Rehabilitation Medicine, University of British Columbia, T325-2211, Wesbrook Mall, Vancouver, British Columbia, Canada V6T 2B5.

SR Harris, PhD, PT, FAPTA, is Associate Professor, School of Rehabilitation Medicine, University of British Columbia, and Faculty Clinical Associate, Therapy Department, Sunny Hill Hospital for Children.

JL Gregson, BSc, PT, is Physical Therapist, Positioning Assessment Unit, Sunny Hill Hospital for Children.

D Field, BSc, OT, is Occupational Therapist, Positioning Assessment Unit, Sunny Hill Hospital for Children.

This research project was approved by the Clinical Screening Committee for Research and Other Studies Involving Human Subjects, University of British Columbia. It was supported by Grant #89-50, British Columbia Medical Services Foundation. A preliminary report of the project was presented at the Seventh International Seating Symposium, Memphis, Tenn, February 20–22, 1991.

Adaptive seating has been used increasingly over recent years as a therapeutic modality to improve postural control and functional performance[1–4] and to assist in the prevention of musculoskeletal contractures, deformities,[5] decreased respiratory function,[6] and pressure sores.[7] The number of individuals requiring specialized seating is not known. One of the most comprehensive surveys of seating needs was conducted in the Dundee district of Scotland.[8] Based on referrals elicited from hospital and community health professionals and agencies, self-referral by disabled persons, and direct assessment of 400 referred subjects, it was estimated that an average of 4.6 individuals per 1,000 persons in the total population surveyed (N=204,000) had seating problems. Older subjects with problems arising from stroke, arthritis, and general frailty constituted by far the largest group of inadequately seated subjects. Persons with cerebral palsy and associated disorders constituted the next largest diagnostic group. The latter group exhibited the most complex seating problems.

Attempts have been made to determine the nature and cost of specialized seating provided by the many seating clinics in North America. A survey of 320 members of the Wheeled Mobility and Seating Special Interest Group of the Association for the Advancement of Rehabilitation and Assistive Technologies generated a 13% response rate.[9] Respondents represented 43 seating centers from 22 states and 3 Canadian provinces. This relatively small percentage of respondents reported a total volume cost of $7,000,000 annually for new seating systems. Boenig et al state,

> Adding volume from re-evaluations of seating and considering that our survey sample is a small segment of seating practitioners and suppliers in the United States and Canada, it is apparent that seating continues to grow as a significant area of rehabilitation treatment and equipment.[9(p10)]

Based on our experience in the children's seating clinic of Sunny Hill Hospital for Children (Vancouver, British Columbia, Canada), the cost of individual seating systems ranges from approximately $400 to $5,000 and may require replacement at 2- to 4-year intervals. Mobility bases, such as strollers or wheelchairs, could add a further $1,000 to $10,000 per individual. These costs do not include the professional time for assessment and follow-up.

As in many other areas of rehabilitation, the capacity to measure the success of seating system applications has not kept pace with the widespread and increasing use of this modality. The need for reliable and valid measurements to assess the effects of

adaptive seating has become increasingly evident.

At a consensus conference on the efficacy of physical therapy in the management of cerebral palsy held in 1990, Campbell identified postural effects as potentially important outcomes of therapy, but noted that "clinically feasible tools for assessing postural alignment, control and stability are not currently available."[10(p139)] She urged the development of such tools for use as outcome measures in future efficacy research.

As the costs and sophistication of seating systems increase, so does the pressure from third-party payers to justify seating selections. Reliable and valid seating assessment measurements would increase accountability in developing individualized prescriptions for seating and would allow physical therapists to test clinical assumptions regarding anticipated seating outcomes. Furthermore, the development of standardized seating assessment tools would facilitate communication across different centers.

New concepts of motor control must be incorporated into the development of seating assessment instruments. Whereas earlier theories regarded posture as a static state representing summed responses of stretch reflexes, current thinking suggests a primary function of posture is the integration of movements into coordinated action sequences.[11] Thus, movement and posture are believed to be tightly integrated rather than separately controlled. This hypothesis suggests a comprehensive assessment of seating system outcomes should not be confined to assessment of postural alignment, but should include an assessment of the effects of changes of alignment on functional outcomes, such as control of the trunk and upper extremities, swallowing, and respiration, and on prevention of pressure sores. At Sunny Hill Hospital for Children, we are in the process of incorporating assessment of both alignment and function into a measure that could serve as an evaluation instrument for adaptive seating out-

comes. The purposes of this article are to review the literature on seating assessments and to report on the development and pilot testing of the Seated Postural Control Measure (SPCM) and the Level of Sitting Scale (LSS).

Literature Review

The research literature on assessment of postural control and seating can be divided into two broad areas: (1) measures requiring complex instrumentation and (2) clinical evaluation scales.

Use of Measures Requiring Complex Instrumentation

The most commonly measured variable in postural control studies is the amount of postural sway. Usually, sway characteristics are described on the basis of movements of the center of pressure recorded in force-plate studies. Riach and Hayes[12] used this technique to describe the maturation of postural sway in young children. Sway characteristics in sitting are now being studied in adults who have incurred a brain injury[13] and in children with cerebral palsy.[14] Investigators at the Hugh MacMillan Rehabilitation Centre (Toronto, Ontario, Canada) have used a postural tracking system to monitor children's seated stability on horizontal and anteriorly tilted seats.[15]

If postural movement strategies are to be effective in returning the center of body mass to a position within the support base, the timing of muscle contractions is important. Delay in the onset of muscle responses can result in instability if the center of body mass moves outside the limits of stability before an effective corrective force can be generated by appropriate muscles.[16] The correct sequencing of muscle responses is also important to ensure appropriate alignment of the multiply linked body segments.[16]

These aspects of muscle coordination have been studied by examining electromyographic (EMG) and force-plate responses to perturbations of standing subjects. Such studies have been reported for newly standing children (ie, children during development of independent standing balance),[17] children with cerebral palsy,[18] and children with Down syndrome.[16] Woollacott and colleagues[19] described the development of motor coordination patterns in children without neuromotor disabilities, aged 3 months to 10 years, while standing and, in some subjects, while seated.

Other researchers have used videography in studying the development of postural control for sitting. In an unpublished study, Harbourne and colleagues[20] digitized movement trajectories from videotapes of infants who were at the "presitting" and "propped sitting" levels of development. The infants were manually supported in erect sitting and were videotaped while the support was withdrawn. The movement trajectories as well as EMG recordings demonstrated progressively organized movement control strategies in the children with more experience in sitting. In other unpublished studies,[21,22] no significant effects of supported versus unsupported seating on speed and smoothness of reaching were found in six children with spastic cerebral palsy and in five 4- to 5-month-old infants without neuromotor disabilities. The investigators in those studies caution that, because of small sample sizes and large individual variability, the effect of trunk support on function remains unclear. Reports in peer-reviewed publications of this and other research will add to our ability to use these and other findings. Further investigation of these findings is clearly important for providers of adaptive seating.

Effects of seated positioning on resting EMG activity have been described for nondisabled subjects[23,24] and for subjects with cerebral palsy.[25-27] Although nondisabled adults showed decreased back muscle activity as the orientation of the backrest was inclined posteriorly,[23] children with mild to moderate cerebral palsy showed the least muscle activity with a vertical backrest.[25] In another study,[26] children with cerebral palsy

who could sit independently had increased lordosis and increased activity of the lumbar extensor muscles when they sat on seats with an anterior tilt as compared with horizontal seats. These findings contrast with those for nondisabled adults in which anterior seat tilt led to decreased EMG activity recorded at the vertebral levels of T-10 and L-3.[24] These contrasting findings, however, possibly indicate beneficial effects of anteriorly tilted seats. The children with cerebral palsy, by reducing the excessive lumbar flexion associated with their posture on horizontal seats, sat more erect, and the adults with lessened back muscle activity demonstrated increased sitting tolerance. In a pilot study of eight subjects with severe spastic quadriplegia,[27] there were no consistent EMG patterns across the subjects in response to seating system changes in orientation of the backrest or seat-to-back angle. Although responses to position change (ie, significantly increased or reduced EMG activity in one or more muscles) were evident, they appeared to be unique to individual subjects.

In examining the effects of different inclinations of the seat backrest while maintaining a 90-degree seat-to-back angle, Nwaobi[28] found that children and adolescents with cerebral palsy could use their upper extremities to activate a switch significantly faster when positioned in a vertical orientation compared with 15 degrees of anterior incline and 15 and 30 degrees of posterior incline. When the effects of varying hip flexion angles (backrest maintained in the vertical plane while the seat angle was manipulated) or upper-extremity function were measured in similar groups of subjects, however, conflicting results were reported by Seeger et al[29] and Nwaobi et al.[30] Seeger et al found no effects of varying hip angles on response time, whereas Nwaobi et al found performance time optimal with hip flexion at 90 degrees.

Use of Clinical Evaluation Scales

Several clinical evaluation scales for assessing the effectiveness of seating systems have been described recently. According to Kirshner and Guyatt,[31] a clinical evaluation scale should include all items assumed likely to be affected by the intervention. Thus, items on speed and accuracy of independent wheelchair mobility should be included, even though not all children will attain independent mobility. Each item should have a sufficient number of defined levels in order to detect clinically meaningful change. The scale should also be reliable and feasible to administer in the clinical setting. Whereas the following scales are clinically feasible to administer, they have shortcomings that limit their value to clinicians.

Questionnaires to assess the caregivers' retrospective perceptions of subjects' behavioral changes after use of seating systems were described by Hulme and colleagues in 1983[32] and more recently by Murphy.[33] Although the behavioral information was valuable, these questionnaires did not directly assess changes in performance. An assessment instrument based on direct observations by therapists was also described by Hulme and associates.[34,35] This instrument was used to code various seated behaviors, including controlled sitting posture, head control, reaching, grasping, eye tracking, drinking, eating, sitting support, and alertness. The items were coded by two to six defined levels of task achievement or by multiple timed trials. The authors described interrater reliability of 80% agreement for this instrument, but they did not report test-retest reliability. Probabilistic statistical analysis of reliability was not reported. We believe the time required for administration of this instrument (ie, 60–90 minutes) makes it impractical for routine clinical use.

A seven-level developmental scale of sitting ability, the Level of Sitting Ability Scale (LSAS), has been described for use in prescription of adaptive seating systems as well as for use in assessing outcomes of adaptive seating programs.[36,37] Instructions for administration of the LSAS and explanation of ability level definitions are not available. Information on the reliability and validity of measurements obtained with this scale have not been reported.

In light of the limitations of current clinical evaluation scales for assessing the effects of adaptive seating, our objective was to develop a scale that can be used to detect clinically meaningful change across the full spectrum of age and postural abilities of children. The remainder of this article discusses the initial development of the scale and pilot testing of reliability on the SPCM and a modified version of the LSAS.

Development of the Seated Postural Control Measure

In selecting potential test items for this scale, we reviewed currently available measurement tools such as the Gross Motor Function Measure,[38] the Assessment of Behavioral Components: Analysis of Severely Disordered Posture and Movement in Children with Cerebral Palsy,[39] the Movement Assessment of Infants,[40] the Posture and Fine Motor Assessment of Infants,[41] and the Peabody Developmental Motor Scales.[42] Although this review was helpful in establishing a format for the scale, items specifically related to postural alignment in sitting were lacking. Thus, new items were generated in consultation with local physical therapists and occupational therapists experienced in seating. Eventually, we limited the measure to assessment of sitting behaviors in two domains: (1) static postural alignment and (2) functional movement. Though we believe these are not the only adaptive seating outcomes of importance, they are the outcomes most consistently considered during the prescription process.

The first drafts of the alignment and function items were mailed to seven external seating experts* for their opinions on the face and content validity, comprehensiveness, clarity, and clinical feasibility of the items. Based on the input received, the items were modified frequently over several months. Informal trials by our seating clinicians with children of different ages and abilities also led to some modifications.

Description of the Seated Postural Control Measure

The existing pilot version of the SPCM has two sections. One section examines postural alignment and consists of 22 items; the other section examines functional movement and consists of 12 items. The SPCM can be administered and scored in 20 minutes or less.

In the alignment section, graphic representations and written descriptions of postures are used to facilitate learning and administration of the measure. We define the "90-90-90" position (erect head and trunk with hip, knee, and ankle joints at right angles) as normal alignment and arbitrarily define three increasing angular deviations from this position as representing mild, moderate, and severe degrees of abnormal alignment for each body segment. An ordinal scale of 0 to 3 is used to score each segmental posture. A given deviation, whether to the right or the left, would receive the same score. Visual observation and palpation are the only methods used to estimate postural alignment. Figures 1 and 2 show examples of alignment items.

At the beginning of the assessment, the child is placed in the seat in what the assessing therapist considers an optimal position. Verbal encouragement (without manual support) to maintain a correct posture is given. The child's postural alignment is ob-

served in the following order: (1) anterior view, (2) lateral view, and (3) superior view. If the seating system is adjustable, the child is evaluated with the system in the configuration usually adopted by the child when actively engaged in tasks such as school work. The rater records body-segment positions by selecting the score that represents the position closest to that observed. If the observed angle is midway between two scores, the score representing the most abnormal posture is selected. If the child frequently changes position, the score estimated to represent the posture most frequently sustained is selected.

Each of the items in the function section consists of four levels, with higher grades representing better task achievement (from zero to completion). The items assess head and trunk control, reaching, grasping and releasing objects, opening and closing a screw-lid jar, manipulation of small objects, and mobility (operation of the child's wheelchair). Appendix 1 presents examples of items from the function section of the SPCM. Equipment required for measuring function items includes a portable tray, a stopwatch, and materials such as a toy block, dice, and a pen. The portable tray is placed horizontally at approximately waist height. If the child's seating system includes a tray, the portable tray rests on the system tray. All means of encouraging the child's optimal response other than manual assistance or support are permissible. A maximum of 1 minute is allowed for motivating the child and completing each item. If more than one attempt is made, the best performance is scored.

Modification of the Level of Sitting Ability Scale

We planned to use the LSAS as an index of the need for adaptive seating. Such an index would also be useful in future studies of the concurrent validity and responsiveness of the SPCM. For example, we might hypothesize that scores on the SPCM would be correlated with scores on the

---

*Experts, from Canada and the United States, were either clinical coordinators of seating clinics, authors of books on adaptive seating, or executive members of professional adaptive seating organizations.

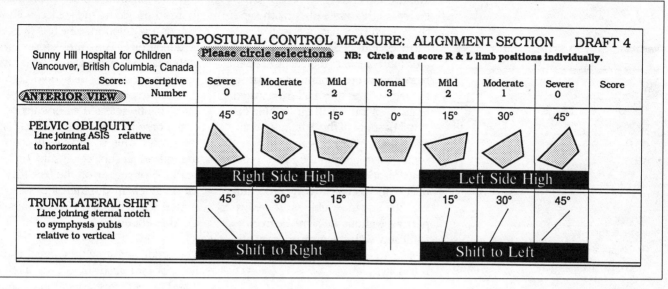

Figure 1. *Descriptive and numerical score categories of Seated Postural Control Measure alignment section items are based on arbitrarily selected angular deviations of a reference line from the normal alignment in erect sitting. (ASIS=anterior superior iliac spine.)*

LSAS. When we examine whether SPCM scores respond over time in children who have undergone significant clinical change, we would be able to determine whether such responsiveness is similar for children with different degrees of need for adaptive seating. We therefore modified the LSAS to clarify definitions of scale levels and renamed it the Level of Sitting Scale. The LSS is described in Appendix 2.

Pilot Study

We conducted a pilot study to assess the interrater and test-retest reliability of the SPCM items and the LSS scores.

Subjects

The original sample of 45 children included all clients of the Positioning Assessment Unit at Sunny Hill Hospital for Children who were from the Greater Vancouver Regional District, who were less than 19 years of age, and for whom we had informed consent. The study was approved by the Clinical Screening Committee for Re-

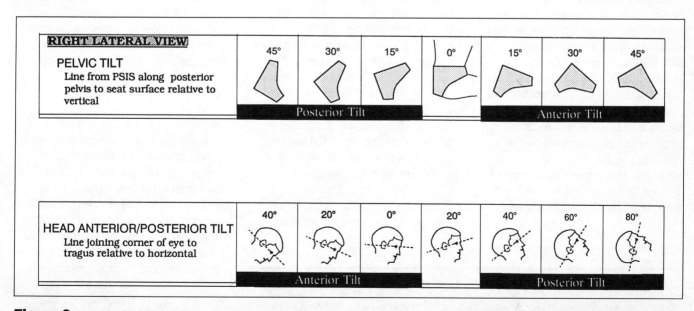

Figure 2. *Examples of items from Seated Postural Control Measure alignment section. (PSIS=posterior superior iliac spine.)*

Table 1. *Characteristics of Subjects (N=40)*

Variable	N
Sex	
Male	22
Female	18
Age (y)	
<3	6
3–5	8
6–9	5
>9	21
Medical diagnosis	
Cerebral palsy	
Spastic quadriplegia	15
Diplegia	2
Triplegia	1
Hemiplegia	1
Brain injury	7
Meningomyelocele	2
Muscle disease	3
Developmental delay	2
Other	7
Ability to understand verbal instructions (opinion of rater)	
Yes	19
No	21

search and Other Studies Involving Human Subjects at the University of British Columbia (Vancouver, British Columbia, Canada). All subjects were nonambulatory and users of seating systems prescribed prior to initiation of the study. The sessions with the first 4 subjects were scheduled as practice trials, and their scores were not included in the data analysis. An additional subject did not participate because of her inability to attend during scheduled session times. The mean age of the remaining 40 subjects was 9.06 years, with a range of 1.67 to 18.5 years. Table 1 presents the characteristics of the subjects.

Raters

The two raters were an occupational therapist (DF) and a physical therapist (JLG). Each rater had at least 5 years' experience in pediatrics, including 2 or more years in the adaptive seating field. They were generally familiar with the measure, as they had participated in its development. Their training consisted of study of the Administration Guidelines, informal administration of some of the items in the raters' regular practice, and supervised (by SEF) conduct of the complete study procedure with the first four subjects. Therefore, persons without the same degree of familiarity with the measure may not be able to obtain the same degree of reliability.

Procedure

Data were collected over a 6-week period. Subjects attended two assessment sessions, which were approximately 3 weeks apart. We assumed that a 3-week interval would be adequate for the raters to forget scores from the first assessment and that the children would not undergo significant clinical change between sessions.

Both the LSS and the SPCM were administered to subjects at each of the two assessment sessions. Each rater independently administered the LSS while the other rater was outside of the testing room. The SPCM was then administered by each rater to the subjects in two different conditions: (1) sitting with their prescribed seating system (condition 1) and (2) sitting without their prescribed seating system (condition 2). The rationale for administering the SPCM under both seating conditions was that we proposed to use the SPCM to compare alignment and function outcomes under both conditions.

If children were not independent sitters (ie, if they scored lower than

5 on the LSS), they were provided with Tumbleform Feeder Seats[†] for condition 2. We used this procedure to avoid providing the subject with "hands–on" support, which is difficult to standardize. The Tumbleform seats with a lap belt were placed on a modified wheeled base[‡] that could be reproducibly oriented in space. The raters jointly selected an orientation of the base judged to be optimal for the safety, comfort, and function of the individual subjects. If subjects scored 5 or higher on the LSS, they sat on a bench with their feet supported while the SPCM was administered in condition 2.

The order of testing (alignment and function) for each subject was alternated between test conditions. The order of test conditions was alternated in successive subjects. For each subject, this sequence was maintained in the second session. Both raters assessed and independently scored the alignment items simultaneously. One rater administered the function items while the other rater observed, and each rater independently scored the items. The same rater administered the functional items to a given subject at both sessions, and the administering rater was alternated for successive subjects.

Subjects attended in pairs for sessions of approximately 2 hours' duration. This procedure allowed for rest periods and repositioning of subjects between administration of the LSS and the SPCM under the two test conditions.

Data Analysis

Interrater and test-retest reliability for SPCM and LSS items were assessed by examination of agreement tables. The percentage of agreement (number of agreements/total observations×100) and the Kappa statistic were used as indexes of estimated reliability. The Kappa statistic reflects the percentage of agreement not attributable to chance alone.[43,44] Kappa values will be low, even if percentage of agreement is high, if the observed scores for an item fall mainly in one cate-

[†]JA Preston Corp, 60 Page Rd, Clifton, NJ 07012.

[‡]MOSS II Modular Orthotic Seating System, Otto Bock Orthopedic Industry, 4120 Hwy 55, Minneapolis, MN 55422.

gory. In this case, there is a greater probability that chance alone is responsible for agreement. Haley and colleagues,[45] in assessing reliability of the Movement Assessment of Infants,[40] interpreted Kappa values as follows: poor, if less than .40; fair to good, if .40 to .74; and excellent, if .75 or higher. We chose a Kappa value of .40 as our minimum level of acceptable reliability. The percentage-of-agreement statistic is included in Tables 2 through 4 because of its frequent use in the literature.

Results

Seated Postural Control Measure

Interrater reliability. Across the two seated conditions and the two test sessions, the overall mean of the item Kappa coefficients was .45 for the alignment section and .85 for the function section (Tab. 2). Within the four data sets, the number of alignment items with Kappa values under the acceptable level of .40 ranged from 6 to 12 out of a possible 22 items. In the function section, only 1 of 12 items had a Kappa value of less than .40. There were 5 alignment and 11 function items with Kappa values of .40 or better across all four data sets.

Test-retest reliability. Across the two seated conditions and two raters, the overall mean of the item Kappa coefficients was .35 for the alignment section and .29 for the function section (Tab. 3). Within the four data sets, the number of alignment items with Kappa values under the acceptable level of .40 ranged from 11 to 15 out of a possible 22 items. The number of function items with Kappa values less than .40 ranged from 8 to 10 out of a possible 12 items. Only one alignment and one function item had a test-retest Kappa value of .40 or better across all four data sets.

Level of Sitting Scale

The mean Kappa value for interrater reliability over the two test sessions was .60, with mean agreement of

69%. The mean Kappa value for test-retest reliability across the two raters was .55, with mean agreement of 64%. The results are presented in Table 4.

Discussion

Seated Postural Control Measure

Neither interrater nor test-retest reliability appeared to be consistently better between seating conditions, raters, or test sessions. As shown in Tables 2 and 3, percentage-of-agreement values for items were generally higher than Kappa values. This finding reflects the fact that the Kappa statistic corrects for chance agreement.

The low Kappa values for interrater agreement were likely due to a combination of three factors: lack of standardized use of the measure, inaccurate observations by raters, and fluctuations in the subjects' behaviors. Clarity of item definitions and test guidelines or the amount of rater training, for example, may not have been adequate to ensure standardized administration of the measure. The ability of trained therapists to observe and accurately detect small angular deviations while children are positioned in their seating systems may also explain the limited reliability of the alignment items.

In a clinical study of cervical spine motion, Youdas et al[46] reported only poor to fair interrater reliability for both goniometric and visual estimation measurements in patients with orthopedic disorders of the cervical spine. Measurement of spinal alignment, as in our study, is further hampered when children are positioned in closely fitted seating systems, because simple measuring instruments such as goniometers, inclinometers,[47] scoliometers,[48] flexible rulers,[49] and the Schöber method[50] cannot be utilized. Williams and Callaghan,[51] however, reported that physical therapists produced results of similar accuracy when measuring a shoulder joint angle with visual estimation and three types of standard goniometers. In an-

other recent study in a clinical setting, visual estimates of knee range of motion yielded interrater intraclass correlation coefficients of >.80.[52] Thus, there is some support in the literature for therapists consistently estimating positions for the large peripheral joints. Even though therapists commonly differentiate among mild, moderate, and severe deviations from normal spinal posture, however, it has not yet been demonstrated that this can be done reliably. Although the raters in our study assessed alignment of body segments almost simultaneously for the interrater comparisons, some children were unable to sit quietly and frequently moved during the assessment. Moreover, these were the children likely to have less constraint built into their seating systems.

Poor test-retest results, especially those for the function section, were not likely due to the clinical condition of the subjects undergoing change in the short interval between tests. Subject behaviors, however, might well have changed, in part because of the subjects' familiarity with the procedures on the second visit. By examining within-subject change scores for one data set, we investigated whether there was a consistent trend toward higher or lower scores on the second test. The maximum possible change in item scores was 3. The mean within-subject change score between tests ranged from −0.09 to 0.23 for alignment items and from −0.14 to 0.17 for function items. The direction of change scores between tests indicated worse alignment on the second test for 15 of 22 alignment items. The direction of change scores for function items was evenly divided between positive and negative change.

We intend to examine change scores more thoroughly before designing the next version of the SPCM. This examination will help us determine whether there were any consistent patterns of change scores that could be attributed to the seating conditions, raters, or test sessions. Several alternatives will also be considered.

Table 2. *Interrater Reliability of the Seated Postural Control Measure: Kappa Values and Percentages of Agreement*

Item No.	Description	C1, T1[a] Kappa	%	C1, T2[b] Kappa	%	C2, T1[c] Kappa	%	C2, T2[d] Kappa	%
Alignment Items									
A1	Pelvic obliquity	.52	73.7	.44	71.4	.36	63.2	.31	57.1
A2	Trunk lateral incline	.51	83.8	.84	94.3	.52	70.3	.39	67.6
A3	Shoulder height	.35	65.8	.30	62.9	.42	70.3	.46	73.5
A4	Head lateral tilt	.52	77.8	.60	82.9	.43	67.6	.54	76.5
A5	Hip right rotation	.24	57.9	.37	65.7	.60	77.8	.58	77.1
A6	Hip left rotation	.66	81.6	.54	74.3	.75	86.1	.68	82.9
A7	Pelvic tilt	.55	73.7	.32	62.9	.31	50.0	.26	48.5
A8	Lumbar curve	.08	48.6	.54	77.1	−.02	32.4	.06	37.1
A9	Thoracic curve	.28	57.9	.41	71.4	.30	56.8	.26	54.3
A10	Trunk anterior-posterior incline	.49	73.0	.50	74.3	.59	73.7	.52	71.4
A11	Head anterior-posterior tilt	.24	66.7	.46	73.5	.39	60.5	.31	57.6
A12	Hip right flexion/extension	.42	80.6	.77	94.3	.37	68.4	.26	62.9
A13	Hip left flexion/extension	.31	75.0	.77	94.3	.53	76.3	.33	65.7
A14	Knee right flexion/extension	.37	78.9	.62	91.4	.76	89.5	.75	91.4
A15	Knee left flexion/extension	.42	81.6	.52	91.4	.47	76.3	.62	85.7
A16	Ankle right dorsiflexion/plantar flexion	.31	89.5	1.00	100.0	.73	86.8	.70	88.6
A17	Ankle left dorsiflexion/plantar flexion	.25	86.5	.87	97.1	.77	89.5	.61	85.7
A18	Pelvic rotation	.43	67.6	.30	61.8	.20	56.8	.29	57.1
A19	Trunk rotation	.49	76.3	.12	60.0	.07	52.6	−.05	42.9
A20	Head rotation	.59	86.5	.61	88.6	.53	77.8	.44	77.1
A21	Hip right adduction/abduction	.47	69.4	.53	73.5	.63	77.1	.36	58.8
A22	Hip left adduction/abduction	.32	59.5	.21	54.3	.67	81.1	.27	55.9
	Mean	.40	73.3	.53	78.1	.47	70.0	.41	67.1
Mean across all data sets		Kappa: .45		Percentage of agreement: 72.1					
Function Items									
F1	Head up anterior-posterior	.16	89.5	.16	74.3	.46	84.2	.21	68.6
F2	Head up midline	.90	86.8	.90	94.3	.54	70.3	.82	88.2
F3	Trunk move anterior-posterior	.85	91.9	.85	91.2	.81	88.9	.91	94.3
F4	Trunk move rotation	.95	87.9	.95	97.1	.79	88.2	.87	91.4
F5	Arm lift	.92	92.1	.92	94.3	.57	67.6	.89	91.4
F6	Grasp block	.95	97.4	.95	97.1	.92	94.6	1.00	100.0
F7	Grasp raisin	.96	97.3	.96	97.1	.88	91.9	1.00	100.0
F8	Manipulate jar	1.00	94.7	1.00	100.0	.84	89.2	.92	94.3
F9	Manipulate pen	.89	100.0	.89	94.1	.89	94.3	1.00	100.0
F10	Manipulate dice	.95	94.7	.95	97.1	.90	94.4	1.00	100.0
F11	Wheelchair mobility speed	1.00	94.4	1.00	100.0	1.00	100.0	1.00	100.0
F12	Wheelchair mobility accuracy	1.00	100.0	1.00	100.0	.91	96.9	.79	92.6
	Mean	.88	93.9	.88	94.7	.79	88.4	.87	93.4
Mean across all data sets		Kappa: .85		Percentage of agreement: 92.6					

[a]C1, T1=condition 1 (sitting with prescribed seating system), test 1.

[b]C1, T2=condition 1, test 2.

[c]C2, T1=condition 2 (sitting without prescribed seating system), test 1.

[d]C2, T2=condition 2, test 2.

Table 3. *Test-Retest Reliability of the Seated Postural Control Measure: Kappa Values and Percentages of Agreement*

Item No.	Description	C1, R1[a] Kappa	%	C1, R2[b] Kappa	%	C2, R1[c] Kappa	%	C2, R2[d] Kappa	%
Alignment Items									
A1	Pelvic obliquity	.16	57.1	.43	68.6	.08	45.5	.11	42.4
A2	Trunk lateral incline	.77	91.2	.63	88.6	.18	47.1	.35	63.6
A3	Shoulder height	.44	71.4	.44	74.3	.44	67.6	.30	66.7
A4	Head lateral tilt	.41	72.7	.51	79.4	.35	63.6	.41	69.7
A5	Hip right rotation	.35	62.9	.02	48.6	.44	68.8	.32	64.7
A6	Hip left rotation	.29	60.0	.07	48.6	.27	59.4	.26	58.8
A7	Pelvic tilt	.22	57.1	.36	62.9	.33	53.3	.16	40.6
A8	Lumbar curve	−.00	58.8	.32	60.0	.15	44.1	.14	41.2
A9	Thoracic curve	.24	65.7	.23	54.3	.20	48.5	.46	64.7
A10	Trunk anterior-posterior incline	.39	67.6	.45	71.4	.48	67.6	.77	85.3
A11	Head anterior-posterior tilt	.44	72.7	.55	79.4	.50	67.6	.50	72.7
A12	Hip right flexion/extension	.12	70.6	.46	85.7	.59	79.4	.61	79.4
A13	Hip left flexion/extension	.09	67.6	.40	82.9	.70	85.3	.61	79.4
A14	Knee right flexion/extension	.53	85.7	.31	82.9	.62	85.3	.60	82.4
A15	Knee left flexion/extension	.68	91.4	.37	85.7	.46	79.4	.62	82.4
A16	Ankle right dorsiflexion/plantar flexion	.21	85.7	.48	94.3	.50	76.5	.66	85.3
A17	Ankle left dorsiflexion/plantar flexion	.10	79.4	.37	91.4	.66	85.3	.70	88.2
A18	Pelvic rotation	.28	60.6	.13	54.5	.16	47.1	.17	53.1
A19	Trunk rotation	.04	51.4	.16	65.7	−.03	44.1	.17	61.8
A20	Head rotation	.24	73.5	.19	74.3	.18	61.8	.45	76.5
A21	Hip right adduction/abduction	.25	55.9	.34	60.0	.39	57.6	.23	52.9
A22	Hip left adduction/abduction	.56	74.3	.25	58.8	.39	60.6	.34	61.8
	Mean	.31	69.7	.34	71.5	.36	63.4	.41	67.0
Mean across all data sets		Kappa: .35		Percentage of agreement: 67.9					
Function Items									
F1	Head up anterior-posterior	−.15	3.2	−.03	2.9	−.21	7.4	−.03	0.0
F2	Head up midline	−.08	35.5	−.11	34.4	.03	40.6	−.13	32.3
F3	Trunk move anterior-posterior	.41	60.0	.32	51.5	.33	50.0	.25	40.6
F4	Trunk move rotation	.42	65.7	.20	46.7	.28	53.1	.25	45.2
F5	Arm lift	.24	45.7	.37	54.3	.15	35.5	.45	59.4
F6	Grasp block	.33	50.0	.35	50.0	.26	42.4	.25	41.2
F7	Grasp raisin	.29	42.9	.31	44.1	.17	30.3	.19	29.4
F8	Manipulate jar	.36	57.1	.37	57.1	.23	46.9	.43	60.6
F9	Manipulate pen	.38	57.1	.31	51.5	.23	46.9	.27	45.5
F10	Manipulate dice	.34	60.0	.32	60.0	.38	60.6	.44	63.6
F11	Wheelchair mobility speed	.63	82.4	.59	81.3	.77	92.6	.77	92.3
F12	Wheelchair mobility accuracy	.49	78.1	.49	77.4	.72	92.3	.32	77.8
	Mean	.31	53.1	.29	50.9	.28	49.9	.29	49.0
Mean across all data sets		Kappa: .29		Percentage of agreement: 50.7					

[a]C1, R1=condition 1 (sitting with prescribed seating system), rater 1.

[b]C1, R2=condition 1, rater 2.

[c]C2, R1=condition 2 (sitting without prescribed seating system), rater 1.

[d]C2, T2=condition 2, rater 2.

Table 4. *Reliability of Level of Sitting Scale*

	No. of Subjects	Kappa	Percentage of Agreement
Interrater			
Test 1	38	.58	68.4
Test 2	35	.62	68.6
Test-retest			
Rater 1	34	.54	64.7
Rater 2	33	.55	63.6

Items in both sections of the SPCM are being reviewed by our seating clinicians with the purpose of improving clarity of items and deleting the most unreliable items, particularly when the item content is not essential. An educational module for more standardized training of raters will be developed. Reduction of item levels, from four levels to three levels, will also be considered if acceptable reliability is not achieved in the next clinical trial. We will also determine whether reliability is enhanced when testing total SPCM scores, alignment and function section scores, and scores for relevant clusters of items such as all alignment items of the pelvis or trunk, all grasp items, and so on. Once acceptable reliability of the SPCM is attained (our goal is a Kappa value of ≥.40 for each item), we will determine whether the instrument can be used to detect significant clinical change, as may occur, for exam-

ple, in children following recovery from injury or following treatment interventions. This will be done initially by using serial administrations of the measure on children following acute brain injury, because these children are likely to show more rapid change in status than children with cerebral palsy. Changes in clinical status will be monitored to determine whether the changes are accompanied by changes on the SPCM.

Level of Sitting Scale

Considering the interpretation of Kappa levels,[45] the LSS reliability estimates were fair to good. The majority of disagreements, between raters or between tests, were by only one level. There was disagreement by more than one level in a maximum of four subjects across the two data sets. We anticipate that better standardization of administration procedures will enhance the interrater reliability of the LSS. It will then be used in studies of concurrent validity of the refined SPCM.

The generalizability of the reliability results reported in this article is limited on three counts. First, the two raters were involved in development and critique of the measures and thus were not subject to the same motivations/biases a rater from another center may have had. Second, although each rater independently administered the SPCM to one half of the subject sample, the presence of the other rater may have influenced inter-

actions with the subjects. Third, the raters had special knowledge about the SPCM and interaction with the test developer. In addition, we did not use a weighted Kappa. We used the Kappa statistic to analyze agreement. This statistic does not take into account the magnitude of disagreement and treats all disagreements equally.

Conclusions

There is a great need in physical therapy for standardized measurement instruments that can be used to evaluate therapeutic outcomes and to aid clinical decision making. Currently, a clinical observation tool that can reliably define posture and motor performance under either of the test conditions in this study (ie, seated with or without postural support) is not available. The pilot SPCM is clinically feasible to administer in 20 minutes or less and has face and content validity, according to external seating experts. We believe there is potential for acceptable reliability after further refinement of this measure.

Acknowledgments

We thank Lynne Balfour, OT, Adrienne Falk Bergen, PT, Doreen Dewes, PT, Eric Ferguson, PT, Jessica Presperin, OT, Elaine Trefler, OT, and Diane Ward, OT, for participating as external seating experts in developing the SPCM. We also thank the staff of the Positioning Assessment Unit, Sunny Hill Hospital for Children, for sharing their clinical expertise, Christopher Dumper for assistance with the computer analysis, and Ruth Milner for statistical consultation.

Appendix 1. *Sample Items from the Function Section of the Seated Postural Control Measure*

1. *Lifts head upright and maintains position for 3 seconds*

If child's head is not flexed forward prior to test, instruct or assist child to do so. Upright position of the head is defined as that position in which central gaze is directed along the horizontal plane.

0. Does not initiate head lift

1. Initiates head lift

2. Lifts head, does not attain upright position, but holds position for 3 seconds

3. Lifts head upright and maintains position for 3 seconds

3. *Leans forward, touches toy with preferred wrist or hand, re-erects*

Small toy placed on board at child's midline at a distance of 1½ times "arm length" anterior to the trunk midline.

0. Does not lean forward and re-erect

1. Leans forward, but does not touch toy

2. Leans forward, touches toy, but does not re-erect

3. Leans forward, touches toy, re-erects

6. *Reaches forward, grasps and releases toy with preferred hand*

Small toy placed on board an "arm length" anterior to the trunk midline.

0. Does not touch toy

1. Touches toy with palm or fingers

2. Grasps toy and lifts it off board for 3 seconds

3. Releases toy into large container placed conveniently by therapist

8. *Removes and replaces lid of screw–lid jar*

Jar placed on board anterior to child's midline at any location that accommodates child's attempts to grasp jar.

0. Does not touch jar

1. Places one or both hands on jar

2. Unscrews and removes jar lid

3. Replaces jar lid and screws it closed

10. *Places dice in jar, one at a time, with preferred hand, in 30 seconds*

Place dice and jar on board as indicated by paper guide immediately in front of child. Request child to place dice into jar, one at a time, using one hand, as fast as possible. If at end of time period child has picked up a die but not completed placing it in the jar, give credit for that die.

0. Does not place any dice in jar

1. Places 1 die

2. Places 2 to 5 dice

3. Places 6 dice

12. *Moves wheelchair forward 10 ft*[a] along 8-ft-wide corridor, turns right or left 90 degrees, and passes through 33-in[b] doorway

Allow one practice trial to ensure child understands the task. Maximum of 60 seconds allowed for completion of the task.

0. Does not move wheelchair forward 10 ft without bumping into walls

1. Moves wheelchair forward 10 ft, but does not initiate a turn

2. Moves wheelchair forward 10 ft and turns to face doorway

3. Moves wheelchair forward 10 ft, turns, and passes freely through doorway

[a] 1 ft=0.3048 m.

[b] 1 in=2.54 cm.

Appendix 2. *Pilot Version of Level of Sitting Scale*

The seven levels of sitting ability are based on the amount of support required to maintain the sitting position and, for those children who can sit independently without support, the stability of the child while sitting.

Test Conditions:

Child is in "sitting position" at edge of a high mat or bench with feet unsupported.

Definition of "sitting position":

1. The child's hips and lower trunk can be flexed sufficiently so that the trunk (defined by a line joining T-1 and sacrum) is inclined at least 60 degrees above the horizontal plane.

2. The child's head is either neutral with respect to the trunk or flexed.

3. The position can be maintained for a minimum of 30 seconds with due regard for the comfort and safety of the child.

Level	Descriptor	Definition
0	Unplaceable	Child cannot be placed in sitting or cannot be held in sitting by one person
1	Supported from head downward	Child requires support of head, trunk, and pelvis to maintain sitting position
2	Supported from trunk downward	Child requires support of trunk and pelvis
3	Supported at pelvis	Child requires support only at the pelvis
4	Maintains position, does not move	Child maintains sitting position independently if he or she does not move limbs or trunk
5	Shifts trunk forward, re-erects	Child, without using hands for support, can incline trunk at least 20 degrees anterior to the vertical plane; re-erects
6	Shifts trunk laterally, re-erects	Child, without using hands for support, can move one or both hands to the side of his or her body and can recover balance after inclining the trunk at least 20 degrees to one or both sides of midline

References

1 Bergen AF, Presperin J, Tallman T. *Positioning for Function: Wheelchairs and Other Assistive Technologies.* Valhalla, NY: Valhalla Rehabilitation Publications Ltd; 1990:3–6.

2 Ward D. *Positioning the Handicapped Child for Function.* 2nd ed. Chicago, Ill: Phoenix Press; 1984.

3 Henderson B, compiler. *Seating in Review: Current Trends for the Disabled.* Winnipeg, Manitoba, Canada: Otto Bock Orthopedic Industry of Canada Ltd; 1989.

4 Taylor S, Trefler E. Decision making guidelines for seating and positioning children with cerebral palsy. In: Trefler E, ed. *Seating for Children with Cerebral Palsy.* Memphis, Tenn: University of Tennessee; 1984:55–76.

5 Letts M, Rang M, Tredwell S. Seating the disabled. In: Bunch WH, Keagy R, Kritter AE, et al, eds. *Atlas of Orthotics.* 2nd ed. St Louis, Mo: CV Mosby Co; 1985:440–486.

6 Nwaobi OM, Smith PD. Effect of adaptive seating on pulmonary function of children with cerebral palsy. *Dev Med Child Neurol.* 1986;28:351–354.

7 Crenshaw RP, Vistnes LM. A decade of pressure sore research: 1977–1987. *J Rehabil Res Dev.* 1989;26:63–74.

8 Bardsley GI. The Dundee Seating Programme. *Physiotherapy.* 1984;70:59–63.

9 Boenig B, Reger SI, Little J. *Survey of Seating Delivery Systems in the United States and Canada.* Report of SIG 09, RESNA, Washington, DC, 1989.

10 Campbell SK. Efficacy of physical therapy in improving postural control in cerebral palsy. *Pediatric Physical Therapy.* 1990;2: 135–140.

11 Reed ES. Changing theories of postural development. In: Woollacott MH, Shumway–Cook A, ed. *Development of Posture and Gait Across the Life Span.* Columbia, SC: University of South Carolina Press; 1989:3–24.

12 Riach CL, Hayes KC. Maturation of postural stability in young children. *Dev Med Child Neurol.* 1987;29:650–658.

13 Ferguson-Pell M, Snow J. A system for monitoring trunk control and head position during a reaching task for persons with head trauma. In: *Proceedings of the International Conference of the Association for Advancement of Rehabilitation Technology; June 24–30, 1988; Montreal, Quebec, Canada;* pp 116–117.

14 McClenaghan BA. Sitting stability of selected subjects with cerebral palsy. *Clinical Biomechanics.* 1989;4:213–216.

15 Reid DT, Sochaniwskyj A, Milner M. An investigation of postural sway in sitting of normal children and children with neurological disorders. *Physical & Occupational Therapy in Pediatrics.* 1991;11:19–35.

16 Nashner LM, Shumway-Cook A, Marin O. Stance posture control in select groups of children with cerebral palsy: deficits in sensory organization and muscular coordination. *Exp Brain Res.* 1983;49:393–409.

17 Shumway-Cook A, Woollacott MH. Dynamics of postural control in the child with Down syndrome. *Phys Ther.* 1985;65:1315–1322.

18 Forssberg H, Nashner LM. Ontogenetic development of postural control in man: adaptation to altered support and visual conditions during stance. *J Neurosci.* 1982;2:545–552.

19 Woollacott MH, Debu B, Mowatt M. Neuromuscular control of posture in the infant and child: is vision dominant? *Journal of Motor Behavior.* 1987;19:167–186.

20 Harbourne RT, Guiliani C, MacNeela JC. A kinematic and electromyographic analysis of the development of sitting posture in infants. *Phys Ther.* 1989;69:370. Abstract.

21 Gross AL. The effects of a supported seating position on upper extremity control in children with spastic cerebral palsy. *Physical & Occupational Therapy in Pediatrics.* 1989; 9:143. Abstract.

22 Clary-Trimm BL. The effect of proximal support on upper extremity reaching. *Physical & Occupational Therapy in Pediatrics.* 1991; 10:134. Abstract.

23 Andersson BJ, Ortengren R, Nachemson AL, et al. The sitting posture: an electromyographic and discometric study. *Orthop Clin North Am.* 1975;6:105–120.

24 Soderberg GL, Blanco MK, Cosentino TL, Kurdelmeier KA. An EMG analysis of posterior trunk musculature during flat and anteriorly inclined sitting. *Hum Factors.* 1986;28:483–491.

25 Nwaobi OM. Effects of body orientation in space on tonic muscle activity of patients with cerebral palsy. *Dev Med Child Neurol.* 1986; 28:41–44.

26 Milner M, Lotto W, Koheil R, et al. *Dynamic Positional and Electromyographic Monitoring of Sitting Posture.* Toronto, Ontario,

Canada: Rehabilitation Engineering Department, The Hugh MacMillan Medical Centre; 1987. Annual report.

27 Fife SE, Roxborough LA, Cooper D, et al. Tonic electromyographic activity in seated subjects with spastic quadriplegia: a pilot study. In: *Proceedings of the Fourth International Seating Symposium, "Challenges '88: Seating the Disabled"; February 18–20, 1988; Vancouver, British Columbia, Canada*; pp 16–20.

28 Nwaobi O. Seating orientations and upper extremity function in children with cerebral palsy. *Phys Ther*. 1987;67:1209–1212.

29 Seeger BR, Caudrey DJ, O'Mara NA. Hand function in cerebral palsy: the effect of hip flexion angle. *Dev Med Child Neurol*. 1984; 26:601–606.

30 Nwaobi O, Hobson D, Trefler E. Hip angle and upper extremity movement time in children with cerebral palsy. In: *Proceedings of the Eighth Annual RESNA Conference; June 24–28, 1985; Memphis, Tenn*; pp 39–41.

31 Kirshner B, Guyatt G. A methodological framework for assessing health indices. *J Chronic Dis*. 1985;38:27–36.

32 Hulme JB, Poor R, Schulein M, Pezzino J. Perceived behavioral changes observed with adaptive seating devices and training programs for multihandicapped, developmentally disabled individuals. *Phys Ther*. 1983;63:204–208.

33 Murphy TE. The positioner chair: a classroom chair for children with a forward tilting seat. In: *Proceedings of the Fifth International Seating Symposium, "Seating the Disabled"; February 16–18, 1989; Memphis, Tenn*; pp 23–28.

34 Hulme JB, Gallacher K, Walsh J, et al. Behavioral and postural changes observed with use of adaptive seating by clients with multiple handicaps. *Phys Ther*. 1987;67:1060–1067.

35 Hulme JB, Shaver J, Acher S, et al. Effects of adaptive seating devices on the eating and drinking of children with multiple handicaps. *Am J Occup Ther*. 1987;41:81–89.

36 Green E. Assessment and measurement of sitting ability. In: *Proceedings of the International Seating Conference; September 12–16, 1988; Dundee, Scotland*. Abstract 33.

37 Mulcahy CM, Pountney TE, Nelham RL. Adaptive seating for the motor handicapped: problems, a solution, assessment and prescription. *Physiotherapy*. 1988;74:531–536.

38 Russell DJ, Rosenbaum, PL, Cadman DT, et al. The Gross Motor Function Measure: a means to evaluate the effects of physical therapy. *Dev Med Child Neurol*. 1989;31:341–352.

39 Hardy MA, Kudar S, Macdonald JA. *Assessment of Behavioral Components: Analysis of Severely Disordered Posture and Movement in Children with Cerebral Palsy*. Springfield, Ill: Charles C Thomas, Publisher; 1988.

40 Chandler LS, Andrews MS, Swanson MW. *The Movement Assessment of Infants: A Manual*. Rolling Bay, WA: Movement Assessment of Infants; 1980.

41 Case-Smith J. *Posture and Fine Motor Assessment of Infants: Research Edition*. Rockville, Md: American Occupational Therapy Foundation; 1988.

42 Folio MR, Fewell RR. *Peabody Developmental Motor Scales and Activity Cards (PDMS)*. Allen, Tex: DLM Teaching Resources; 1983.

43 Fleiss JL. *Statistical Methods for Rates and Proportions*. 2nd ed. New York, NY: John Wiley & Sons Inc; 1980.

44 Haley SM, Osberg JS. Kappa coefficient calculation using multiple ratings per subject: a special communication. *Phys Ther*. 1989;69: 970–974.

45 Plewis I, Bax M. Cited by: Haley SM, Harris SR, Tada WL, Swanson MW. Item reliability of the Movement Assessment of Infants. *Physical & Occupational Therapy in Pediatrics*. 1986; 6:21–39.

46 Youdas JW, Carey JR, Garrett TR. Reliability of measurements of cervical spine range of motion: comparison of three methods. *Phys Ther*. 1991;71:98–106.

47 Bendix T, Biering-Sorensen F. Posture of the trunk when sitting on forward inclining seats. *Scand J Rehabil Med*. 1983;15:197–203.

48 Amendt LE, Ause-Ellias KL, Eybers JL, et al. Validity and reliability testing of the Scoliometer®. *Phys Ther*. 1990;70:108–117.

49 Frey JK, Tecklin JS. Comparison of lumbar curves when sitting on the Westnofa Balans® Multi-Chair, sitting on a conventional chair, and standing. *Phys Ther*. 1986;66:1365–1369.

50 Miedaner JA. The effects of sitting positions on trunk extension for children with motor impairment. *Pediatric Physical Therapy*. 1990; 2:11–14.

51 Williams JG, Callaghan M. Comparison of visual estimation and goniometry in determination of a shoulder joint angle. *Physiotherapy*. 1990;76:655–657.

52 Watkins MA, Riddle DL, Lamb RL, Personius WJ. Reliability of goniometric measurements and visual estimates of knee range of motion obtained in a clinical setting. *Phys Ther*. 1991; 71:90–97.

Assessment of Lower-Extremity Alignment in the Transverse Plane: Implications for Management of Children with Neuromotor Dysfunction

The authors present nine clinical assessment procedures designed to detect factors contributing to transverse-plane structural and joint alignment abnormality in children with neuromotor dysfunction. Where applicable, each assessment is accompanied by a discussion of the normal features of pediatric lower-extremity torsional and rotational alignment; limitations of the assessment procedures as regards reliability, specificity, and age-related normative findings; and clinical management suggestions. The authors urge clinical evaluators to expand the existing knowledge base. [Cusick BD, Stuberg WA. Assessment of lower-extremity alignment in the transverse plane: implications for management of children with neuromotor dysfunction. Phys Ther. 1992;72:3–15.]

Beverly D Cusick
Wayne A Stuberg

Key Words: *Lower extremity, general; Neuromotor disorders, general; Orthopedics, general; Pediatrics, evaluation.*

Children with chronic neuromotor dysfunction commonly exhibit deviations in transverse-plane (torsional and rotational) alignment of the pelvis and lower extremities (Fig. 1). Abnormal weight bearing and muscle action and shortened soft tissues impose forces that combine to impede and impair normal maturation of torsional and rotational features of skeletal structure and joint alignment. Unlike children with normal neuromotor status, most children who lack normal neuromuscular function do not develop efficient mechanisms to compensate for these structural abnormalities.[1] Alignment problems generally worsen with increasing age.[2–19]

The clinician should base management decisions on findings gained through a combination of gait analysis, posture evaluation, and a thorough biomechanical assessment.[3,17,20,21] To determine whether a clinical biomechanical finding indicates the presence of pathology, a clinician must identify and acknowledge normal maturational changes in skeletal architecture and joint configuration as they are currently understood.[1] We believe that research is needed to establish adequate norms and to evaluate the efficacy of interventions.

The purpose of this article is to raise the therapist's awareness of certain biomechanical components that can influence lower-extremity transverse-plane alignment and function and of the need to expand the existing body of research pertaining to the significance of clinical findings. Following a brief review of terminology, we present nine clinical biomechanical assessment procedures. The discussion pertaining to these assessments covers normative data, normal maturational changes in structural and joint configuration, limitations of the procedures as regards reliability and validity issues, and clinical management implications of assessment results.

Terminology

Rotation—a movement of one or both joint segments in a plane that is perpendicular to the axis of the motion.[22,23] Medial rotation and lateral rotation occur when a joint segment is rotated toward and away from midline, respectively, around a vertical axis.

BD Cusick, MS-CCT, PT, is Clinical Specialist, Lucille Packard Children's Hospital at Stanford, 725 Welch Rd, Palo Alto, CA 94304. She also teaches, consults, and is involved in private practice. Address all correspondence to Ms Cusick at 415 Velarde St, Mountain View, CA 94041 (USA).

WA Stuberg, PhD, PT, is Director of Physical Therapy, Meyer Rehabilitation Institute, Associate Professor, Division of Physical Therapy Education, and Assistant Professor, Department of Anatomy, University of Nebraska Medical Center, 600 S 42nd St, Omaha, NE 68198-5450.

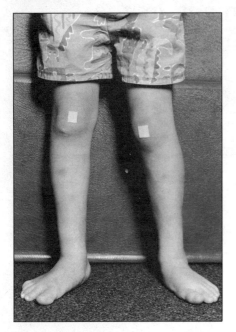

Figure 1. *Malalignment, characterized by medially rotated patellae (left more than right), positive foot progression angle, and bilateral foot pronation.*

Torsion—a structural, osseous state of twist in a bone along its longitudinal axis.[24] "Femoral antetorsion" and "medial femoral torsion" are synonymous terms describing a femur that bears a medial twist of the distal-on-proximal ends.[3,25,26] "Femoral retrotorsion" and "lateral femoral torsion" are also synonymous terms that describe a deformity ranging from a lack of normal medial torsion to a true lateral twist of the distal-on-proximal ends of the femur.[3,25,26] Clinical tibiofibular torsion describes a state of twist, either medial or lateral, in the long axis of the tibiofibular unit.

Version—"The act or process of turning something or changing direction."[24(p1830)] For example, the femoral head and neck are described as anteverted when the head lies anterior to the frontal plane and retroverted when the head lies posterior to the frontal plane. Version and torsion are not identical, although they may occur together. Version describes

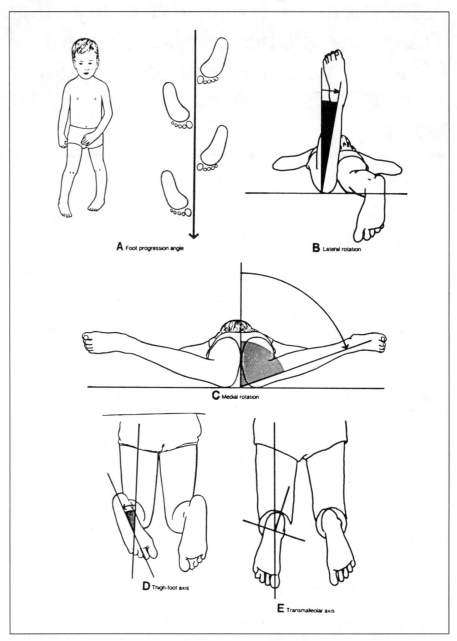

Figure 2. *Staheli's "Rotational Profile": (A) foot progression angle; (B) hip lateral rotation; (C) hip medial rotation; (D) thigh-foot angle; (E) transmalleolar axis-thigh angle.*

a position in space relative to a plane. Torsion describes a twist in structure.

Genicular position—an abnormality in the relative ranges of medial or lateral axial tibiofibular rotation with the knee joint flexed 90 degrees.[25]

Clinical Biomechanical Assessment Procedures

At least 13 biomechanical factors can be cited as contributing to lower-extremity malalignment in the transverse plane: (1) pelvic rotation in the transverse plane[7]; (2) immature acetabular anteversion[19,27–32]; (3) soft tissue restriction of hip joint medial or lateral rotation mobility[19,25,33–35]; (4) abnormal magnitude of femoral torsion*; (5) abnormal activity of the

---

*References 4, 7, 19, 21, 25, 26, 33, 36–45.

medial hamstring muscles[3,4,21,36,39,46]; (6) medial or lateral genicular position[23,25,43,47]; (7) abnormal magnitude of tibiofibular torsion[†]; (8) abnormal transverse-plane alignment of the talar body within the ankle mortise[49,50]; (9) persistent talar neck adduction relative to the talar body[38]; (10) abnormal foot pronation, resulting in midtarsal joint abduction[36,45,51–53]; (11) abnormal foot supination, resulting in midtarsal joint adduction[21,52,53]; (12) metatarsus adductus[37,44,45]; and (13) overpull of the abductor hallucis muscle ("searching toe").[54,55] We refer the reader to the cited references for information that is beyond the scope of this article.

We present a battery of nine assessment procedures that constitute a general screening. The battery features elements of Staheli's "Rotational Profile," which includes foot progression angle (FPA), medial and lateral hip rotation mobility with the hips extended, thigh-foot angle, transmalleolar axis (TMA)-thigh angle, and foot configuration (Fig. 2).[9,44,45,55–58] We have expanded Staheli's profile by adding pelvic rotation in the transverse plane, Ryder's test for femoral torsion, axial tibiofibular rotation mobility, and tibiofibular torsional status with the knee joint extended.

The assessment process is begun by observing the foot progression angle (FPA) to provide a basis for investigating specific components of limb structure and joint mobility. The remaining eight tests proceed from proximal to distal body segments.

General Alignment

Test 1—foot progression angle.
This test helps determine the angle formed by the foot and the line of forward progression. Abnormal FPA is commonly described as a gait deviation characterized by toeing-in or toeing-out beyond the normal mean.

Procedure. The therapist dusts the soles of the child's feet with chalk and obtains a series of footprints. We measure FPA as the angle formed by the longitudinal bisection of the foot and the line of progression (Fig. 2). The longitudinal bisection of the foot normally falls between the center of the plantar heel and the second and third metatarsals.[59] We obtain at least six measurements for each foot and calculate the average FPA. Toeing-in is indicated by a negative value, and toeing-out is indicated by a positive value.

Norms. Normative studies[60,61] have shown a mean FPA of 4 to 10 degrees in infants, children, and adults. The variability is greatest in children younger than 2 years of age.[60,61]

Limitations. Replicability of findings is hindered by the problem of establishing a precise reference for the line of progression, as few children walk in a purely straight line. Pronation and supination foot deformities induce compensatory lateral and medial deviations, respectively, of the axis of the forefoot relative to that of the hindfoot. We use the longitudinal bisection of the hindfoot to measure FPA in children with neuromotor dysfunction. The orientation of the hindfoot bisection to the sagittal plane offers a closer manifestation of proximal rotary and torsional influences on foot alignment than does that of the bisection of the compensating forefoot. The longitudinal forefoot bisection divides the second and third metatarsals.

Clinical implications. Toeing-in, which typically occurs in fewer than 30% of infants without neuromotor dysfunction, usually resolves by the age of 4 years.[40,47,48] An FPA of −1 to −10 indicates a mild abnormality, an FPA of −10 to −15 degrees indicates a moderate abnormality, and an FPA beyond −15 degrees indicates a severe abnormality. Adults rarely exhibit a nega-

tive FPA.[40,43,47,48,62] Children without neuromotor dysfunction who show persistent toe-in gait typically show no evidence of functional deficit.[63] A positive FPA exceeding 15 degrees imposes abnormal pronatory forces on the foot structures, as weight is borne abnormally on the medial aspect of the midfoot.[53]

Motion analysis reveals the occurrence of lateral rotation of the femur and, to a greater degree, the tibia during the mid-stance and propulsion phases of gait in all children, including early walkers.[40,64] As the ligaments of the knee joint and foot gain integrity, these stance-phase lateral torque forces descending on the foot evidently induce spontaneous correction of toeing-in.[1,51]

Children with abnormal muscle activity or myelomeningocele often demonstrate an abnormal magnitude of FPA.[4,7,36,39,40,65] Abnormal FPA in children with cerebral palsy depletes stability in the early stance phase of gait; necessitates that double-support stance begin prematurely; and reduces normal acceleration, velocity, and step length.[36] The components that contribute to abnormal FPA are discussed in the context of the remaining tests.

Proximal Alignment Features

We urge therapists to observe the postural alignment of each knee joint and patella relative to the sagittal plane of the limb. If the knee axis and patella align medially in quiet stance, we look for pelvic rotation, soft tissue restriction on lateral hip rotation, and evidence of abnormally increased medial femoral torsion (see tests 2–4). If medial deviation increases in gait, we assess hamstring muscle length[4,39] using the popliteal angle test as described by Jones and Knapp[21] and Rang et al.[16] If the patella and knee axis align laterally, we look for restriction on medial hip rotation mobility and femoral retrotorsion (see tests 3 and 4).

[†]References 7, 9, 19, 23, 25, 36, 44, 47, 48.

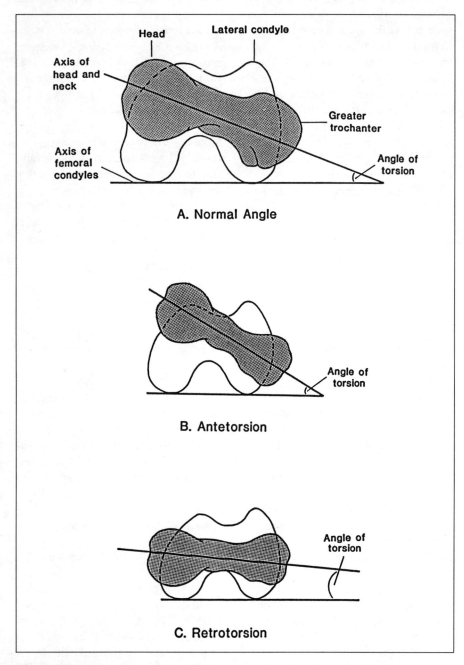

Labels in figure:
Head
Lateral condyle
Axis of head and neck
Greater trochanter
Axis of femoral condyles
Angle of torsion

A. Normal Angle

Angle of torsion

B. Antetorsion

Angle of torsion

C. Retrotorsion

Figure 3. *Proximal and distal reference axes for femur of an adolescent (unshaded) and an adult (shaded): (A) normal mean antetorsion (12°–20°); (B) abnormal or immature antetorsion (>20°); (C) femoral retrotorsion (<12° antetorsion).*

Test 2—pelvic rotation. As the child stands and walks, we observe pelvic rotation in the transverse plane and note whether the right or left anterior superior iliac spine is anterior to a frontal-plane reference line.

Norms. The pelvis ideally aligns on the frontal plane.[66(p144)]

Clinical implications. If abnormal rotation is evident, the acetabulum on the anterior side may consequently be more anteverted than the acetabulum on the posterior side. Thus, the femur on the anterior side might falsely appear to be medially rotated.[19,30] Acetabular anteversion normally diminishes with skeletal maturation.[30,32,67,68] Persistence of structurally increased acetabular anteversion can cause toeing-in when femoral torsion is normal, or it can occur in conjunction with increased femoral antetorsion.[19,30] We know of no clinical test to determine acetabular orientation. Radiographic confirmation is needed.

Test 3—Ryder's test. The magnitude of femoral torsion is measured as the angle formed by the transverse-plane intersection of the femur's proximal reference axis (PRA) and distal reference axis (DRA). The PRA bisects the femoral head and greater trochanter, and the DRA lies parallel to the posterior aspects of the femoral condyles and is known as the transcondylar axis (TCA).

Femoral antetorsion is evident when the TCA is placed on the frontal plane and the femoral head lies anterior to the frontal plane (Fig. 3). Femoral retrotorsion is evident when the TCA is placed on the frontal plane and the femoral head lies less than 10 to 12 degrees anterior to the frontal plane (Fig. 3).[25,26,43] The orientation of these axes to each other can only be estimated on clinical examination using Ryder's test, which features palpation of the position of the greater trochanter while rotating the femur.[4,19,25]

Procedure. Position the child prone, supine, or sitting with the knee flexed to 90 degrees. The findings should be consistent in all positions, as they should represent the bony configuration. The examiner holds the leg proximal to the ankle and rotates the hip while palpating the anterior and posterior borders of the greater trochanter. When the trochanter reaches the most lateral position in the arc, we presume that the femoral neck and head are aligned on or near the frontal plane (Figs. 4, 5). We then measure the resulting position of hip rotation.

We use a straight line connecting the mid-patella and the mid-ankle as the DRA.[69] If measuring with a goniometer, we use the table surface as the PRA (frontal plane) and subtract the resulting value from 90. We prefer to use a 7.62-cm-diameter (3-in-diameter), gravity-driven angle

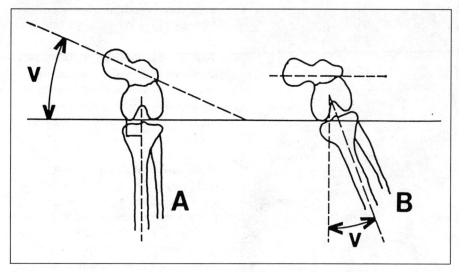

Figure 4. *Skeletal representation of Ryder's test in context of increased left medial femoral torsion: (A) When the distal reference axis (DRA) of the tibia is aligned on the sagittal plane, the greater trochanter lies posterior to the frontal plane; (B) when the proximal reference axis of the greater trochanter and the femoral neck is aligned on the frontal plane, the distal DRA of the tibia deviates laterally to represent a position of hip medial rotation. (V-angle of femoral torsion.)*

finder,[‡§] adapted by holding an extended straightedge against the shorter side of the angle finder (Fig. 5). The angle finder offers a vertical-plane reference, which is a gravitational constant.

Norms. The magnitude of medial femoral torsion at birth approaches a mean of 40 degrees. Thereafter, the mean torsion angle reduces to 31 degrees at age 2 years, decreases to 25 degrees by age 8 years, and drops rapidly to the adult mean of 16 degrees between ages 14 and 16 years.[5,70] Stuberg and colleagues[71] reported mean medial rotation values of 10 to 13.5 degrees (SD=3.3°=3.9°) obtained by three testers on a group of 17 subjects, aged 3 to 22 years.

Limitations. Age-related reliability coefficients and normative data for Ryder's test results have not been established. Stuberg et al[71] used a different goniometric technique from the one we

suggest and showed a mean intertester difference of approximately 3 degrees. Reliability improved with the testers' clinical experience. Thickness of soft tissues overlying the greater trochanter can affect the precision of palpation. Age-related torsional normative values for computed tomography (CT) or magnetic resonance imaging (MRI) findings have not been established or validated against measurements on anatomic specimens.

Clinical implications. Given the current available data comparing CT results with both Ryder's test results and measurements taken on an anatomic femur specimen, one can presume that the femur is twisted medially approximately 20 degrees more than the measured hip rotation value indicates.[7,71,72] For example, 5 degrees of lateral rotation (the distal leg deviates medially) represents a femur with approximately 15 degrees of medial torsion, whereas 5 degrees of medial rotation (the distal leg deviates later-

ally) suggests the presence of approximately 25 degrees of medial torsion.

Children with spastic cerebral palsy exhibit increased femoral antetorsion,[‖] as do many children with myelomeningocele.[19,73] These children typically show persistent hip flexion contractures, with a concurrent lack of adequate extension and lateral rotation forces crossing the proximal femoral shaft.[1,3,38] Habitual sleep and play postures, such as W-sitting, correlate with persistence of femoral antetorsion.[19,41,43,74,75] Staheli[45] has described a malalignment syndrome that causes awkward gait and chondromalacia in children with normal neuromotor function. This syndrome is characterized by increased femoral antetorsion, which persists into adolescence with compensatory, excessive lateral tibiofibular torsion. Correction would require femoral and tibial derotational osteotomy. Because the most rapid decline in femoral antetorsion normally occurs during the first 4 years postnatally,[70] we advise the pediatric clinician to intervene early to gain biomechanically efficient limb alignment before this malalignment syndrome evolves in children with neuromotor deficits.

No radiologic or anatomic studies have documented the effects of twister cables, antirotation braces, exercises, orthoses, splints, or shoes on the existing degree of femoral or tibial torsion.[5,25,38,41,47,57,74,76] Twister cables are not recommended for femoral antetorsion, as they may promote excessive lateral tibiofibular torsion or rotation.[38] Until research proves that exercise, positioning, and orthoses offer no benefit, we base our management recommendations on the principle that the application of correct forces is required for optimum skeletal modeling before the skeleton ossifies[6,11,12] and on findings relating habitual limb positioning to torsional abnormality. For children with adequate innervation, from birth to 8 years of age, we recommend multiple daily repetitions of resisted hip extension and lateral rotation, the reduction of hip and knee flexion and femoral medial rotation postures in stance and gait, the im-

[‡]Macklanburg Duncan Inc, Oklahoma City, OK 73118.

[§]Model AF100, Dasco Pro Inc, 2215 Kishawaukee St, Rockford, IL 61101.

[‖]References 2, 5, 7, 9, 10, 13, 14, 18, 41, 70.

pracondylar femoral derotational osteotomy, undertaken for 11 children with spastic cerebral palsy, aged 7 to 15 years ($\overline{X}$=9.5).[19]

Test 4—hip rotation mobility test.
Another way to assess femoral torsional status and to evaluate soft tissue extensibility is to measure passive hip medial rotation and lateral rotation (Fig. 2).

Procedure. The therapist positions the child prone with knees flexed 90 degrees and tibias vertical. Keeping the pelvis level, the therapist allows the feet to fall apart from each other until gravity stops the motion. Range of motion (ROM) is measured using the same DRA landmarks as described for the Ryder's test (see test 3 and Fig. 5). To measure lateral rotation mobility, the pelvis is gently kept level, and the therapist laterally rotates each hip 10 to 20 times to reduce any influence of soft tissue restriction.[19]

The therapist identifies soft tissue effects on rotation by noting whether the magnitude of ROM changes with the hip and knee flexed 90 degrees (sitting).[19,25] Evidence of abnormal femoral torsion is supported when the same findings are obtained with the hip flexed and extended.[25]

Norms. Lateral rotation contracture normally limits medial rotation mobility in infancy.[35,77] As the contracture reduces, medial rotation increases. At age 24 months, medial rotation exceeds lateral rotation by an average of 7 degrees.[77] A normative study of medial rotation findings for school-aged children showed a mean approximating 40 to 50 degrees (range=15°–65°), whereas the mean lateral rotation value approached 70 degrees before age 1 year and decreased to approximately 45 degrees (range= 25°-65°) from age 5 years through mid-adulthood. This study examined between 11 and 28 children in age groups of 1 year each greater than 1 year.[61]

Limitations. Reliability studies for measurements obtained from medial rotation/lateral rotation tests on chil-

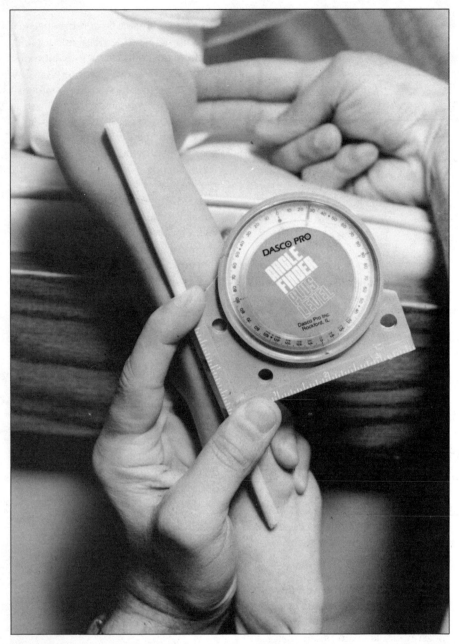

Figure 5. *Ryder's test for femoral torsion. Palpate the greater trochanter and align it in its most lateral position. Use the adapted angle finder to measure hip rotation. Landmarks: mid-patella and mid-ankle.*

provement of lateral and posterior weight transfer skills over the feet, and the institution of a consistent positioning program. Because abnormal foot pronation deformity is believed to promote medial rotation of the proximal limb structures,[52,53] we protect the foot from pronating abnormally by serial casting to gain full ankle dorsiflexion mobility (minimum of 10°) and by combining the consistent use of appro-

priate splints or orthoses with weight transfer training.

The general opinion among orthopedists is that femoral derotation osteotomy is the only effective treatment for antetorsion for children aged 7 years and older.[5,7,19,39,63] Tachdjian[19] and Staheli[45] discuss criteria for osteotomy for the neurologically normal child. Hoffer et al[7] report good results and minimal complications following sudren have not been published, nor have medial rotation/lateral rotation findings been validated using CT or MRI analysis of torsion. This test cannot be used to identify abnormal femoral torsion in children less than age 2 years because of persistence of normal intrauterine lateral rotation contracture of the hip joint.[35,40,77] If lax ligaments allow abnormally increased medial rotation and lateral rotation mobility, the findings cannot be used to discern torsional status. We believe the medial rotation/lateral rotation test cannot be used to distinguish femoral torsion from abnormal acetabular anteversion or retroversion. We use Ryder's test as an adjunct to the medial rotation/lateral rotation test, and we repeat the medial rotation/lateral rotation test in the sitting position.

Clinical implications. Clinically significant medial femoral torsion is evident when medial rotation is greater than 60 degrees and lateral rotation is less than 25 degrees.[38,44,45] Limitation of lateral rotation range is the principal finding.[19] If medial rotation/lateral rotation findings corroborate those obtained with the Ryder's test, we try to manage torsional deformity as suggested for the Ryder's test (see test 3). If soft tissue limitation becomes evident, we use positioning, soft tissue mobilization techniques, and exercises to gain mobility.

Distal Limb Features

If the hindfoot FPA is negative and the patella aligns on the sagittal plane, we look for a medial genicular position, excessive activity or shortening of the medial hamstring and popliteus muscles, medial tibiofibular torsion, or a combination of these factors (see tests 5–8).[25,42,50,54,78] If the forefoot FPA is negative, we look for evidence of increased talar torsion,[38] foot supination, or forefoot adductus (see tests 5, 6, and 9). If the patella aligns either medially or normally and the hindfoot FPA is abnormally positive, we look for a lateral genicular position or excessive lateral tibiofibular torsion, or both (see tests 5–8). If a line bisecting the forefoot deviates laterally on the hindfoot, we evaluate for foot pronation, which is characterized by midtarsal joint dorsiflexion and abduction (see test 9).

Test 5—thigh-foot angle test. Staheli[44,45,57] uses this test to assess tibiofibular torsional status. We suggest instead that it is a composite test of axial tibiofibular rotation position, tibiofibular torsion, subtalar joint alignment, and foot configuration (ie, adduction, supination, pronation, and so forth).

Procedure. The therapist positions the child prone with the knee flexed 90 degrees, the tibia vertical, and the ankle dorsiflexed to 0 degrees. As this test is used to evaluate structures distal to the femur, we believe the position of proximal femoral rotation or hip abduction is not relevant. We hold the foot in the subtalar joint neutral position (neither supinated nor pronated) and use the bisection of the plantar surface of the hindfoot only as the DRA to eliminate forefoot deviations as a factor in measurement. We measure the angle formed by the bisecting line of the thigh (PRA) and the longitudinal axis of the hindfoot (DRA) (Fig. 2). Medial deviation (adduction) of the foot results in a negative value; lateral deviation (abduction) produces a positive value.

Norms. The range of normal findings is wide, especially during infancy.[61] Through age 2 years, the mean angle lies between 0 and −10 degrees (range=−25°–20° at birth). The angle gradually increases to a mean of 10 degrees (range=−5°–30°) from middle childhood on.[61]

Limitations. Normative clinical data represent small age-specific study groups of 11 to 28 children.[61] Reliability data are not available for this test, nor are validity data available for comparisons of thigh-foot angles and tibiofibular torsion CT or MRI findings for children of more than 9 months' gestational age.[49] Age-related normative data for CT and MRI findings are also not available. The thigh-foot angle results might reveal factors that falsely indicate the presence of medial tibiofibular torsion, such as normal infantile hyperextensibility of the knee joint ligaments and capsule, which interferes with stabilizing and identifying the rotary position of the proximal tibia[42]; normal neonatal medial rotation bias of the knee joint ligaments and capsule[79]; medial hamstring and popliteus muscle activity or shortening[25]; release of the screw-home mechanism with knee flexion, which allows medial axial tibiofibular rotation to occur[25,66,80,81]; or persistence of medial genicular position attributable to habitual sleep or play postures. Talar torsion or medial rotation of the talar body in the ankle mortise might position the well-aligned foot in medial rotation under the tibia and fibula.[49,50] We believe this factor accounts primarily for the failure of Badelon et al[49] to find a correlation between the thigh-foot angle test and the status of anatomic tibiofibular torsion in fetal cadaver specimens.

Clinical implications. Staheli[57] states that, if the thigh-foot angle is greater than −5 degrees (child's age unspecified), medial tibial torsion is present. We use the thigh-foot angle as a global indicator of change rather than as a reliable or valid indicator of tibiofibular torsion. We supplement this test with the axial tibiofibular rotation test (see test 8), the TMA-thigh angle test (see test 6), and examination of tibiofibular torsion status with the knee joint extended (see test 7) before proposing a management program.

Test 6—the transmalleolar axis-thigh angle test. The TMA-thigh angle moves the scope of assessment to the segment proximal to the subtalar joint.[9,19,45,55,61]

Procedure. The therapist positions the child prone with the knee and ankle flexed 90 degrees and the tibia vertical. We locate the anterior-posterior (AP) malleolar bisections and mark a line joining them on the plantar surface of the foot, representing the TMA. We also mark a perpendicular line from the TMA posteriorly on the heel. This perpendicular line is the DRA. The PRA is the long bisection of the posterior thigh. We measure the

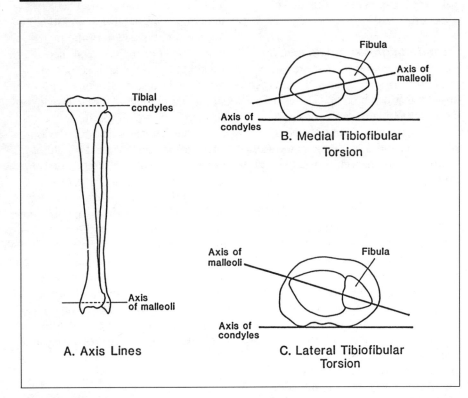

Figure 6. *(A) Proximal and distal reference axes for tibiofibular (TF) torsion; (B) medial TF torsion; (C) lateral TF torsion.*

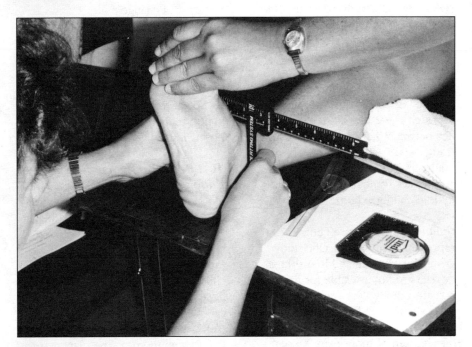

Figure 7. *Measure the width between the malleolar bisections by carefully aligning the measuring device (photo shows a medial-lateral caliper) on both the transverse and frontal planes. Do not take a diagonal width measurement.*

#References 23, 25(p103), 34(p326), 62(p311), 82(p308).

angle formed by the PRA and DRA (Fig. 2).

Norms. The normative values for TMA-thigh angle are higher than those for thigh-foot angle by approximately 10 degrees.[61] The mean TMA-thigh angle at birth is about 0 degrees (range=−30°–20°), gradually increasing to approximately 20 degrees (range=0°–45°) during and after middle childhood.[61] In our opinion, these normative values, when compared with those for thigh-foot angle, reveal evidence of a normal medial rotation of the foot under the malleoli.

Limitations. The same reliability and validity issues discussed in reference to the thigh-foot angle test pertain to the TMA-thigh angle test. "Pseudolack of malleolar torsion" describes a low orientation of the TMA to the frontal plane that might falsely suggest medial tibiofibular torsion.# Although a rather high incidence (30%) of toe-in gait has been reported for infants without neuromotor dysfunction,[48] Rosen and Sandick found "a surprising lack of true [internal] TF torsion"[23(p854)] among 2-year-old children who exhibit a toe-in gait.

Clinical implications. We advise using the TMA-thigh angle to measure change, rather than to indicate tibiofibular torsion in children with neuromotor deficits. We evaluate axial tibiofibular rotation and torsion with the knee extended before intervening. Computed tomography provides the most accurate impression of torsional status, but age-related normative data are not yet available.

Test 7—tibiofibular torsion test in knee extension. Tibiofibular torsion is measured clinically as the angle (DRA) formed by the intersection of a frontal-plane bisection of the knee joint (PRA) and a line bisecting the medial and lateral malleoli (TMA). On CT scans, the frontal-plane bisection of the proximal tibial condyles forms the PRA (Fig. 6). After aligning the PRA on the frontal plane, medial tibiofibular torsion is evident when the medial malleolus lies posterior to the frontal plane. Lateral tibiofibular tor-

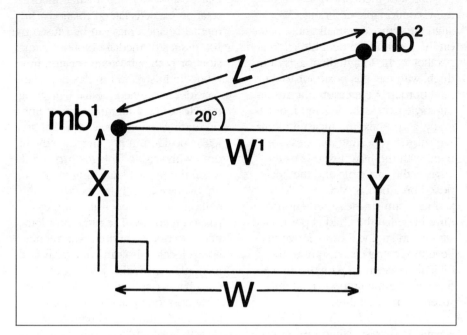

Figure 8. *Calibrating tibiofemoral torsion. (X=distance between malleolar bisection (mb¹) and surface. Y=distance between malleolar bisection (mb²) and surface. W=width between malleolar bisections, measured parallel with the transverse and frontal planes. W¹ represents the frontal plane, connects mb¹ and Y, and lies parallel to line W. Z=transmalleolar axis (TMA), connecting mb¹ and mb². The angle formed by the intersection of lines W¹ and Z indicates that the TMA is oriented 20° to the frontal plane.)*

sion is evident when the lateral malleolus lies posterior to the frontal plane.

The collateral and cruciate ligaments and the popliteus muscle become taut with the knee extended, locking the fully extended mature knee joint against transverse- and frontal-plane motions.[42,83,84] Given that the knee joint ligaments are intact and not hyperextensible, and that the extensibility of the knee joint capsule allows full knee extension to occur, we believe that extending the knee joint to measure tibiofibular torsional status secures the proximal tibia against rotating and reduces measurement error.

Procedure. The therapist positions the child sitting or supine on a firm table surface with the knee fully extended and the ankle and foot hanging off the table edge. The table surface represents the frontal plane of the limb and serves as the PRA for this test. The therapist then places the knee joint axis on the frontal plane by flexing the knee a few times in the pure

sagittal plane. An assistant supports the knee at 0 degrees of extension, stabilizing it against rotating.

We rotate the tibiofibular unit medially and laterally under the stabilized distal femur. If the joint allows more than 10 degrees of rotation, we carefully align the tibial tuberosity and tibial crest on the sagittal plane and have the assistant stabilize the tibia. The assistant then dorsiflexes the ankle on the sagittal plane to the comfortable end-range and holds the ankle in that position.

We mark a dot on the AP bisection of the medial and lateral malleoli (mb¹ and mb²). We also measure the distance (X and Y) between each malleolar bisection (mb) and the table surface. Holding a medial-lateral caliper on both the transverse and frontal planes, we measure the width (W) between the malleoli (Fig. 7). All three measurements are transferred onto graph paper, using W as the baseline and setting X and Y at each end of the baseline (Fig. 8). We draw

a horizontal line (W¹) from the top of the shorter mb line to the longer mb line, parallel to the baseline. Another line (Z), connecting the dots at mb¹ and mb² and representing the TMA, is drawn. A goniometer is used to measure the angle formed by Z and W¹. We believe lateral tibiofibular torsion is evident when the medial mb line is longer than the lateral mb line and is recorded as a positive value. Medial tibiofibular torsion occurs when the lateral mb line is longer than the medial mb line and is recorded as a negative value.

Norms. Existing normative values vary in magnitude, having been obtained using a variety of anatomical landmarks and knee joint positions.[23,48,49,85–89] We refer the reader to cited references for details. Because McCrea[25] measures tibiofibular torsional status with the knee joint extended, we report his stated normative values, as follows: −5 to 10 degrees in infancy, 10 to 15 degrees by age 2 years, and 20 to 30 degrees by age 5 to 7 years through adulthood. Jakob et al[89] found a mean tibiofibular torsion of 30 degrees in adult cadavers, measuring with the knee joint extended. Badelon et al[47] assessed fetal cadavers and found a mean anatomical angle of 20 degrees (range=10°–32°) at 9 months' gestational age, suggesting that the tibiofibular unit might achieve a mature magnitude of lateral torsion at birth. If so, the reported normative values for infants and very young children may be affected by medial genicular position.

Limitations. Reliability coefficients and age-related, normative values for the tibiofibular torsion assessment procedure described are not established. Age-related normative values do not exist for CT or MRI measurements of tibiofibular torsion.

If the knee joint cannot be fully extended, the screw-home mechanism cannot operate to secure the proximal tibia. If the lateral malleolus is abnormally enlarged, as often occurs with supination deformity, the width of the ankle might be misrepresented.

Clinical implications. If true medial tibiofibular torsion is present in young children, it usually improves spontaneously, whereas lateral tibiofibular torsion often worsens.[45] Valmassey (RL Valmassey; personal communication; June 28, 1991) and various authors[25,40,43,90] suggest intervening early to reduce a significant, negative FPA, using serial casting, night splinting bars, and counterrotation devices. The criteria for using such interventions, however, are not specified. Radiologic studies are needed to ascertain the efficacy of these interventions. It is likely that these interventions actually impose lateral rotation on soft tissues within the knee joint, as they do not secure the proximal tibia.[43,47] The immediate and long-term biomechanical influences of these interventions on tibiofibular torsion and knee joint status have not been investigated.[45,47]

Staheli[45,58] has reported suggested guidelines for surgical osteotomy for children with normal neuromotor status. For children with cerebral palsy, abnormal lateral tibiofibular torsion may be a greater biomechanical problem than medial tibiofibular torsion. Õunpuu et al[65] recommend supramalleolar derotational osteotomy for children with cerebral palsy who show evidence of increased tibiofibular lateral torsion. They claim results that show improved sagittal-plane gait features at the knee and ankle after reducing the mean FPA from 31.8 to 11.5 degrees.

Test 8—axial tibiofibular rotation test.
We believe this test helps to distinguish axial rotation mobility and alignment from tibiofibular torsional status. Maximum axial rotation occurs with the knee joint flexed between 60 and 90 degrees.[91] Infants normally exhibit 20 to 30 degrees of rotary mobility with the knee joint extended.[42,92]

Procedure. The therapist positions the child prone with the knee flexed 90 degrees, the tibia vertical, and the ankle flexed to 0 degrees. Refer to the illustration for thigh-foot angle in Figure 2 for landmarks of measurement. Holding the foot and malleoli

as a stable unit, we rotate the leg, ankle, and foot medially to the maximum comfortable end-range. We align the arms of a small goniometer on the longitudinal heel bisection and parallel to the longitudinal axis of the thigh, with the axis posterior to the heel border. We measure the resulting angle, rotate the leg and foot laterally, and repeat the measurement. We suggest repeating the measurement with the hips flexed over the edge of the mat table and the knees flexed on a bench. McCrea[25] describes a similar measurement procedure in which the child is positioned sitting and supine; however, we believe the reference axes are more difficult to ascertain with this procedure, thus impeding potential measurement replicability.

Norms. McCrea's[25] clinical experience suggests that children without neuromotor dysfunction under age 3 years, positioned sitting with hips and knees flexed 90 degrees, show a normal medial rotation-to-lateral rotation ratio of between 1:1 and 1:2, with normal findings of 45 to 65 degrees for medial rotation and 45 to 95 degrees for lateral rotation.[25] By age 3 to 4 years, the knee joint typically gains integrity, and rotation range decreases.[42,92] An unpublished study, lacking specification of reference axes, revealed that the mean total range of axial tibiofibular rotation in women without neuromotor dysfunction approached 40 degrees (SD=8°), with a lateral rotation-to-medial rotation ratio of approximately 2:1. Axial tibial rotation with the knee extended was 0 degrees.[93] Other authors report unsubstantiated values ranging from 10 degrees of medial and lateral rotation[80,81] to 30 degrees of medial rotation and 45 degrees of lateral rotation.[79,94]

Limitations. Reliability studies and studies to determine age-specific pediatric normative values have not been undertaken for this test. Clinical judgment must rest on the merits of reported clinical experience. Correlation has not been established between axial tibiofibular rotation mobility and FPA or between axial tibiofibular rotation and foot deformity.

Clinical implications. A medial genicular position is evident when medial rotation exceeds lateral rotation. The medial rotation bias can be caused by soft tissues or medial tibiofibular torsion, or both.[25] If lateral rotation mobility diminishes in hip flexion, then consider shortened medial hamstring muscles to be a limiting factor. Clinical findings often reveal a medial genicular position in preschool-aged children with spastic diplegia, particularly when the medial hamstring muscles are overactive and shortened and the child habitually kneel-sits with legs rotated medially. The same problem often occurs in children with meningomyelocele who can voluntarily control only the medial (and not the lateral) hamstring muscles. We believe early positioning and night splinting to maintain full medial hamstring muscle ROM and to gently rotate the leg laterally under the flexed knee may reduce the functional problems relating to this medial rotational bias. Gait studies and radiographic assessments are needed to evaluate the structural and functional effects of these interventions.

Medial hamstring muscle lengthening has been shown to produce a significant and perhaps pathological increase in FPA in children with spastic cerebral palsy over age 4 years.[3,44] The resulting stability of the tibiofemoral articulation was not evaluated.

We find that children with hemiparesis who exhibit equinovarus deformity at the foot and ankle often reveal increased lateral axial tibiofibular mobility. The rigid, supinating foot imposes lateral rotation forces on the tibiofibular unit during the stance phase of gait. We suggest reducing this deforming strain by gaining dorsiflexion and pronation mobility through progressive casting, use of night splints and orthoses, or, if casting yields no gain of mobility, surgical intervention.[1,95]

Test 9—foot configuration.
Consider the shape of the foot as a factor affecting FPA when proximal factors are normal.

Procedure. The therapist positions the child prone to allow a view of the plantar surface of the foot. We stabilize the foot in the subtalar neutral position of maximum congruity (ie, neither supinated nor pronated) and view the plantar surface. We align the arms of a small goniometer on the longitudinal bisection of the heel and parallel with a line bisecting the second and third metatarsals.

Norms. The ideal hindfoot/forefoot angle is 0 degrees.[53,59,88,96]

Limitations. Reliability and validity tests are needed for this procedure. Age-related normative values have not been established.

Clinical implications. Metatarsus adductus and supination or pronation deformities affect the FPA.[45] A straight foot positioned in adduction (medial rotation) under a normally aligned femur and TMA suggests the presence of increased talar torsion or medial rotation of the talar body within the ankle mortise.[38,49,50]

In young children with spastic diplegia who bear excessive weight on the medial forefoot, we often see foot pronation deformity, characterized by an abducted forefoot on an adducted hindfoot. The lateral forefoot deviation masks a negative hindfoot FPA. In this case, we believe that when the foot is supported in proper alignment with an orthosis, toeing-in appears or worsens. Clinicians should alert caretakers to this possibility prior to intervening to protect the foot pronation deformity from progressing, as caretakers usually perceive toeing-in as a more serious problem than progressive foot pronation.

As children with spastic diplegia grow beyond preschool age, some develop lateral tibiofibular rotation and torsion as well as foot pronation, which increases the hindfoot FPA.[27] The medial knee joint ligaments and capsule become overstretched by abnormal loading forces.[19,27,38,53,54,78] Having identified the presence of shortened triceps surae muscles, we work to reduce foot pronation and strain on

the knee joint and tibiofibular unit by (1) gaining ankle dorsiflexion mobility with serial casting or stretch splinting, or surgery if these measures fail; (2) applying appropriate orthoses or splints to maintain ideal foot alignment; and (3) facilitating lateral/posterior weight transfers over the foot.[1,95,97]

Because the forefoot adducts on the hindfoot in individuals with foot supination deformity, the hindfoot FPA might be more positive than that of the forefoot. We reduce the supination deformity with serial casting and the use of orthoses as needed to achieve a more normal FPA.[1,95,97]

Summary

The field of biomechanical analysis as it applies to children with neuromotor deficits is clearly in its infancy. The clinical assessment procedures presented in this article require further research to establish their validity and reliability for children with and without neuromotor dysfunction. Large-scale normative studies should follow, recording coincidental measures of the FPA. Sophisticated radiographic techniques should be used to determine the efficacy of commonly prescribed splinting apparatuses and therapeutic exercise programs. Such studies would contribute greatly to our understanding of the functional significance and management of transverse-plane biomechanical factors for children with neuromotor dysfunction.

References

1 Cusick BD. *Progressive Casting and Splinting for Lower Extremity Deformities in Children with Neuromotor Dysfunction.* Tucson, Ariz: Therapy Skill Builders; 1990.

2 Beals RK. Developmental changes in the femur and acetabulum in spastic paraplegia and diplegia. *Dev Med Child Neurol.* 1969;11:303–313.

3 Bleck EE. *Orthopedic Management of Cerebral Palsy.* Philadelphia, Pa: JB Lippincott Co; 1987.

4 Chong KC, Vojnic CD, Quanburg AO, Letts RM. The assessment of internal rotation gait in cerebral palsy: an electromyographic gait analysis. *Clin Orthop.* 1978;132:145–149.

5 Fabry G, MacEwen GD, Shands AR. Torsion of the femur. *J Bone Joint Surg [Am].* 1973;55:1726–1738.

6 Frost HM. *Intermediary Organization of the Skeleton.* Boca Raton, Fla: CRC Press; 1986.

7 Hoffer MM, Prietto C, Koffman M. Supracondylar derotational osteotomy of the femur for internal rotation of the thigh in the cerebral palsied child. *J Bone Joint Surg [Am].* 1981;63:389–393.

8 Kasser JR, MacEwen GD. Examination of the cerebral palsy patient with foot and ankle problems. *Foot Ankle.* 1983;4:135–144.

9 King HA, Staheli LT. Torsional problems in cerebral palsy. *Foot Ankle.* 1984;4:180–184.

10 Laplaza FJ, Root L, Tassanawipas A, Burke S. Femoral torsion and neck-shaft angles in patients with cerebral palsy. *Dev Med Child Neurol.* 1989;31:27. Abstract.

11 LeVeau BF. Developmental biomechanics and the principles of growth. In: Wilson JM, Davis IA, eds. *Orthopedic Aspects of Developmental Disabilities.* Chapel Hill, NC; University of North Carolina Press; 1980:1–27.

12 LeVeau BF, Bernhardt DB. Developmental biomechanics: effect of forces on the growth, development, and maintenance of the human body. *Phys Ther.* 1984;64:1874–1882.

13 Lewis FR, Samilson RR, Lucas DB. Femoral torsion and coxa valga in cerebral palsy. *Dev Med Child Neurol.* 1964;6:591–597.

14 Majestro TC, Frost HM. Cerebral palsy: spastic internal femoral torsion. *Clin Orthop.* 1971;79:44–56.

15 Mann R. Biomechanics in cerebral palsy. *Foot Ankle.* 1983;4:114–119.

16 Rang M, Silver R, de la Garza J. Cerebral palsy. In: Lovell WW, Winters RB, eds. *Pediatric Orthopaedics.* 2nd ed. Philadelphia, Pa: JB Lippincott Co; 1986:345–396.

17 Samilson RL, Dillin L. Postural impositions on the foot and ankle from trunk, pelvis, hip, and knee in cerebral palsy. *Foot Ankle.* 1983;4:120–127.

18 Staheli LT, Duncan WR, Schaefer E. Growth alterations in the hemiplegic child. *Clin Orthop.* 1968;60:205–212.

19 Tachdjian MO. *Pediatric Orthopedics.* 2nd ed. Philadelphia, Pa: WB Saunders Co; 1990.

20 Hoffer MM, Perry J. Pathodynamics of gait alterations in cerebral palsy and the significance of kinetic electromyography in evaluating foot and ankle problems. *Foot Ankle.* 1983;4:128–134.

21 Jones ET, Knapp DR. Assessment and management of the lower extremity in cerebral palsy. *Orthop Clin North Am.* 1987;18:725–738.

22 Cole TM, Tobis JS. Measurement of musculoskeletal function. In: Kottke FJ, Lehmann JF, eds. *Krusen's Handbook of Physical Medicine and Rehabilitation.* 4th ed. Philadelphia, Pa: WB Saunders Co; 1990;20–71.

23 Rosen H, Sandick H. The management of tibiofibular rotation. *J Bone Joint Surg [Am].* 1955;37:847–855.

24 *Dorland's Illustrated Medical Dictionary.* 27th ed. Philadelphia, Pa: WB Saunders Co; 1988:1830.

25 McCrea JD. *Pediatric Orthopedics of the Lower Extremity: An Instructional Handbook.* Mount Kisco, NY: Futura Press; 1985.

26 Smith C, Fuller E. *Biomechanics III—Syllabus.* San Francisco, Calif: California College of Podiatric Medicine.

27 Feltz WL. The prenatal development of the human femur. *Am J Anat.* 1954;94:1–44.

28 Lloyd-Roberts GC, Harris NH, Chrispin AR. Anteversion of the acetabulum in congenital dislocation of the hip: a preliminary report. *Orthop Clin North Am.* 1978;9:89–95.

29 McKibbin B. Anatomical factors in the stability of the hip joint in the newborn. *J Bone Joint Surg [Br].* 1970;52:148–159.

30 McSweeney A. A study of femoral torsion in children. *J Bone Joint Surg [Br].* 1971;53:90–95.

31 Stanisavljevic S. Congenital dysplasia, subluxation, and dislocation of the hip in stillborn and newborn infants. *J Bone Joint Surg [Am].* 1963;45:1147–1158.

32 Watanabe RS. Embryology of the human hip. *Clin Orthop.* 1974;98:1–26.

33 Engel GM, Staheli LT. Natural history of torsion and other factors influencing gait in childhood. *Clin Orthop.* 1974;99:12–17.

34 Hlavac HF. Major considerations in the clinical evaluation of the lower extremity. In: Sgarlato T, ed. *A Compendium of Podiatric Biomechanics.* San Francisco, Calif: California College of Podiatric Medicine; 1971:321–344.

35 Pitkow RB. External rotation contracture of the extended hip. *Clin Orthop.* 1975;110:139–145.

36 Gage JR. An overview of normal and cerebral palsy gait. *Neurosurgery: State of the Art Reviews.* 1989;4:379–401.

37 Alexander I. Evaluation of in-toeing in children. In: *The Foot: Examination and Diagnosis.* New York, NY: Churchill Livingstone Inc; 1990:149–160.

38 Bleck EE. Developmental orthopaedics, III: toddlers. *Dev Med Child Neurol.* 1982;24:533–555.

39 Sutherland DH, Schottstaedt ER, Larsen LJ, et al. Clinical and electromyographic study of seven spastic children with internal rotation gait. *J Bone Joint Surg [Am].* 1969;51:1070–1082.

40 Sutherland DH. *Gait Disorders in Childhood and Adolescence.* Baltimore, Md: Williams & Wilkins; 1984.

41 Swanson AB, Greene PW, Allis HD. Rotational deformities of the lower extremity in children and their clinical significance. *Clin Orthop.* 1963;27:157–174.

42 Valmassy RL. Biomechanical evaluation of the child. In: Ganley JV, ed. *Symposium on Podopediatrics.* Philadelphia, Pa: WB Saunders Co; 1984;563–579.

43 McDonough MW. Angular and axial deformities of the legs of children. In: Ganley JV, ed. *Symposium on Podopediatrics.* Philadelphia, Pa: WB Saunders Co; 1984:601–620.

44 Staheli LT. Torsional deformity. *Pediatr Clin North Am.* 1977;24:799–811.

45 Staheli LT. The lower limb. In: Morrissy RT, ed. *Lovell and Winter's Pediatric Orthopaedics.* 3rd ed. Philadelphia, Pa: JB Lippincott Co; 1990;1:741–766.

46 Sullivan RC, Krzyzanowski JA, Harris GF. Rotational changes in the lower limbs following distal medial hamstrings surgery for cerebral-palsied children. *Dev Med Child Neurol.* 1986;28:107. Abstract.

47 Scoles PV. Lower extremity development. In: Scoles PV. *Pediatric Orthopedics in Clinical Practice.* 2nd ed. Chicago, Ill: Year Book Medical Publishers; 1988:82–121.

48 Hutter CG, Scott W. Tibial torsion. *J Bone Joint Surg [Am].* 1949;31:511–518.

49 Badelon O, Bensahel H, Folinais D, Lassale B. Tibiofibular torsion from the fetal period until birth. *J Pediatr Orthop.* 1989;9:169–173.

50 Ritter MA, DeRosa GP, Babcock JL. Tibial torsion? *Clin Orthop.* 1976;120:159–163.

51 Jordan RP, Cusack J, Resseque B. Foot function and its relationship to posture in the pediatric patient with cerebral palsy and other neuromotor disorders: course materials and lecture notes. Symposium, presented by Langer Biomedical Group, sponsored by the Neurodevelopmental Treatment Association; May 20–22, 1983; New York, NY.

52 Oatis CA. Biomechanics of the foot and ankle under static conditions. *Phys Ther.* 1988;68:1815–1821.

53 Root ML, Orien WP, Weed JH. *Normal and Abnormal Biomechanics of the Foot: Clinical Biomechanics.* Los Angeles, Calif: Clinical Biomechanics Corp; 1977: vol 2.

54 Kumar SJ, MacEwen GD. Torsional abnormalities in children's lower extremities. *Orthop Clin North Am.* 1982;13:629–639.

55 Staheli LT. Torsional deformity. *Pediatr Clin North Am.* 1986;33:1373–1381.

56 Staheli LT, Engel GM. Tibial torsion. *Clin Orthop.* 1972;86:183–186.

57 Staheli LT. Rotational problems of the lower extremities. *Orthop Clin North Am.* 1987;18:503–512.

58 Staheli LT. Torsion: treatment indications. *Clin Orthop.* 1989;247:61–66.

59 Aharonson Z, Voloshin A, Steinbach TV, et al. Normal foot-ground pressure pattern in children. *Clin Orthop.* 1980;150:220–223.

60 Scrutton D. Footprint sequences of normal children under five years. *Dev Med Child Neurol.* 1969;11:44–53.

61 Staheli LT, Corbett M, Wyss C, King H. Lower extremity rotational problems in children. *J Bone Joint Surg [Am].* 1985;67:39–44.

62 Sgarlato T. *A Compendium of Podiatric Biomechanics.* San Francisco, Calif: California College of Podiatric Medicine; 1971:311.

63 Staheli LT, Clawson DK, Hubbard DD. Medial femoral torsion: experience with operative treatment. *Clin Orthop.* 1980;146:222–225.

64 Sutherland DH, Olshen R, Cooper A, Dale D. The development of mature gait. *J Bone Joint Surg [Am].* 1980;62:336–353.

65 Õunpuu S, Andrews M, Gage JR. The effects of internal tibial derotation osteotomy on the gait of children with cerebral palsy. *Dev Med Child Neurol.* 1989;31(suppl 59):8. Abstract.

66 Hoppenfeld S. *Physical Examination of the Spine and Extremities.* East Norwalk, Conn: Appleton-Century-Crofts; 1976:144, 186–189.

67 Dega W. Richerche anatomiche e meccaniche sull'anca fetale rivolte a chiarire l'etiologia e la patogenisi della lussazione congenita. *Chir Organi di Movimento.* 1933;18:425–505.

68 Ogden JA. *Skeletal Injury in the Child.* Philadelphia, Pa: Lea & Febiger; 1982:16–40.

69 Forero N, Okamura LA, Larson MA. Normal ranges of hip motion in neonates. *J Pediatr Orthop.* 1989;9:391–395.

70 Shands AR, Steele MK. Torsion of the femur: a follow-up report of the use of the Dunlap method for its determination. *J Bone Joint Surg [Am].* 1958;40:803–816.

71 Stuberg WA, Koehler A, Wichita M, et al. Comparison of femoral torsion assessment using goniometry and computerized tomography. *Pediatric Physical Therapy.* 1989;1(3):115–118.

72 Murphy SB, Simon SR, Kijewski PK, et al. Femoral anteversion. *J Bone Joint Surg [Am].* 1987;69:1169–1176.

73 Carroll NC. Assessment and management of the lower extremity in myelodysplasia. *Orthop Clin North Am.* 1987;18:709–724.

74 Crane L. Femoral torsion and its relation to toeing-in and toeing-out. *J Bone Joint Surg [Am].* 1959;41:421–428.

75 Knight RA. Developmental deformities of the lower extremities. *J Bone Joint Surg [Am].* 1954;36:521–526.

76 Knittel G, Staheli LT. The effectiveness of shoe modifications for intoeing. *Orthop Clin North Am.* 1976;7:1019–1025.

77 Phelps E, Smith LJ, Hallum A. Normal ranges of hip motion of infants between nine and 24 months of age. *Dev Med Child Neurol.* 1985;27:785–792.

78 Kling TF. Toe in, toe out. *Emer Med.* March 1986:32–46.

79 Wilkins KE. Bowlegs. *Pediatr Clin North Am.* 1986;33:1429–1438.

80 Grimsby O. *Fundamentals of Manual Therapy: A Course Workbook.* 2nd ed. Vagsbygd, Norway: Sorlandets Fysikalske Institutt A/S; 1980.

81 Schafer RC. *Clinical Biomechanics: Musculoskeletal Actions and Reactions.* 2nd ed. New York, NY: Marcel Dekker Inc; 1987.

82 Tax HR. *Podopediatrics,* 2nd ed. Baltimore, Md: Williams & Wilkins; 1985.

83 Kisner C, Colby LA. The knee. In: Kisner C, Colby LA. *Therapeutic Exercise Foundations and Techniques.* 2nd ed. Philadelphia, Pa: FA Davis Co; 1990:345–356.

84 Warren R, Arnoczky SP, Wickiewicz TL. Anatomy of the knee. In: Nicholas JA, Hershman EB, eds. *The Lower Extremity and Spine in Sports Medicine.* St Louis, Mo: CV Mosby Co; 1986:657–694.

85 Le Damany P. La torsion des tibias, normale, pathologique, experimentale. *J de l'Anat Phys.* 1909;45:598–615.

86 Wynne-Davies R. Talipes equinovarus: a review of eighty-four cases after completion of treatment. *J Bone Joint Surg [Br].* 1964;46:464–476.

87 Dupius PV. La torsion tibiale. In: *Son Interet Clinique: Radiologique et Chirurgical.* Paris, France: Masson et Cie; 1951:3–68.

88 Root ML, Orien WP, Weed JH, Hughes RJ. *Biomechanical Examination of the Foot.* Los Angeles, Calif: Clinical Biomechanics Corp; 1971: vol 1.

89 Jakob RP, Haertel M, Stussi E. Tibial torsion calculated by computerized tomography and compared to other methods of measurement. *J Bone Joint Surg [Br].* 1980;62:238–242.

90 McCollough NC. Orthotic management. In: Lovell WW, Winter RB, eds. *Pediatric Orthopaedics.* 2nd ed. Philadelphia, Pa: JB Lippincott Co; 1986:1038–1039.

91 Larson RL. Physical examination in the diagnosis of rotary instability. *Clin Orthop.* 1983;172:38–44.

92 Valmassy RL. *Normal and Abnormal Development of the Lower Extremity in the Infant: Treatment of Common Pediatric Musculoskeletal Disorders—Course Syllabus.* San Francisco,

Calif: California College of Podiatric Medicine; 1990.

93 Mossberg K, Smith LK. Axial rotation of the knee in adult females. Cited in: Lehmkuhl LD, Smith LK. *Brunnström's Clinical Kinesiology,* 4th ed. Philadelphia, Pa: FA Davis Co; 1983:292.

94 Weber D, Agro M, eds. *Clinical Aspects of Lower Extremity Orthotics.* Oakville, Ontario, Canada: Elgan Enterprises; 1990.

95 Cusick BD. *Serial Casts: Their Use in the Management of Spasticity-Induced Foot Deformity.* Rev ed. Tucson, Ariz: Therapy Skill Builders; 1990.

96 Seibel MO. *Foot Function: A Programmed Text.* Baltimore, Md: Williams & Wilkins; 1988.

97 Rang M, Wright M. What have 30 years of medical progress done for cerebral palsy? *Clin Orthop.* 1989;247:55–60.

Lower-Extremity Surgery for Children with Cerebral Palsy: Physical Therapy Management

The purpose of this article is to discuss physical therapy for children with cerebral palsy who undergo orthopedic surgery. Children with spasticity (increased tone) often undergo surgical procedures to increase the length of the hip, knee, and ankle musculature in an attempt to improve musculoskeletal alignment and functional abilities. Presurgical assessment of posture and movement to determine potential for change in function and postsurgical management are discussed. Intervention immediately following soft tissue surgery at the hips and knees and intervention at the time of cast removal for those children immobilized in a hip spica cast are reviewed. Specific postsurgical management protocols related to immobilization in splints/casts, positioning, and treatment activities are presented. [Harryman SE. Lower-extremity surgery for children with cerebral palsy: physical therapy management. Phys Ther. 1992;72:16–24.]

Susan E Harryman

Key Words: *Cerebral palsy, surgery; Lower extremity, hip/knee; Orthopedics, general; Orthotics/splints/casts, lower extremity; Pediatrics, treatment.*

The clinical management protocols discussed in this article were initiated in 1971 and gradually modified and refined during the ensuing 20 years. The protocols were established in conjunction with orthopedic surgeons serving the Cerebral Palsy Clinic at the Kennedy Institute for Handicapped Children in Baltimore, Md, and are currently used with children receiving physical therapy services at this facility. Surgical procedures for these children are carried out at the Johns Hopkins Hospital or the Children's Hospital in Baltimore.

Numerous reports[1–5] describe lower-extremity surgical procedures in children with cerebral palsy. The majority of these reports discuss surgical techniques or musculoskeletal status prior to and following surgery. Little has been written on presurgical physical therapy assessments or physical therapy management following orthopedic surgery. Recently, there have been reports describing specific physical therapy interventions following hamstring and gracilis muscle releases[6]; for children with spastic diplegia undergoing adductor tenotomy, psoas muscle transfer, femoral osteotomy, and hamstring muscle lengthening[7]; following surgery for knee dysfunction[8]; and following procedures at the hip or knee.[9,10] In only one report[6] is there a discussion of physical therapy management during the postoperative period. The objective of this article is to stimulate further clinical discussion and research related to the most efficacious treatment of children with cerebral palsy.

Soft tissue surgical procedures at the hip and knee that are commonly performed on children with cerebral palsy include adductor tenotomy, with or without anterior division obturator neurectomy[3,11,12]; adductor transfer to the ischium[10,12]; psoas muscle release or lengthening[3,10]; hamstring muscle lengthening, release, or transfer[8]; and distal rectus femoris muscle transfer or release.[3,8] Following any of these soft tissue procedures, as well as following pelvic or femoral osteotomies, children with cerebral palsy should receive physical therapy.

The management protocol discussed in this article includes presurgical assessment, intervention in the period immediately following soft tissue surgery at the hip or knees, and intervention at the time of cast removal for

SE Harryman, MS, PT, is Director of Physical Therapy, Kennedy Institute for Handicapped Children, 707 N Broadway, Baltimore, MD 21205 (USA), and Instructor, Department of Pediatrics, Johns Hopkins School of Medicine, Baltimore, MD 21218. Address correspondence to Ms Harryman at the first address.

those children immobilized in a hip spica cast.

Presurgical Assessment

Decisions regarding orthopedic surgical procedures in children with cerebral palsy should be made, in conjunction with the family, by a professional team who has known the child for a period of time.[5,6] For some conditions, such as progressive hip subluxation, the timing and choice of procedures may be limited.[3] Often, however, the potential for surgical intervention has been present for months before surgery is scheduled. This allows the therapist and family to plan for the procedure. In addition, important decisions related to postoperative management of positioning and therapy needs should always be open for discussion by the team and family.

Improved musculoskeletal alignment is the most obvious expected result of most surgeries on the soft tissues of children with cerebral palsy. Other areas of anticipated change include quality of posture and movement, function, access to the environment, and ease of management by caregivers. Postsurgical improvement in the quality of posture and movement frequently produces immediate improvement in skills such as sitting[6] and serves as a basis for improved developmental function over an extended period of time. Functional changes in mobility may occur, not only in ambulation, but also in other areas such as in transfers to and from the wheelchair. Children with severe disabilities are likely to be easier to manage during daily care activities following orthopedic surgery. I believe that reduction in pain and deformity and increased tolerance to handling and positioning facilitate improvement in the general quality of family life. Children who are postoperatively able to be placed in and maintain more symmetrical postures in their seating system, as discussed by Hoffer,[3] exhibit improved head, trunk, and upper-extremity control. This improved control may, in turn, lead to increased interaction with the environment

through improved ability to use motorized wheelchairs, computers, augmentative communications systems, and environmental control units.

The evaluation techniques used in examining any patient with orthopedic problems, including analysis of walking patterns and documentation of passive and active range of motion (ROM), should be used with all children who have cerebral palsy. Instrumented gait analysis, if a gait laboratory is available, provides an assessment of muscle function to assist in planning surgical procedures.[3,8,14–16] In the population of children with cerebral palsy, in order to delineate which factors interfere with function, the assessment should include analyses of developmental activities and underlying automatic movement reactions.

My experience suggests certain children with cerebral palsy respond particularly well to intensive physical therapy in the immediate postoperative period, showing more mature expression of equilibrium reactions. These responses may then serve as a basis for functional improvement. For children who stabilize in abnormal patterns utilizing increased flexor, extensor, or adductor tone prior to surgery, new means are needed for maintaining posture and coordinating movement following surgery. The presurgical analysis of rolling, sitting, and crawling activities, in addition to walking, assists in determining those patterns of movement that utilize increased tone and that may be interfering with freedom of movement.

Automatic movement reactions, particularly equilibrium, should be assessed during developmental activities and should include determination of the reactions' presence or absence, factors interfering with their expression, and potential for their improved expression following surgery. All components of equilibrium, including the positioning and movement of the head, shoulders, trunk, pelvis, and extremities, should be examined. Lower-extremity components, including weight shift through the pelvis, stabilization at the

pelvis and hip, and countermovements against gravity of the pelvis and hip, can be analyzed during developmental activities such as rolling, reaching in the prone and sitting positions, sitting transitions, pulling to a standing position, and cruising (ie, walking sideways along a support). The important countermovement of hip abduction combined with extension should be assessed during both self-initiated and imposed weight shift in a variety of positions and, if necessary, in conjunction with handling techniques to reduce abnormal tone. For example, rotation of the pelvis relative to the trunk and of the femur relative to the pelvis immediately prior to facilitating weight shift may provide a temporary reduction in tone and allow optimal expression of hip abduction. Only with careful analysis of these components of equilibrium can the potential to facilitate improved function be explored.

The presurgical physical therapy assessment should provide sufficient information to determine potential for change in function, target areas for intervention, set postsurgical expectations, and determine treatment strategies. Those children in whom pelvic and lower-extremity components of equilibrium reactions can be elicited in a structured therapy session, but not spontaneously expressed in functional activities, should be considered as candidates for intensive therapy in the postsurgical period. I believe that children who show compromised expression of equilibrium reactions at the pelvis and hips secondary to increased tone, combined with abnormal postural alignment of the lower extremities secondary to muscle shortening, are particularly amenable to physical therapy intervention immediately following orthopedic surgery.

Once the physical therapist and the orthopedist have completed their respective evaluations, surgical procedures and definitive postsurgical expectations should be discussed. The physical therapy contribution related to potential for improved function in posture and movement will assist in selection and timing of procedures as well as in planning optimal postsurgical management. Recommendations should then be shared with the family and a postsurgical management plan formulated. The child's current seating systems should be assessed jointly by the orthopedist and the physical therapist with the expectation that surgery may necessitate equipment adaptations. Molded chair inserts that were adequate prior to surgery will probably no longer be satisfactory because of improved symmetry of the spine, pelvis, and hips. Seat depths often need adjustment following femoral varus osteotomy, and lateral supports for the trunk, pelvis, or femur may need repositioning following surgery at the hips. Following hamstring muscle surgery, the leg and foot supports may need to be replaced or adjusted because of a different position of the knee at rest in the chair. Specific steps must be taken to ensure that a plan is in place for appropriate adapted seating in the immediate postoperative period. The need for orthoses or other positioning devices following surgery must also be anticipated during the planning period.

Postsurgical Management—Adductor Releases

Potential Areas for Improvement

This management protocol assumes that surgery will be performed on the adductor muscles, with or without surgery to the psoas muscle. Surgical intervention to the psoas muscle is more variable. Hip adduction is one component of the tonic extensor pattern (which includes hip extension, adduction, and internal rotation; knee extension; and plantar flexion) and is frequently observed in children with cerebral palsy. The presurgical sitting posture on a flat surface often is characterized by a posterior pelvic tilt, with compensatory trunk flexion and a narrow adducted base of support. Many children habitually assume a spontaneous W-sitting posture, considered to be a compensation for increased extensor tone across the pelvis and hips, in which the legs are maintained in a flexed position by the weight of the body. Although W-sitting

is a stable and functional posture, it limits the use of the pelvis and precludes the use of countermovements of the lower extremities to assist in maintenance of balance. Presurgical patterns of movement include limited or absent weight shifting through the pelvis; limited or absent countermovements of the lower extremities; limited or absent disassociation of movement between the trunk and the pelvis, between the pelvis and the femur, and between the lower extremities; and compensatory patterns of flexion and adduction in an attempt to maintain stability.

Surgical intervention to the adductor muscles appears to interrupt a tonic extensor pattern that is often present presurgically. This intervention allows the child to use more normal patterns of posture and movement at the pelvis and hips. Decreased extensor tone at the pelvis and hips allows the pelvis to be placed in a neutral position in sitting, that is, with the pelvis perpendicular to the supporting surface. This, in turn, allows the trunk to be extended over the pelvis. The child's ability to maintain hip abduction ultimately provides a more stable base of support than was possible prior to surgery. With postoperative treatment, increased mobility of the pelvis relative to the trunk and the femur relative to the pelvis, improved hip abduction, and a newfound ability to combine hip abduction with hip extension all may lead to functional improvements in sitting stability, sitting transitions (movement in and out of sitting), and mobility. Prior to surgery, standing and walking are usually compromised by a narrow adducted base of support, which may be accompanied by compensatory flexion at the hips and knees. In my experience, improved lateral stability at the pelvis and hips combines with improved hip extension to frequently lead to significant improvement in lower-extremity weight-bearing activities. In addition, the improved lateral stability of the hip combined with improved hip abduction is helpful in arresting or decreasing hip dysplasia.

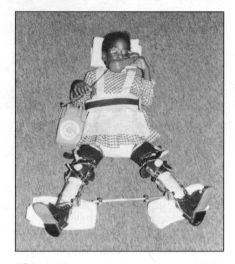

Figure 1. *Abduction orthosis used with short, tone-inhibiting leg casts.*

Splints/Casts

Children who are candidates for the type of early mobilization that is increasingly being reported in the literature[6,8–10,14,17] are placed in orthoses that are removed only for daily physical therapy. The specific orthosis used is dependent for the most part on the choice of the orthopedic surgeon. All orthoses extend proximally over the pelvis to the midtrunk for maintenance of symmetry and are adjustable in relation to amount of hip abduction, hip rotation, and knee extension. The orthoses extend distally to the foot and are usually worn in conjunction with short, nonremovable, "tone-inhibiting" leg casts (Fig. 1). At the end of 6 weeks, the orthoses are removed during the day, but continue to be used at night for a minimum of 6 to 12 months.[2,3,6,14] Children who are not candidates for early mobilization because of severity of involvement, marked hypertonicity, nonavailability of physical therapy services, or osteotomies in conjunction with soft tissue procedures are placed in a hip spica cast. Postsurgical management of these children is discussed at the end of this article.

Positioning

Structured positioning protocols are established for each child during the

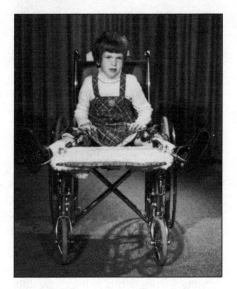

Figure 2. *Chair position in abduction orthosis.*

6 weeks immediately following surgery.[5,6,8,9,18] The prone position is used at night and initially during the day, except when the child is eating meals. In my experience, the abducted position of the hips following surgery often stimulates flexion of the hips and knees, particularly in the first few days following surgery. The accompanying abnormal flexor activity during this period is best controlled in the prone position, which, in conjunction with the orthosis, limits hip flexion. If necessary, tone-reducing medication may be used.[14] If the psoas muscle has been lengthened or released, the tendency toward hip flexion may be reduced, but the prone position is still preferred for maintaining the improved range of hip extension.

A wheelchair that has been adapted for use with abduction orthoses is used for meals, usually beginning on the third postoperative day. The pelvis is positioned as close to neutral as possible in the chair. The back of the chair is reclined as necessary to seat the pelvis in contact with the chair and allow the trunk to be positioned directly over the pelvis. By the seventh postoperative day, the pelvis can usually be maintained in a neutral position, with the seat-to-back angle at 90 degrees (Fig. 2). By the end of the

second week, during non–therapy-related activities, the chair is used most of the day, with 2 to 3 hours of prone positioning interspersed during the day. Children who exhibit increased hip flexor activity or limitations in hip extension may need increased time in the prone position or more frequent position changes.

Supported standing, with the child positioned with the hips in abduction and with the hips and knees in extension, is initiated with the use of the prone stander, on which the child can be secured in an optimal position. The prone stander is used for a minimum of 1 hour daily, usually beginning in the second week; the amount of daily use depends on the degree of influence of increased extensor activity. Orthoses are removed, but short leg casts are worn during use of the prone stander.

Treatment Activities

Treatment activities begin on the third postoperative day.[6] The initial focus of treatment is to develop tolerance for supported movement without eliciting abnormal patterns. Normal movement patterns such as symmetrical hip flexion are encouraged, and therapeutic handling techniques are used to inhibit the abnormal movement patterns that are present presurgically and the abnormal flexor activity that is often seen postsurgically. The handling techniques, which reduce abnormal muscle activity, are not the primary focus or goal of treatment, but are used to prepare the child to maintain postures and to execute movements in the most normal manner possible.

I believe that all treatment should be based on the principle of the neurodevelopmental approach, with initial emphasis on weight-shifting activities in the prone position to assist the child in spontaneously using the movements of abduction with extension as part of the equilibrium reactions. These weight-shifting activities may be performed on a moving surface such as a therapy ball or during facilitated active movements such as when reaching in

a prone position or rolling. During prone activities on the ball, the initial expected response is maintenance of hip abduction to oppose the presurgical adduction response. Weight shifting through the pelvis is encouraged to elicit a countermovement of the pelvis, which will later be accompanied by a countermovement of hip abduction with extension.

Handling techniques used during rolling from a supine to a prone position have the ability to facilitate disassociated movement between the lower extremities, between the femur and the pelvis, and between the pelvis and the trunk. For example, emphasis is placed on initiating movement with hip flexion of the leading lower extremity rather than bilateral hip flexion when rolling from a supine to a prone position. Weight shifting through the pelvis, requiring disassociation of the pelvis from the trunk, with active hip extension and abduction, requiring disassociation of the femur from the pelvis, is emphasized as the transition to a prone position is completed. During rolling from a side-lying or prone position to a supine position, hip abduction, hip extension, and active movement of the pelvis on the trunk are stressed.

Supported sitting is initiated on the third postoperative day. Initial emphasis is placed on achieving an erect trunk over a neutral pelvis and maintaining posture with trunk extension, hip flexion, and knee extension. To develop optimal control of the trunk over the pelvis, most children require considerable practice in this new posture. Weight-shifting activities in both a long-sitting position and a sitting position with the hips and knees flexed to 90 degrees are introduced as soon as a stable midline posture can be maintained. Weight shifting is usually encouraged through active reaching while the child is seated on a stable surface, I believe, because the various components of equilibrium can be more easily isolated on a stable surface than on a moving surface such as the therapy ball. Self-initiated movement is also more readily incorporated into functional activities in the sitting position in contrast to maintenance of posture on a moving surface, which has minimal functional purpose in daily life. Emphasis during weight-shifting activities is placed on facilitating trunk elongation in contrast to lateral trunk flexion on the weight-bearing side, rotating the trunk relative to the pelvis, and achieving countermovement against gravity of the pelvis combined with hip abduction and extension. Movements into and out of a sitting position, especially from a prone to a sitting position, are used to obtain active rotation of the trunk relative to the pelvis, weight shift through the pelvis, disassociation of movement between the femur and pelvis, and active hip abduction and extension.[9]

Supported standing activities are introduced through use of the prone stander, usually during the second postoperative week. Children who were ambulatory prior to surgery will also begin standing activities with a walker. When hip abduction with hip and knee extension can be maintained while standing with a walker, weight-shifting activities are introduced. To facilitate weight shifting through the pelvis, emphasis is placed on reaching activities, trunk elongation in contrast to lateral trunk flexion on the weight-bearing side, maintenance of hip extension on the weight-bearing side, and hip abduction on the unweighted side. Weight shifting through the pelvis, disassociation of movement between the femur and pelvis, and active hip abduction in an extended position can also be encouraged through cruising. The therapist should ensure that the child's pelvis is parallel to the supporting surface to achieve hip abduction rather than hip flexion and that the trunk and pelvis are free from the supporting surface to achieve weight shift through the pelvis and hips without support of the pelvis and trunk. Moving between sitting and standing postures provides an opportunity for the child to control hip and knee extension while maintaining hip abduction. Assuming a standing posture through one-half kneeling requires disassociation of movement between the lower extrem-

ities as well as more refined pelvic stability.

Ambulation activities are initiated when hip abduction with relative hip and knee extension can be maintained during weight-shifting activities while standing at a support. In our facility, all children, even those who are freely ambulatory prior to surgery, begin ambulation with an assistive device to ensure the best postural alignment and control. Walking is usually initiated with the use of a posterior walker to facilitate hip extension.[6] The use of quad canes, progressing to single-point canes if the child is able, is begun as soon as possible after surgery to improve lateral hip stability.

Six weeks following surgery, the orthoses are no longer used during the day, although their use is continued at night. Close monitoring of posture and movement patterns by the therapist is necessary for the next 2 to 3 weeks as the child gradually returns to a less structured therapy protocol; is free to move in the environment; and increases participation in school, play, and daily living activities. In my experience, a majority of the children who receive therapy in the immediate postoperative period will be functionally stable sitters when orthoses are removed during the day. I believe that children who were walking prior to surgery will usually be ambulatory with improved quality of posture and movement. Walking speed and distance, at this time, will usually be decreased in comparison with the presurgical status because of decreased endurance and the need to adapt to new patterns of movement, but should gradually improve as lateral hip stability continues to improve.

Postsurgical Management— Soft Tissue Surgery at the Knees

Potential Areas for Improvement

The management protocol outlined is designed for children who have surgical releases of the hamstring muscles, with or without surgery to the rectus

femoris or psoas muscle. Before surgery, because of the tightness of the hamstring muscles, the child sits with posterior pelvic tilt and a resultant compensatory flexion of the trunk. The tilt is increased when the child is placed in a long-sitting position, but the posterior pelvic tilt usually is present in sitting with the hips and knees flexed to 90 degrees (ie, the "90/90" position) as well. The majority of children will have learned to habitually maintain a W-sitting posture in which the legs are maintained in a flexed position by the weight of the body. Although the child may have successfully used this posture to maintain a stable sitting position prior to surgery, this posture prevents the lower extremities from contributing to equilibrium reactions when the child sits or moves from the sitting position. Following surgery, the increased length of the hamstring muscles allows the child to achieve and maintain a neutral position of the pelvis during sitting. The trunk can then be extended over the pelvis. The lower extremities, as a result, are free to move separately from the pelvis, and there is increased ROM at both the hips and the knees. I find that children frequently demonstrate dramatically improved sitting posture after surgery, and this improved posture leads to independent sitting with increased stability and function within the first 2 to 3 weeks following surgery.[6]

Prior to surgery, standing is usually compromised by knee flexion with compensatory hip flexion or plantar flexion. I have observed that ambulatory children usually walk with short stride lengths and show knee flexion during mid-stance and terminal stance and decreased endurance attributable to inefficiencies in gait. During the normal gait cycle, the knee provides energy conservation throughout stance by minimizing the vertical excursion of the body's center of mass.[14] This is accomplished by knee flexion during the loading response, with progressive extension during mid-stance and terminal stance. Maintenance of knee flexion in children with cerebral palsy, therefore, results in increased energy consumption.[14]

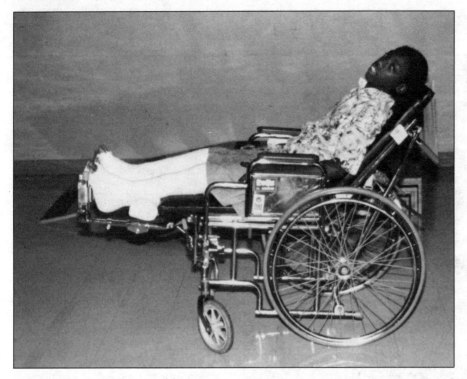

Figure 3. *Reclined sitting in long leg casts following hamstring muscle surgery.*

Lengthening of the hamstring muscles, combined with surgical intervention for the rectus femoris or psoas muscle, if necessary, allows for a qualitatively more normal posture with hip and knee extension. This improved posture, in turn, leads to improved stability, function, and efficiency in standing and walking.

Following surgery, children with quadriplegia and little or no equilibrium reactions will often be able to maintain the pelvis in neutral within their seating system, even when they cannot achieve unsupported sitting. The neutral position of the pelvis allows for improved trunk extension with potentially improved head and upper-extremity control.

Splints/Casts

Following surgery, children are placed in long leg casts or short, tone-inhibiting leg casts with knee-ankle-foot orthoses (KAFOs) for a period of 6 weeks. The immobilization method depends on the preference of the orthopedist. Those children whose knees cannot be fully extended during

surgery are usually placed in plaster casts and may undergo serial casting[8,18] during the initial immobilization period. The use of removable orthoses, whenever possible, is recommended to allow early mobilization and active involvement of the knee. Knee-ankle-foot orthoses continue to be used at night for a minimum of 6 to 12 months.

Positioning

Following hamstring muscle surgery, positioning should be designed to achieve the full length of the hamstring muscles, such as would be needed for long sitting with the pelvis in neutral. I believe alternate positioning should support combining hip extension as needed for standing activities with knee extension. Supported sitting for meals is usually initiated in an adapted wheelchair on the third postoperative day. Seating after surgery (Fig. 3) usually requires a reclined chair,[6,8] so that the pelvis will be in contact with the chair back and the trunk will be directly over the pelvis. Within the limits of comfort, the angle of inclination is gradually

reduced. In our experience, this reduction usually results in a neutral position of the pelvis within 7 to 10 days following surgery. The neutral pelvic position in the chair should be maintained either with pelvic straps (Fig. 4) or by securing the child in the chair using the foot plates (Fig. 5). Older children who have had long-standing contractures may require a longer period of time to achieve a neutral position.

The prone position is used at night.[6] The prone position is also the initial primary position used during the day, and it is used for varying amounts of time, depending on the status of the hip flexors. If the hip flexors have been released or lengthened, or if they are tight, the maintenance of hip extension is important to allow for optimal positioning of the hips and lumbar spine when the child stands and walks. Positioning in the prone stander is usually initiated at the end of the first postoperative week. The angle of inclination should be reduced if the child is experiencing hip flexion spasms when attempting to maintain an antigravity position.

By the end of the second week, the long-sitting position,[5,6,8] with the pelvis in neutral and the hips flexed and abducted, is used for a minimum of 6 hours daily. The prone position is used 1 to 2 hours daily, and the prone stander is used a minimum of 1 hour daily. The remaining hours are individualized for each child, depending on the factors mentioned.

Treatment Activities

Treatment activities begin on the third postoperative day, and, as with hip surgery, the initial focus is on increasing tolerance to supported movement without eliciting flexor spasms or abnormal patterns of posture and movement. Therapeutic handling techniques to inhibit abnormal movement patterns are used to prepare the child to maintain posture and execute movement in the most normal pattern possible. As with soft tissue releases at

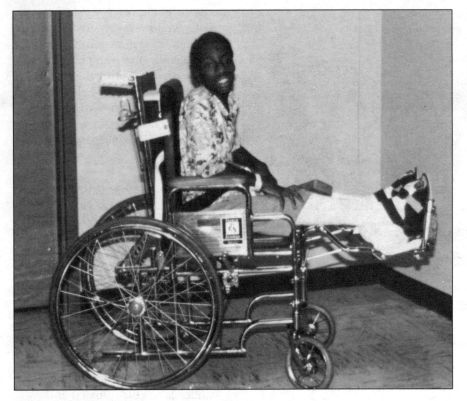

Figure 4. *Neutral pelvic position maintained by foot pedals.*

lengthening often experience considerable difficulty in adapting to a new standing posture with their knees extended. Prior to surgery, hip flexion has frequently been used as a compensatory posture. Following surgery, the child may attempt to use hip flexion in conjunction with knee extension and increased lumbar lordosis, which is a stable posture and precludes the need to grade movement between flexion and extension of the hips and knees.

With the child, standing activities are used to achieve and maintain hip extension, in combination with hip abduction and knee extension. Treatment activities focus on weight shifting through the pelvis to maintain hip extension on the weight-bearing side, use of the abdominal muscles to support the pelvis and thus decrease lumbar lordosis, and midrange control of the knee as during movement between sitting and standing positions.

Children who were ambulatory prior to surgery usually begin walking with their knees immobilized in extension

the hip, however, handling techniques to reduce tone are not the primary focus or goal of treatment.

Children immobilized in long leg casts will participate in prone and rolling activities that emphasize hip extension to increase hip control and stability. This activity is similar to that discussed in the section related to soft tissue surgery of the hips. If the child is immobilized in orthoses that can be removed during daily physical therapy, graded knee flexion and extension are initiated as well. If surgery has not included the rectus femoris muscle, emphasis is placed on maintaining the length of this muscle, as increased spasticity (hypertonicity) is often observed in the rectus femoris muscle after lengthening of the hamstring muscles.[17] This finding agrees with the finding of Reimers[4] that, in the presence of spasticity, the antagonist functions more strongly following lengthening and weakening of the agonist. Controlled knee extension during movement transitions and in combination with hip extension dur-

ing weight-bearing activities is stressed.

Achieving a neutral position of the pelvis in a sitting position is the focus of numerous activities during therapy. Flexion of the trunk, a habitual presurgical compensatory position for posterior pelvic tilt, usually continues in the immediate postoperative period. Trunk extension over a neutral pelvis must be continually encouraged.[6] Many children require considerable experience in this new posture in order to develop the ability to maintain a midline position of the trunk over the pelvis. If splints can be removed during therapy, 90/90 sitting and movement from a prone to a sitting position can be incorporated into the treatment program. Following hamstring muscle surgery, a neutral pelvic position is more quickly obtained in 90/90 sitting than in long sitting. Sitting with hip and knee flexion, in turn, will allow earlier introduction of weight-shifting activities.

I have found that children who are ambulatory prior to hamstring muscle

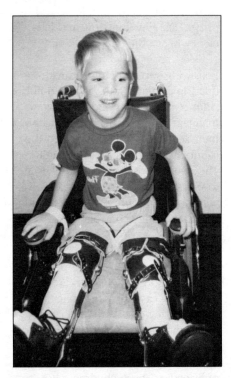

Figure 5. *Neutral pelvic position maintained by pelvic straps.*

within the first postoperative week. If the child uses KAFOs, the orthoses are unlocked during weight-bearing activities, once knee extension can be combined with hip extension during the stance phase of gait. As the ability to maintain midrange control of the knee improves, KAFOs are discontinued and ambulation continues in short, tone-inhibiting leg casts, which are also called "tone-reducing ankle-foot orthoses" (TRAFOs). All children in our facility use a walker or canes to facilitate hip extension until they are sufficiently secure in the new posture such that they do not revert to the presurgical flexion posture of the hips and knees while standing or walking.

At the end of the 6-week period of immobilization, children are usually placed in floor-reaction ankle-foot-orthoses (AFOs), which are rigid AFOs with an anterior shell extending over the proximal tibia. The floor-reaction AFO limits the forward progression of the tibia in mid-stance and assists with maintaining extension of the knee in the first few months following surgery.[8] All children should be closely monitored to determine readiness for improved function with articulated AFOs.[8] I believe that children who have used short leg casts with removable KAFOs during the previous 6 weeks adapt quickly to the floor-reaction AFOs and that children who were ambulatory prior to surgery resume some degree of functional ambulation after 6 weeks, with improved quality of both posture and movement. Children who were immobilized at the knee for the previous 6 weeks often need additional time to regain adequate knee control to return to their previous level of function. According to Gage,[8] improvement can continue for a full year as the child incorporates new muscle length into the walking pattern. With all children, hamstring muscle length is maintained through long sitting, in KAFOs locked at the knees, each day at the time of night brace application.

Postsurgical Management—Immobilization in Hip Spica Cast

Rationale for Hip Spica Cast

Children who are not candidates for early mobilization because of significant involuntary movement, marked hypertonicity, nonavailability of physical therapy services, or osteotomies in conjunction with soft tissue procedures are placed in a hip spica cast.

Positioning

The obvious concerns related to skin integrity, swelling, and circulation must be addressed as well as those more specific to children with cerebral palsy, such as abnormalities in muscle tone. The posture of the head, neck, and upper extremities should be controlled through positioning. Good alignment will help to decrease hypertonus, inhibit fixation patterns, and maintain ROM and function. Support of interaction with the environment for the child in a hip spica cast may require a special mobility device or adaptation of a communication system. Children with significant oral motor disability need ongoing assessment and management of nutritional needs during this period of prolonged immobilization. The presurgical position used for eating is usually not possible because of the hip spica cast, and alternative techniques for feeding the child frequently must be established.

Splints/Casts

Following cast removal, an abduction orthosis is used at night to maintain the surgical result. The orthosis should extend proximally to midtrunk level to control the position of the pelvis and hips.[9] Extension of the orthosis below the knees or to the feet is optional and dependent on the ROM of the knees and feet.

Treatment Activities

Physical therapy is begun on the day of cast removal (ie, about 6 weeks postsurgically). Because increased flexor

activity of the hips and knees is prevalent immediately following cast removal, medication to reduce increased muscle tone is frequently used as an adjunct to treatment and management. Initial emphasis is placed on reducing flexor spasms, establishing positioning, and achieving supported movement during position changes. The prone position, with the lower extremities abducted and extended, is the primary position in the first few days, alternating with supported sitting in an adapted chair for meals. The family or other caregivers must be instructed in handling techniques for controlled movement and postural transitions to reduce the possibility of sudden, uncontrolled flexion, because the supracondylar area of the femur is a common site of fractures in the osteoporotic, nonambulatory child.[3] An appropriate chair is essential and can be temporarily adapted to provide the necessary support on the day of cast removal. The chair should support the improved position of the pelvis and hips and limit knee flexion to help prevent distal femoral fractures.

Approximately 7 to 10 days following cast removal, children usually show no signs of distress during supported movement and are able to tolerate supported sitting for several hours at a time. Children with limited motor development, for whom the goal is supported sitting, have usually at this point completed specific postoperative treatment activities and are ready to return to school. Children who were able to sit or walk presurgically, or have the potential to do so, should continue with therapy, as discussed in the section on adductor releases.

Research Considerations

Although the orthopedic literature is replete with articles related to children with cerebral palsy who undergo orthopedic procedures, little has been documented comparing presurgical function with postsurgical function. Postsurgical ROM,[4,5] radiographic assessments of the hip joint,[2,5,19] descriptions of weight-bearing posture of the lower extremities,[3,5] and ambulatory status[5,7,8] are frequently reported, but this population's postsurgical functional status is less frequently compared with their presurgical functional status. As gait laboratories have become more available, comparative gait analysis has been used to document postoperative change in muscle function and joint angles, assess the surgical results, adjust bracing, and consider additional surgery.[8,14,16]

Physical therapists providing treatment for children with cerebral palsy have an obligation to assist in establishing the most efficacious treatments for these children. A presurgical level of functional performance documented by the physical therapist and expressed in an objective manner provides a baseline for comparison following surgical intervention. Detailed evaluations, established baselines, well-defined treatment strategies, and monitoring of progress are necessary for determining the effectiveness of the therapeutic intervention. In addition to this systematic collection of data, therapists must be willing to share and report results of therapeutic intervention in order to establish the efficacy of physical therapy in children with motor impairment.

Summary

Under optimal conditions, decisions related to orthopedic surgery in children with cerebral palsy should be made, in conjunction with the family, by a team of health professionals who have known the child for a period of time. During a presurgical physical therapy assessment, the therapist should determine potential for change, target areas for postsurgical intervention, determine postsurgical expectations, and delineate initial treatment strategies. Structured positioning protocols and individualized treatment activities must be incorporated into the postsurgical intervention plan. Night splinting and continued monitoring with timely adjustment of the management plan, at least within the first 12 months after surgery, are necessary to support long-term maintenance of the surgical result.

References

1 Bleck EE. *Orthopaedic Management in Cerebral Palsy.* London, England: MacKeith Press; 1987:289–358.

2 Gamble JG, Rinsky LA, Bleck EE. Established hip dislocations in children with cerebral palsy. *Clin Orthop.* 1990;253:90–99.

3 Hoffer MM. Management of the hip in cerebral palsy. *J Bone Joint Surg [Am].* 1986;68: 629–632.

4 Reimers J. Functional changes in the antagonists after lengthening the agonists in cerebral palsy. *Clin Orthop.* 1990;253:35–37.

5 Smith JT, Stevens PM. Combined adductor transfer, iliopsoas release, and proximal hamstring release in cerebral palsy. *J Pediatr Orthop.* 1989;9:1–5.

6 Girolami GL, Hertz K. *Early Mobilization and Postsurgical Management After Hamstring or Gracilis Muscle Release in Children with Cerebral Palsy: Topics in Pediatrics, Lesson 8.* Alexandria, Va: American Physical Therapy Association; 1990.

7 Okawa A, Kajiura I, Hiroshima K. Physical therapeutic and surgical management in spastic diplegia. *Clin Orthop.* 1990;253:38–44.

8 Gage JR. Surgical treatment of knee dysfunction in cerebral palsy. *Clin Orthop.* 1990;253: 45–54.

9 Atkins EM, Harryman SE, Silberstein CE. *Potential for Change Following Orthopedic Surgery (Instructional Course).* Boston, Mass: American Academy for Cerebral Palsy and Developmental Medicine; 1990.

10 Sussman MD. *Orthopedic Management of Cerebral Palsy (Instructional Course).* Boston, Mass: American Academy for Cerebral Palsy and Developmental Medicine; 1987.

11 Jones ET, Knapp R. Assessment and management of the lower extremity in cerebral palsy. *Orthop Clin North Am.* 1987;18:725–738.

12 Wheeler ME, Weinstein SL. Adductor tenotomy: obturator neurectomy. *J Pediatr Orthop.* 1984;4:48–51.

13 Reimers J, Poulsen S. Adductor transfer versus tenotomy for stability of the hip in cerebral palsy. *J Pediatr Orthop.* 1984;4:52–54.

14 Gage JR, Fabian D, Hicks RR, Tashman S. Pre- and post-operative gait analysis in patients with spastic diplegia: a preliminary report. *J Pediatr Orthop.* 1984;4:715–725.

15 Perry J. Distal rectus femoris transfer. *Dev Med Child Neurol.* 1987;29:153–158.

16 Gage JR, Perry J, Hicks RR, et al. Rectus femoris transfer to improve knee function of children with cerebral palsy. *Dev Med Child Neurol.* 1987;29:159–166.

17 Rang M, Silver R, De La Garza J. Cerebral palsy. In: Lovell WW, Winter RB, eds. *Pediatric Orthopedics.* Philadelphia, Pa: JB Lippincott Co; 1986:365.

18 Sharpes CH, Clancy M, Steel HH. A long-term retrospective study of proximal hamstring release for hamstring contracture in cerebral palsy. *J Pediatr Orthop.* 1984;4:443–447.

19 Schultz RS, Chamberlain SE, Stevens PM. Radiographic comparison of adductor procedures in cerebral palsied hips. *J Pediatr Orthop.* 1984;4:741–744.

The Ilizarov Procedure: Limb Lengthening and Its Implications

The purpose of this article is to provide a historical and clinical perspective on the Ilizarov method of external fixation for limb lengthening and deformity correction of the lower extremity. Though relatively new in the United States, the technique has been applied for orthopedic problems with great success for over three decades in Russia and Europe. Physical therapy management is discussed from the preoperative planning phase to removal of the apparatus. [Simard S, Marchant M, Mencio G. The Ilizarov procedure: limb lengthening and its implications. Phys Ther. 1992;72:25–34.]

Key Words: *External fixation, Ilizarov procedure, Orthopedics.*

Stephanie Simard
Mary Marchant
Gregory Mencio

The Ilizarov external fixator is a complex combination of metal rings, threaded rods, and Kirschner wires used for the correction of limb deformities, specifically limb-length inequalities. The fixator is used to create an environment in which distraction osteogenesis takes place. Distraction osteogenesis is a form of direct membranous ossification.[1] A fibrovascular lattice spans the two ends of bone that are undergoing distraction and does so without a cartilage intermediary. Bony trabeculae orient longitudinally in the lattice to form a fibrous-like interzone.[1] This interzone is composed of primitive mesenchymal

cells that differentiate into osteoblasts, which form the bone. Normally, the process of bone growth is controlled by the growth rates of the physes at each end of the bone, whereas in distraction osteogenesis, the rate of lengthening is controlled mechanically by the external fixator.[1] The Ilizarov device has been recently introduced in the United States and has been used successfully with children,[2] but the device is not limited to pediatric use. This article provides an overview of the history, application, advantages, and complications of the Ilizarov external fixator. The rehabili-

tation course of patients who undergo this procedure is also described.

History

The Ilizarov method of external fixation originated during World War II when numerous cases of osteomyelitis and bone deformities occurred.[3] In 1943, Professor Gavriil Abramovich Ilizarov developed a transfixion-wire, circular external fixation system using metal rings, wires, and threaded rods with nuts. This fixation system was initially used for stabilizing fractures and managing difficult bone and soft tissue problems.

Limb lengthening was not a new concept in the 1940s. Codvilla,[3] in 1905, reported the use of this procedure in the English orthopedic literature. Ilizarov, however, refined the method by which bone and soft tissue could regenerate based on a principle called "tension stress." According to Ilizarov, bone and soft tissue, including skin, muscle, and neurovascular structures, will heal and regenerate in a predictable manner under tension. Ilizarov suggested that, with stable

S Simard, BS, PT, was Staff Physical Therapist, Newington Children's Hospital, 181 E Cedar St, Newington, CT 06111, when this article was written. She is currently Staff Physical Therapist and Clinical Coordinator, Greater Hartford Physical Therapy, 85 Gillett St, Hartford, CT 06105 (USA). She is also a student in the Orthopaedic Physical Therapy Master's Degree Program at Quinnipiac College, Hamden, CT. Address all correspondence to Ms Simard.

M Marchant, MAPT, PT, was Staff Physical Therapist, Newington Children's Hospital, when this article was written. She is currently pursuing her doctoral degree in community health at the University of Connecticut, Storrs, CT.

G Mencio, MD, was Assistant Professor of Orthopaedic Surgery, University of Connecticut, Storrs, CT 06268, and Director, Limb Lengthening/Reconstructive Service, Newington Children's Hospital, when this article was written. He is currently Assistant Professor of Orthopaedics and Rehabilitation, Department of Orthopaedics (ND-4207), Vanderbilt University Medical Center, Medical Center North, Nashville, TN 37232.

external skeletal fixation, blood supply preservation, and controlled mechanical distraction, new bone would form within an osteotomy site. By inducing tension stress with the circular external fixator, Ilizarov devised numerous strategies for lengthening limbs while simultaneously correcting associated angular and rotational malalignments, transporting bone segments to fill fracture gaps, and healing nonunited fractures.[4,5]

Purpose and Candidate Selection

When Ilizarov developed this technique, its principal goals were to stabilize long-bone fractures, to correct angular deformities, and to minimize limb-length discrepancies. As this technique has evolved, it has been utilized in the management of a variety of other orthopedic conditions, such as joint contractures and pseudarthroses of long bones (whether congenital or acquired), and in the lengthening of vasculature to avoid amputation secondary to peripheral vascular disease.[6]

Typical goals of Ilizarov external fixator use with children are to lengthen long bones, to correct angular deformities, to provide fixation for fractures, and to facilitate bone growth at sites of nonunion. This article will focus specifically on lengthening and deformity correction of the long bones in the lower extremity, because this is the most common application of the Ilizarov external fixator to date.

Limb-length inequality is a common problem encountered during the growing years and can be caused by a variety of conditions. In the past, poliomyelitis was the most common cause of limb-length inequality[7]; however, the use of prophylactic vaccination has greatly reduced the incidence of poliomyelitis. Today, marked limb-length inequality may result from congenital or developmental abnormalities or from growth arrest of the physes induced by infection or trauma. Malposition of fracture fragments and inflammatory diseases may also contribute to the development of

asymmetries. Minor asymmetries between right and left sides are very common; discrepancies from a few millimeters to 2 cm are observed in approximately two thirds of US Army recruits.[7] Limb-length discrepancies greater than 2 cm often result in pelvic obliquity, scoliosis, alterations in normal walking pattern, and abnormal loading of the hip and patellofemoral joints on the long side, with the attendant risks of premature arthrosis.[8]

We believe that discrepancies less than 2 cm generally are not clinically significant and do not require surgical treatment. Discrepancies between 2 and 6 cm are usually treated by a procedure to shorten the longer limb. For discrepancies greater than 6 cm, the shorter limb can be lengthened or a combined lengthening and shortening procedure can be performed. In very severe discrepancies, amputation of the deficient limb and prosthetic fitting may be appropriate.[8]

Shortening of the longer limb can be achieved by epiphysiodesis, a procedure in which the epiphyseal plates about the knee are surgically obliterated in a skeletally immature patient who has sufficient growth remaining in the shorter limb to accommodate the discrepancy.[8] Alternatively, if there is insufficient growth remaining, the longer limb can be shortened by excising a segment of bone and then stabilizing it with a metal plate or rod.[8]

For patients with larger discrepancies (ie, >6 cm) or those of short stature with lesser discrepancies in whom shortening or epiphysiodesis may not be appropriate, limb lengthening is an option. The advantages of this approach are fairly obvious. By performing a corrective procedure on the abnormal, shorter limb rather than a compensatory procedure on the longer, normal limb, stature is not compromised and body proportions are maintained. The results of limb lengthening can be quite dramatic. Limb lengthening, however, is a much more complex procedure than either the limb-shortening or epiphysiodesis procedure.[9,10]

Surgical Procedure

The basic components of the Ilizarov fixator are smooth and beaded transfixion wires (1.5 or 1.8 mm in diameter), metal rings and arches, threaded rods, and an array of miscellaneous hardware for interconnecting the basic components. The technique for wire insertion includes passing the wire through skin and soft tissue, drilling it through near and far cortices of the bone, and then tapping it through the soft tissue and skin to avoid winding of soft tissue or neurovascular structures around the surgical instrument. The wires are attached to a series of half or full metal rings, which encircle the affected limb, and tensioned to enhance stability. The fixator is completed by connecting the rings with threaded rods aligned colinearly, in the case of straight lengthenings, or at angles by using hinges, if angular deformity correction is planned. The modular design of the system allows for customized assemblage into an almost infinite variety of configurations, making it extremely versatile (Fig. 1).[5,6,11,12]

A corticotomy is then performed through the metaphyseal portion of the bone. This is a special type of osteotomy wherein only the cortex of the bone is cut, leaving intact the periosteal and endosteal blood supplies, which are the most important elements responsible for osteogenesis. The corticotomy is accomplished through a 1-cm incision under fluoroscopic guidance, so as to minimally disrupt the soft tissues enveloping the bone.[11]

After a latency period of 5 to 10 days, distraction is begun by turning the nuts on the threaded rods 0.25 mm four times per day, resulting in a total lengthening of 1 mm a day (Fig. 2). As the distraction proceeds, osteogenesis occurs within the gap (Fig. 3). When the desired limb length has been achieved, the distraction is stopped, but the fixator is not removed to allow consolidation of the new bone. The consolidation phase is generally double the time span re-

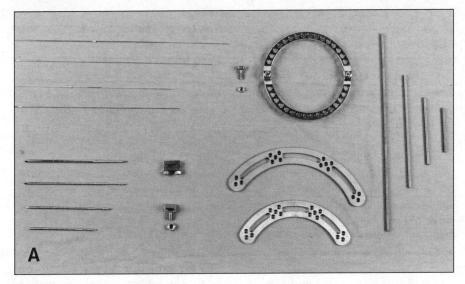

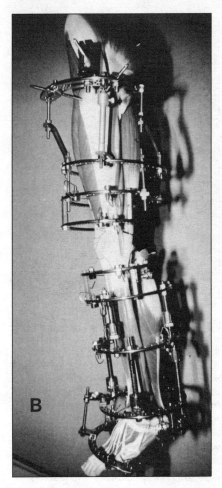

Figure 1. *Ilizarov apparatus hardware: Wires of half pins insert into bone and are then attached to threaded rods (A); modular design allows for customized assemblage into an almost infinite variety of frame configurations (B).*

quired for limb lengthening. Total treatment time using this method averages about 1 month per centimeter of limb lengthened. Although this procedure may seem somewhat protracted, the patient remains ambulatory throughout treatment, can bear full weight on the extremity, is encouraged to participate in low-impact activities (eg, isokinetic training, stationary bicycling, walking on a treadmill), and may swim.[11,12]

Results with this technique can be quite dramatic. Lengthenings of 20% to 30% of the original length of the bone can be achieved (Figs. 4, 5). In contrast to previous methods of limb lengthening (eg, distractional epiphyseolysis, Wagner method, Anderson-Mitchell method), in which bone regeneration was unpredictable and mechanical difficulties with the fixators were common, treatment goals are usually met with the Ilizarov technique and patient satisfaction is almost universal.[13–15]

Advantages

The Ilizarov method has numerous advantages compared with other methods of limb lengthening and deformity correction. First, osteogenesis occurs immediately to bridge the dis-

traction gap. Second, the regenerating bone quickly resembles the already existing bone. Third, the ability to grow new bone exists even in mature bone, making the Ilizarov method effective in adults as well as in children.[2] Another advantage is the modular design of the fixator, which allows each apparatus to be custom-fit for the individual. The use of 1.5- to 1.8-mm pins produces fewer pin-track problems (ie, infection of pin sites) than do conventional methods of limb lengthening, which use larger-diameter (4.5-6.0 mm) half pins. Moreover, the tensioned, smaller-diameter wires are inherently able to withstand dynamic loading of the lengthening segment, which experimentally has been shown to be favorable for fracture gap healing.[16,17]

The circular configuration of the frame enhances stability while ensuring that stress is evenly distributed across the corticomy and distraction gap. This biomechanical combination of frame stability and axial elasticity allows for weight bearing throughout the limb-lengthening and consolidation periods while ensuring osteogenesis across the distraction gap.[16,17]

Complications/Problems

Problems, obstacles, and complications that may arise with the Ilizarov technique during limb lengthening include muscle contractures, joint subluxation, axial deviation, neurological or vascular insult, premature consolidation, delayed consolidation, refracture, pin-site infection, and difficulties with psychological adjustment. According to Paley's classification system, *problems* represent difficulties that do not require operative intervention to resolve and *obstacles* are difficulties that do require operative intervention. *True complications* represent intraoperative injuries and all problems not resolved before the end of treatment.[10] In a study conducted by Paley in 1990, 60 limb segments were treated by the Ilizarov method of limb lengthening. From this sample, there were 35 problems, 11 obstacles, and 27 true complications. Despite these problems, obsta-

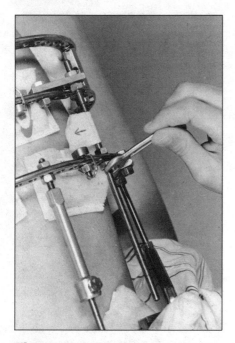

Figure 2. *Rods have 1-mm pitched threads, such that one full turn of the nut distracts or moves the rings closer by 1 mm. Patients perform limb lengthening by advancing the nut one-quarter turn four times daily. Alternatively, graduated telescopic rods with calibrated "clickers" can be used to simplify the process.*

cles, and complications, the goals of surgery were met in 57 of the 60 limb segments treated.[10]

Muscle contractures may occur because of the imbalance between the flexors and extensors on opposite sides of the bone and their resultant inability to accommodate to the distraction of the lengthening limb. Contractures often involve muscles that cross two joints. Range of motion (ROM) may be decreased in all planes of the affected joint. Additionally, there may be significant limitation in one direction because of the overpowering force of a large muscle group. For example, in lengthening of the femur, the hamstrings are the larger muscle group in mass and will therefore offer more resistance to lengthening. Patients with severe muscle contractures 1 year after removal of the fixator may require surgical intervention.[10]

Subluxation may occur in a joint that has preexisting instability or unbal-

anced muscle tension during lengthening. Femoral lengthenings may lead to posterior tibial subluxation secondary to increased stress on the posterior capsule and anterior cruciate ligament from knee hyperextension throughout the stance phase of gait. Patients with joint instability may have the fixator extended to both sides of the joint to prevent subluxation.[10]

As the limb is lengthened, there is a potential risk of angular deformity because of a deviation of the lengthened segment. This deformity may be corrected with a modification of the external hardware or of the amount of daily distraction.

There is a risk of neurological or vascular injury during surgery or distraction, although the surgical procedure is designed to minimize this type of injury. During limb lengthening, patients who are experiencing extreme pain or who demonstrate signs of vascular compromise may have the amount of daily distraction decreased.[18]

Premature consolidation of the lengthening segment may occur before the desired limb length has been achieved, and additional surgical intervention may be necessary. Delayed consolidation may increase the length of time the fixator must be worn. Refracture may also warrant that the fixator remain on for a longer period of time or may indicate the need for additional external support.

Pin-site infection may occur because of poor pin-site care by the patient. The infection must be treated promptly to avoid spreading to other pin sites and to avoid osteomyelitis.[10]

Children who undergo the Ilizarov procedure require support in adjusting to the discomfort, the care, and the loss of independence experienced after surgery. The frustration, anger, and fear felt by the children may manifest in behavior that is difficult to manage. Intervention by a psychologist for behavior management facilitates appropriate ways of coping and

dealing with the child's temporary change in lifestyle.[10]

Physical Therapy Intervention

Preoperative Phase

The preoperative evaluation of a patient who is a candidate for the Ilizarov procedure provides baseline information about the patient's musculoskeletal system and allows for early identification of potential problem areas postoperatively. We believe the preoperative evaluation should include the following:

1. Manual muscle testing of the upper and lower extremities. In the upper extremities, all shoulder, elbow, and wrist motions are tested in order to help determine what piece of adaptive equipment may be the most appropriate for ambulation postoperatively. In the lower extremities, all hip, knee, and ankle motions are tested so that baseline information is obtained. This baseline information is used to predetermine what areas may need emphasis on strengthening or stretching during the rehabilitation process.

2. Assessment of passive ROM of the upper and lower extremities. This assessment is performed to obtain baseline information for comparison postoperatively.

3. Sensation testing of the lower extremities. Sensation of the lower extremities is usually intact to light touch, deep pressure, and pinprick tests prior to surgery. After surgery, there may be alteration in normal sensation for reasons that have been explained previously. This item provides baseline information for postoperative comparison.

4. Girth measurements of bilateral thighs and calves. These measurements provide baseline data for determining the amount of edema in the limb postsurgically.

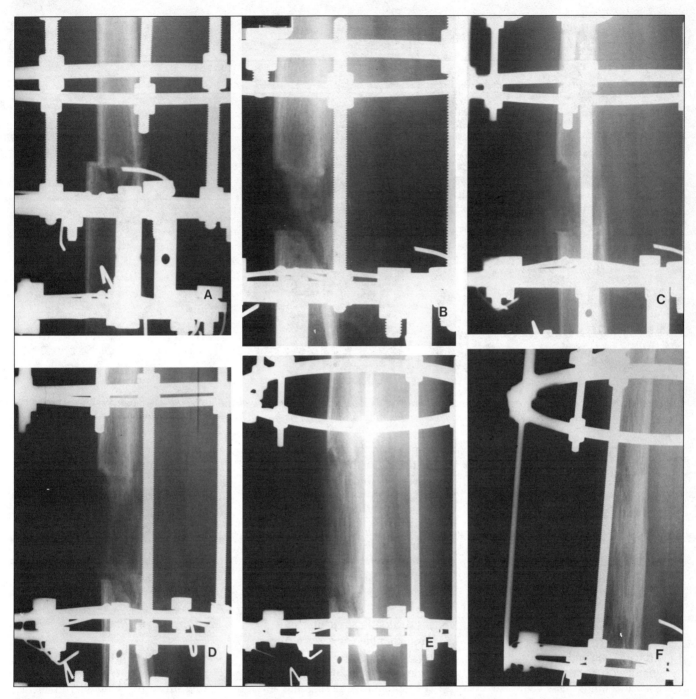

Figure 3. *Radiographs showing limb lengthening via Ilizarov method in a 12-year-old child with right hypoplasia of the femur: initial corticotomy (A), distraction phase with longitudinally oriented trabeculae filling the interzone (B-D), and maturation during the consolidation phase (E-F). Total lengthening was 8.5 cm.*

5. Measurement of shoe lift and leg-length discrepancy. These measurements are used to determine what height the shoe lift will need to be after application of the Ilizarov apparatus.

6. Assessment of joint stability. This is particularly noted at the knee joint, where postsurgical prob-

lems most frequently occur. Varus and valgus ligamentous stress tests are performed, as well as anterior and posterior drawer tests and the Lachman test.

7. Description of bony deformities. These deformities are noted preoperatively so that any effects or changes that the Ilizarov appara-

tus may have on the deformities may be monitored closely after surgery.

8. Postural and gait evaluation. A general assessment of the patient's postural tone and observation of gait serve to identify possible weaknesses in major muscle groups that will need to be partic-

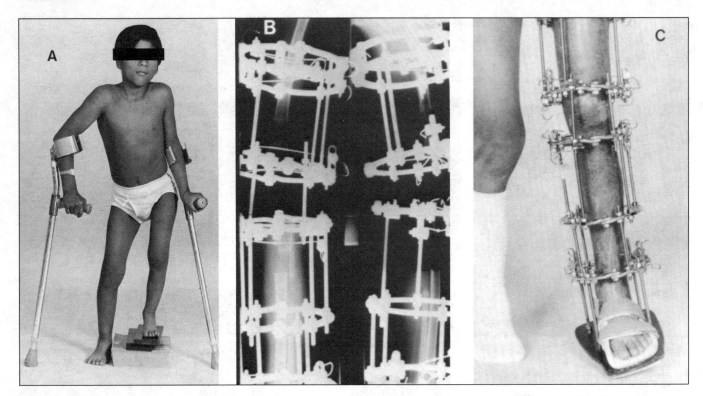

Figure 4. *Child, aged 10 years 6 months, with paralytic shortening of left leg (predicted limb-length discrepancy=7.5 cm) attributable to poliomyelitis (A). Correction by simultaneous lengthening of tibia and femur, with equalization of limb lengths (B, C).*

ularly emphasized during the rehabilitation phase.

9. Assessment of functional mobility skills. This assessment provides baseline data about the patient's ability to ambulate, to ascend and descend stairs, and to move into and out of different positions. It also identifies areas that need to be further developed after surgery.

10. Crutch fitting and instruction in ambulation, including ascending and descending stairs with crutches. This is done so that the patient will be able to learn these skills correctly and so that better carryover is achieved once the Ilizarov apparatus is in place.

11. Instruction in a home exercise program. This instruction is given so that the patient learns to perform the exercises correctly and without substitution, as well as to achieve better carryover postoperatively.

12. Instruction in postoperative positioning and splinting. This instruction is given to improve the patient's and family's carryover after surgery.

13. Instruction in stretching and strengthening exercises to prepare for surgery. The following exercises are included: gluteal sets, straight leg raising, hip abduction in a side-lying position, hip extension in a prone position, knee flexion in a prone position, quadriceps femoris muscle sets, short-arc quadriceps femoris muscle sets, knee flexion and extension in a sitting position, ankle dorsiflexion and plantar flexion, and passive heelcord stretching using a towel or Thera-Band®* in a long-sitting position.

The home exercise program for patients who are candidates for the Ilizarov procedure may include various isometric, active, and passive exercises of muscles crossing the joints above and below the segment being lengthened.[18]

Postoperative Phase

Considerations and precautions.
Precautions postoperatively may vary among surgeons. Generally, a patient is encouraged to begin activities out of bed on the first or second day after surgery. The patient is allowed to begin active-assistive and isometric exercises of the affected limb the first day after surgery. A patient with a lower-extremity Ilizarov external fixator is allowed to bear as much weight as is tolerated the first day after surgery and may begin progressive gait training 2 to 3 days after surgery.[18]

---

*The Hygenic Corp, 1245 Home Ave, Akron, OH 44310.

†The Purdue Frederick Co, 100 Connecticut Ave, Norwalk, CT 06856.

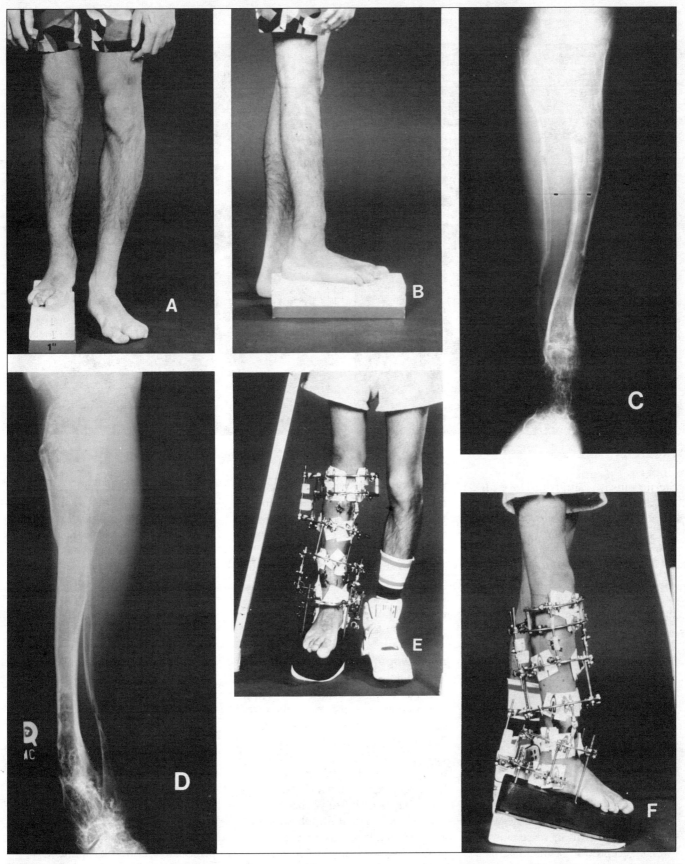

Figure 5. *Sixteen-year-old patient with Ollier's disease, predicted limb-length inequality of 11 cm, and associated multiple-level angular deformities in tibia (A, B). Anterior-posterior radiograph of tibia showing valgus angulation proximally of 30 degrees (C). Lateral radiograph showing distal procurvatum deformity of 30 degrees (D). Postoperative use of Ilizarov frame with hinges to allow gradual correction of both angular deformities, simultaneously (E, F). Note angulation of rings relative to each other, but perpendicular to the long axis of the bone in the plane of the deformity. Anterior-posterior proximal tibia (G). Lateral distal tibia (H). On completion of the angular corrections, rings are parallel to each other (I, J). Hinges have been replaced by threaded rods, and limb lengthening is being performed through the proximal corticotomy (K, L).*

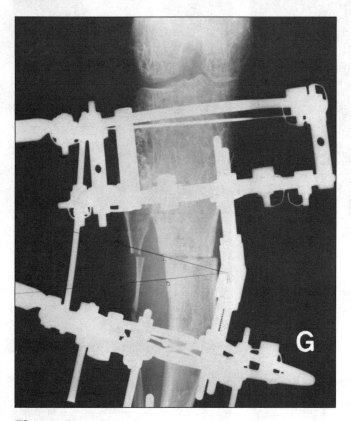

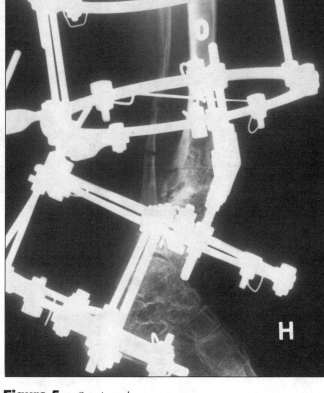

Figure 5. *Continued.*

Figure 5. *Continued.*

Sterile pin-site care, whereby each pin is individually cleansed with Betadine®† solution followed by application of sterile minisponges, is begun on the second day after surgery and is continued for 7 days. The patient may bathe after 8 days, but may not soak the fixator, as this may cause oxidation of the hardware. The patient may swim in a chlorinated pool within 1 to 4 weeks after the surgery, depending on physician preference.[18] Patients are usually hospitalized for 7 to 10 days to ensure limb lengthening is proceeding without complications.

Pre–limb-lengthening stage. Goals of physical therapy management postoperatively are to prevent joint and soft tissue contractures, to decrease pain and edema, to increase ROM of the affected limb, to increase muscle strength, to prevent or minimize gait deviations, and to restore functional mobility and independence.

Pain is a major limiting factor the first week after surgery. The use of modali-

ties in conjunction with medication can be useful for pain management. Edema after surgery can be significant; therefore, patients should be encouraged to begin isometric and active-assistive exercise the first day after surgery. Positioning of the extremity to increase ROM is also encouraged immediately postoperatively and may assist in decreasing joint stiffness.

Limb-lengthening stage. Limb lengthening is usually begun 5 days after surgery. The goals in this stage remain the same as those in the post-operative pre–limb-lengthening stage. Patients may experience increased pain or loss of ROM from the distraction placed on the limb. Patients who have significantly limited ROM at this point may benefit from dynamic splinting, which is the application of force-adjustable splints for the purpose of low-intensity, prolonged stretch.[18]

Following hospital discharge (ie, 7-10 days postsurgery), physical therapy continues three to five times a

week, with emphasis on increasing ROM and muscle strength, monitoring of splinting programs, and monitoring of shoe-lift height for patients with lower-extremity fixators.

Physical therapy techniques that have been used throughout Ilizarov rehabilitation include isokinetic exercise, eccentric exercise, passive exercise on isokinetic equipment, stationary bicycling, walking on a treadmill, electrical stimulation, hydrotherapy, massage, and gross motor developmental activities.[18]

Patients who develop pin-site infections, severe joint stiffness, or joint contractures may need to be readmitted to the hospital. Patients with joint stiffness or contractures may receive intensive physical therapy, possibly in conjunction with manipulation by the physician, followed by splinting or continuous passive motion exercises.

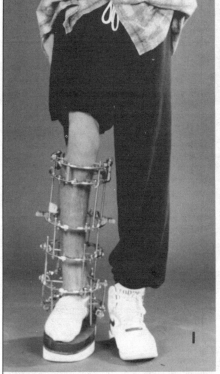
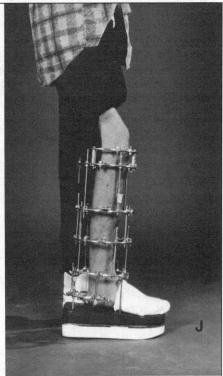
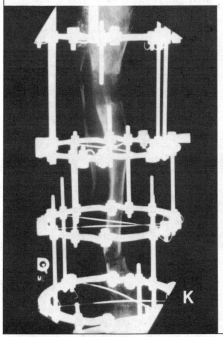
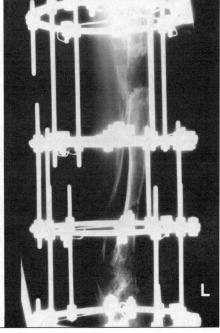

Figure 5. *Continued.*

Consolidation Phase

Goals of physical therapy management after lengthening of the limb is complete are to increase ROM where limited, to increase strength of the affected limb, and to maximize independent function.

Removal of the Fixator

Upon removal of the fixator, the patient's limb may be casted or braced for approximately 1 month to prevent fracture. Goals of physical therapy management during this phase are to maximize ROM, to maximize strength,

to eliminate gait deviations for patients with lower-extremity lengthenings, and to restore functional abilities and independence. Orthotic or prosthetic devices worn preoperatively may require refitting, and patients may require retraining with these devices.

Research

The first study of distraction osteogenesis in humans via the Ilizarov technique was reported by Tajana et al[19] in 1989. The purpose of this study was twofold: (1) to describe the development of the extracellular matrix of the bone created by distraction and (2) to determine the time sequence of morphogenesis. Sixty-four human tibial biopsies were taken at various time frames from the onset of distraction, ranging from 10 days to 24 months. The conclusion yielded by this study was that the process of osteogenesis does not occur in a strict sequential manner, but in stages that overlap. The quality of tissue was not that of a typical homogeneous tissue, but that of a discontinuous, unorganized tissue. The most noteworthy finding of this study was that the phases of osteogenesis resultant from distraction follow a differentiation process that does not include the formation of a cartilaginous model; rather, it is ossification of the direct type.[19]

Another study, conducted by Connolly et al[20] and reported in 1986, had as its main objective to describe animal and clinical investigations of a method of correcting acquired epiphyseal growth deformities, either in length or angularly. The method by which correction was attempted was epiphyseal traction.

Connolly et al[20] conducted their initial animal study, which involved 34 immature dogs from 12 to 16 weeks of age, to determine whether deformity correction achieved initially by epiphyseal traction would have long-lasting effects (ie, until the animals reached skeletal maturity) or would be lost by premature closing of the physis. The initial effect of the limb lengthening on the dogs was a pull-out fracture produced at the junction between the physis and the primary spongiosa of the metaphysis. This separation was consistent in that it began at the posterior part of the femur and progressed anteriorly. The medial and lateral periosteal fibers stretched, but did not rupture, and returned to normal length as the defect healed. This area subsequently filled in with calluslike tissue and later with bony trabeculae.[20]

This study[20] yielded an average of 66% deformity correction across all experimental groups. In 3 of the original 34 cases, the lengthened epiphyseal plate closed prematurely, resulting in a loss of previously gained length. The reasons for this closure were inconclusive; however, the authors hypothesized that compression of the physis or excessively long periods of external fixation may have contributed to the closure.

The methods for limb lengthening and angular deformity correction in the canine model were later applied clinically on humans by the same authors.[20] The first case was that of an 8-year-old boy with a growth deformity of 7 cm in the distal femoral epiphysis secondary to enchondroma. His results were unsatisfactory because the external fixation device was removed prematurely and the lengthened area shortened approximately 2.5 cm before healing completely.

The second patient was an 11-year-old girl with multiple enchondromatosis and a progressively increasing leg-length discrepancy. This trial was also unsuccessful because the external fixation device was removed prematurely secondary to patient discomfort and pin-tract drainage. At growth plate closure 2 years later, the leg-length discrepancy remained at 5 cm as compared with the initial 7 cm.[20]

Although both clinical trials were unsuccessful, the authors[20] felt that the method merits further consideration and application, as the technique allows limb lengthening and angular deformity correction without the need for internal fixation or bone grafting. The authors also concluded that this method is likely to be followed by premature closure of the physis and that this consideration should be kept in mind when treating younger patients.

Implications for the Future

The results of previous limb-lengthening procedures were discouraging because of the unpredictability of regenerated bone formation and mechanical difficulties with the fixators.[15] Technical improvements in the external fixation method and a better understanding of the biological aspects of bone and soft tissue elongation have led to overall improved results with the Ilizarov limb-lengthening procedure. Physical therapy management of a patient with an Ilizarov external fixator, however, may vary among different institutions, and there is no definitive research on the efficacy of physical therapy management with these patients. Continued efforts need to be made for more standardized physical therapy management in order to maximize the benefits of surgery and to ensure improved functional outcomes.

Acknowledgments

We extend special thanks to Cynthia Best, MSPT, PT, Mary Beth Savage, PT, and Dr Harry Kovelman for their valuable contributions to this manuscript; Mary Gail Horelick, JD, PT, Joan Page, MA, PT, and Becky Barrett, PT, for their editorial comments; and Eleanor Fox for her technical assistance.

References

1 Aronson J, Harp J. Factors influencing the choice of external fixation for distraction osteogenesis. In: *External Fixation: Instructional Course Lectures*. Park Ridge, Ill: American Academy of Orthopaedic Surgeons; 1990;39:175–183.

2 Ilizarov GA, Frankel V. The Ilizarov external fixator: a physiologic method of orthopaedic reconstruction and skeletal correction. *Orthopaedic Review*. 1988;17:1142–1154.

3 Codvilla A. On the means of lengthening in the lower limbs, the muscles, and the tissues which are shortened through deformity. *American Journal of Orthopaedic Surgery*. 1905;2:353–369.

4 Browner B, Treharne R. A historical review of the Ilizarov technique. Presented at the Richards Medical Company Convention on Treatment of Pseudarthrosis, Malunions, and Bone Defects; November 15–17, 1989; Houston, Tex.

5 Schwartsman V, McMurray MR, Martin SN. The Ilizarov method: the basics. *Contemporary Orthopaedics*. 1989;6:628–638.

6 Ilizarov GA. The principles of the Ilizarov method. *Bull Hosp Jt Dis Orthop Inst*. 1988;48:1–11.

7 Tachdjian M. *Pediatric Orthopaedics*. Philadelphia, Pa; WB Saunders Co; 1990;4:2850.

8 Moseley CF. Leg length discrepancy. In: Morrissy RT, ed. *Pediatric Orthopaedics*. 3rd ed. Philadelphia, Pa: JB Lippincott Co; 1990;767.

9 Mosca V, Moseley CF. Complications of Wagner leg lengthening and their avoidance. *Orthopaedic Transactions*. 1986;10:462–473.

10 Paley D. Problems, obstacles, and complications of limb lengthening by the Ilizarov technique. *Clin Orthop*. 1990;250:81–104.

11 Newschwander G, Dunst R. Limb lengthening with the Ilizarov external fixator. *Orthopaedic Nursing*. 1989;8:15–21.

12 Paley D. Current techniques of limb lengthening. *J Pediatr Orthop*. 1988;8:73–92.

13 DeBastiani G, Aldegheri R, Brivio L, Trivella G. Chondrodiastasis: controlled symmetrical distraction of the epiphyseal plate. *J Bone Joint Surg [Br]*. 1968;4:550–556.

14 Wagner H. Operative lengthening of the femur. *Clin Orthop*. 1978;136:125–142.

15 DalMonte A, Donzelli O. Comparison of different methods of limb lengthening. *J Pediatr Orthop*. 1988;8:62–64.

16 Aronson J, Boyd C, Harrison B, et al. Mechanical induction of osteogenesis: the importance of pin rigidity. *J Pediatr Orthop*. 1988;8:396–401.

17 Catagni M, Cattaneo R, Tentori L, Villa A. Limb lengthening in achondroplasia by Ilizarov's method. *Int Orthop*. 1988;12:113–179.

18 *Newington Children's Hospital Protocol for Ilizarov Procedures*. Newington, Conn: Newington Children's Hospital; 1990:1–5.

19 Tajana GF, Morandi M, Zembo M. The structure and development of osteogenic repair tissue according to Ilizarov technique in man. *Orthopedics*. 1989;12:515–523.

20 Connolly J, Huurman W, Lipiello L, Pankaj R. Epiphyseal traction to correct acquired growth deformities. *Clin Orthop*. 1986;202:258–268.

Considerations Related to Weight-Bearing Programs in Children with Developmental Disabilities

Standing is a common modality used in the management of children with developmental disabilities. The purpose of this article is to examine the scientific basis for standing programs, with specific emphasis on the known effects of weight bearing on bone development. Guidelines for the use of standing programs are presented, and the supporting rationale is discussed. [Stuberg WA. Considerations related to weight-bearing programs in children with developmental disabilities. Phys Ther. 1992;72:35–40.]

Wayne A Stuberg

Key Words: *Bone development; Child development disorders; Kinesiology/biomechanics, general; Orthopedics, general; Pediatrics, development.*

The use of standing is common to physical therapy management of children with developmental disabilities who are chronologically older than 14 to 16 months of age. Although therapists strive for standing without the use of orthoses or adaptive equipment, external support devices are prescribed when active control is inadequate or absent. A *standing program* refers to the use of orthoses or adaptive equipment to position a child in standing when motor control is inadequate to allow standing without such devices.

Standing programs have been recommended for children who have limited mobility in upright posture, including children with cerebral palsy (CP),[1–3] meningomyelocele,[4] muscular dystrophy,[5] and osteogenesis imperfecta.[6–8] The use of adaptive equipment or orthoses has been an accepted method of providing weight bearing in standing for these children. The efficacy of these standing programs has not been thoroughly examined.

The literature has few data-based studies that outline guidelines for standing programs. Clinicians must judge frequency, duration, and device type when recommending standing programs, and, because no standards exist, decisions are left to the clinician's intuition or experience. The purpose of this article is to examine the basis for standing programs for children with developmental disabilities. Specific emphasis is placed on the effects of weight bearing on bone development. Methodologies for assessing bone development will first be discussed, followed by a review of the factors known to affect bone development. Guidelines for standing programs will then be recommended.

Measurement of Bone Mineral Content/Density

Little is known about the effects of weight bearing on the development of bone in children.[2,3] Measurement of linear growth in bone is possible through the use of standard roentgenograms. Techniques to assess bone mass are single-photon absorptiometry (SPA), dual-photon absorptiometry (DPA), and quantitative computed tomography (QCT).[9] Single-photon absorptiometry detects differential photon absorption between bone and soft tissue to allow calculation of bone mineral content (BMC) and is limited to use at peripheral sites such as the radius. By contrast, DPA, which emits two different gamma energies and permits direct measurement of BMC and bone mineral density (BMD) (ie, the BMC per unit of area scanned), can be used to measure the hip, spine, or total body. Neither SPA nor DPA can discriminate between cortical and trabecular bone. Quantitative computed tomography is used specifically to evaluate trabecular versus cortical BMC.

WA Stuberg, PhD, PT, is Director of Physical Therapy, Meyer Rehabilitation Institute, Associate Professor, Division of Physical Therapy Education, and Assistant Professor, Department of Anatomy, University of Nebraska Medical Center, 600 S 42nd St, Omaha, NE 68198-5450 (USA).

The assessment of modeling changes of bone secondary to standing programs or other loading stimuli is possible through the use of DPA and QCT. Research to assess fracture risk and to determine optimal guidelines for standing programs to maintain joint alignment or facilitate bony development is needed.

Factors Affecting Bony Development

Normal bone growth and development is affected by factors including genetic coding,[10–12] nutrition,[13] appropriate levels of some nutrients and hormones (eg, vitamin D, calcium, estrogen, parathyroid hormone),[14,15] and mechanical loading through weight bearing and muscle tension.[16] In weight-bearing bones, where locomotion efficiency depends in part on bone mass, dynamic strains are essential to maintain bone mass.[14] Dynamic strains are repetitive forces that cause minute deformation of the bone. Activity level has been found to be a major determinant in the development of BMC. Disuse, decreased activity, and non–weight bearing have been shown to precipitate a loss of 0.4% to 0.6% per month in adults without developmental disabilities.[17–19] The early bone loss during disuse has been reported to be primarily in trabecular versus cortical bone because of the rapid metabolic turnover of trabecular bone.[20]

Donaldson and associates[19] studied the effects of a bed-rest program on nondisabled men aged 21 to 27 years. The duration of bed rest was 30 weeks for one subject and 36 weeks for two subjects. Serum calcium levels and BMC were assessed. A 25% to 44% loss of BMC was recorded in the calcaneus from week 12 until the end of the trial. During a 36-week exercise program following termination of bed rest, the subjects recovered BMC at approximately the same rate at which they lost BMC during bed rest. Issekutz and colleagues[17] used a 7-week bed-rest program to study the effects of bed rest on urinary calcium levels in 14 nondisabled male subjects (18-21 years of age). One half of the

subjects exercised while in bed; the other subjects were sedentary. The authors reported that a 1-hour-per-day exercise program, not including weight bearing, was not effective in retarding urinary calcium loss. The researchers, however, did report that other preliminary work demonstrated that 2 to 3 hours of passive standing on a daily basis, used in conjunction with bed rest, was effective in retarding urinary calcium loss.

The effects of mechanical forces on the development and remodeling of the skeleton have been studied extensively for over a century. Wolff's law states that the remodeling of bone occurs in the presence or absence of physical forces, that is, that bone is deposited in sites subjected to adequate force and is resorbed when forces are reduced.[21] Recently, Frost[22] has made significant contributions to the understanding of bone dynamics by introducing the principle of "flexure drift." The principle pertains to the macroarchitectural responses of bone to dynamic bending strain.[22,23] As Frost's principle applies to this article, the important points are

1. The stimulus for remodeling is mechanical strain (deformation), not stress (pressure), and specifically repetitive, dynamic flexure caused by repetitive mechanical loading on the bone.

2. The response will occur to time-averaged, repetitive strains versus single or occasional strains, with the relative rate, frequency, and magnitude of the strain being unknown.

3. Strains must be provided within physiological limits that achieve the desired response (eg, greater strain to induce greater change).

Electrical potentials resulting from repetitive, dynamic strain have been directly measured within bone.[24–26] Wolff's law and Frost's principle of flexural drift, therefore, may be mediated by electrical potentials.[24,25] The electric potentials created during strain of the bone are thought to sig-

nal osteoclastic and osteoblastic cells directly, thus mediating the modeling response. Although the presence of electrokinetic potentials have been recorded in vivo and in vitro, their role in the modeling process has not been fully elucidated.[26]

Specificity of Weight-Bearing Stimulus to Model Bone

Results in Animal Studies

Lanyon and colleagues[15] hypothesized that the first response to loading is a decrease in osteoclastic activity and that only with continued stimuli does osteoblastic activity lead to bone formation. Weight-bearing activities have resulted in increased bone mass and resistance to bending or fracture in animals, including mice,[27–29] roosters,[30] and dogs.[31] Hert and colleagues[32] pioneered a technique of applying known loads to bones in vivo using the rabbit. Rubin and Lanyon[30,33] applied the technique to isolated rooster and turkey ulna preparations using implanted strain gauges. They explored the effect of load duration with static versus intermittent loading and load magnitude on bone mass and architecture. Immobilization with static loading led to rapid and significant bone loss when the load was applied over an 8-week period. This loss was represented by a 15% to 20% reduction in cross-sectional area. These results confirmed the findings of earlier studies.[27,32,34]

Intermittent loading, in contrast to static loading, has been found to retard bone loss. Lanyon and co-workers[15,30,35] studied the effect of intermittent loading at levels measured by in vivo strain gauges during wing flapping on bone loss in rooster and turkey ulnas. They applied intermittent loading for 0, 4, 36, 360, or 1,800 consecutive loading cycles of 0.5 Hz per day for 6 weeks. The four-cycle regimen proved adequate for retarding bone loss, and the 36-cycle regimen demonstrated a 40% increase in BMC, a value that was not significantly improved by the addition of a greater number of loading cycles.

Rubin and Lanyon[36] also examined the effect of load magnitude by varying the strain load from 15% to 100% of physiologic levels at a constant load frequency of 100 consecutive daily reversals over an 8-week period. Maintenance of original bone area was achieved with a strain load corresponding to 30% of strain levels ascertained during wing flapping. Strains greater than 30% showed an incremental increase in the amount of bone deposited, with the greatest amount recorded following the highest strain.

Results in Human Studies

Weight bearing has been described as a key component in decreasing the likelihood of osteoporosis in nondisabled adults.[37-39] The effects of weight bearing and exercise on BMD have been documented in studies of osteoporosis in postmenopausal women.[40-43] The results of these studies consistently showed increased BMD as a benefit of weight bearing and exercise.

In a study of 64 male athletes who participated in full-scale physical exercise programs versus 39 nondisabled, age-matched, sedentary male subjects, Nilsson and Westlin[44] reported athletes to have greater BMD. Bone mineral density is task related, with greater densities recorded in weight lifters and football players than in runners or swimmers.[45,46] Activity-related differences in BMD within an individual demonstrate the importance of mechanical loading in the development of BMD. An example is the significantly higher BMC in the dominant wrist than in the nondominant wrist of professional tennis players.[47]

No studies describing the effects of standing programs on bone modeling for children with developmental disabilities have been published. Research is currently underway, however, in a group of 20 children with CP who are nonambulatory and using standing programs in their educational settings.[48,49] Preliminary results indicate that BMD is significantly less

in nonambulatory children with severe to profound CP than in children who are nondisabled. Bone mineral density measurements of the patella, tibial plateau, and supracondylar femur of children with CP demonstrate values of one third to one half of those of age-matched peers without disabilities.[48] Additionally, use of a standing program of 60 minutes' duration four or five times per week appears to result in increased BMD measurements.[49] Reduction of BMD was observed upon removal of the standing program for even a short period of time (ie, summer break) or when the standing program had an average duration of 30 minutes and a frequency of three times per week.[49]

Acetabular development appears to be dependent on articulation of the femoral head in the acetabulum and is promoted through weight bearing.[50-54] The findings of Phelps[50] have been substantiated by Howard et al[53] and Samilson et al[54] regarding the significant role of weight bearing on the development of the acetabulum in children with CP. The use of standing programs to enhance acetabular development appears valid. The justification for the use of standing programs to facilitate acetabular development is particularly strong for children with CP, as hip dysplasia is typically not present at birth in these children.[50,53,54]

Clinical Implications

Children who are known or suspected to have decreased bone mass or bone density should be considered candidates for standing programs. If the results of animal studies of the effect of mechanical loading on bone are applicable to humans (and the similarities across species suggest the assumption may be valid), then important implications can be drawn from these studies about standing programs in children with developmental disabilities. Although specific guidelines for selected disabilities are included in the "Additional Considerations" section later in the article, I believe the following guidelines can

be used as a general framework in prescribing a standing program.

Guidelines for Standing Programs

Amount of weight bearing in standing. Results of research using the turkey ulna indicate that strain loads as small as 15% to 30% may have a sparing effect if the loading frequency is adequate.[33] Maximal strain levels were established by direct strain-gauge measurements of the turkey ulna during vigorous wing flapping.[35] The strain level to stimulate bone modeling in children has not been ascertained. If we assume, however, that the force exerted through the lower extremities during standing is within the range to stimulate bone homeostasis and possibly deposition, then standing programs may be an effective stimulus to bone development in children.

The amount of weight bearing that a child is receiving in standing should be ascertained if the goal of the program is to stimulate bone development. The type of orthosis or adaptive equipment used by a child can become important if the equipment redistributes the vertical load by supporting the torso or lower extremities. For example, a child tilted 50 degrees from vertical on a prone stander with the child's arms supported may be placing only one half of the body weight through the legs.[55] Miedaner[55] and Curtis[56] have both reported that widely used standing devices such as prone or supine standers allow loading of up to 70% to 75% of body weight if the devices are adjusted near vertical. I suggest that therapists check for the amount of vertical loading by placing a scale or pressure gauge under the child's feet. In using orthoses, such as knee-ankle-foot orthoses or any orthotic device that supports the legs or torso, the pressure on the bottom of the foot in the brace should be measured.

Standing duration. Duration of the standing program is variable, dependent on whether the goal is bone development, acetabular development,

or contracture management. A standing program of 2 to 3 hours per day for adults has been reported to retard bone resorption.[17,57,58] Preliminary work I have conducted indicates that a duration of at least 60 minutes, in conjunction with a frequency of four or five times per week, is needed to retard bone loss in children with CP who are nonambulatory.

Phelps[50] recommends beginning weight-bearing programs as early as 12 to 16 months of age in children with CP who are at risk for hip dislocation. Phelps reports using a protocol of 3 hours daily with no more than 1 hour at a time. The report by Phelps, however, is anecdotal, without objective outcome measures.

Standing programs of approximately 45 minutes' duration, three times daily, are also reported to control contractures of the lower extremity and to facilitate bone development in children with CP,[1] muscular dystrophy,[59] and meningomyelocele.[60] Specific guidelines to control contractures in children with spastic CP have been advocated by Tardieu and colleagues[61] and include elongation of the muscle for at least 4 hours daily.

Standing frequency. According to animal studies, if loading is near physiologic levels, then a frequency of only four loading cycles per day over a period of 2 weeks would be needed to maintain and possibly stimulate additional bone formation.[30] The duration of the loading cycle was 0.5 seconds for the animal model experiment.[35] Perhaps these four cycles could be carried out in a single session; however, the practice advocated by researchers thus far is daily standing or standing for a minimum of four times per week.[49,50,59,60]

Smith[62] has recommended a three-times-per-week frequency of weight bearing for elderly adults to retard osteoporosis. Based on a review of current practice and animal studies, I believe that children should participate in a standing program at least four or five times per week for a duration of about 60 minutes to facilitate

bone development. Standing at a frequency of two or three times daily for a duration of 45 minutes should be considered as an adjunct to a positioning program to control lower-extremity flexion contractures.

Additional Considerations

Chronological age, as opposed to developmental age, is the most common criterion for the use of standing programs chosen by many orthopedists, with the standing program beginning when the child is approximately 12 to 16 months of age.[50,51] Developmental age may be a more appropriate criterion for the use of a standing program for some children, particularly when orthopedic management goals do not preclude postponing the onset of standing. Additionally, standing without appropriate postural support may be detrimental to the child with spasticity, regardless of the age criterion used. Standing equipment should provide correct anatomical alignment of the torso and lower extremities. As most standing devices (eg, a prone or supine stander) do not typically provide distal control, splints or orthoses should be considered.

Monitoring of children's nutritional programs by a dietitian or nutritionist is recommended, particularly for children who are significantly below the normal range on the growth curve or who have osteoporosis. Inadequate dietary intake of calcium or other nutrients required for development of bone mass and bone density will have a detrimental effect, regardless of the appropriateness of the standing or activity program.[38,41]

The use of standing programs for children who have high-lumbar or thoracic meningomyelocele is encouraged by several researchers.[63–65] Rosenstein et al[66] have reported a direct relationship among ambulatory status, lesion level, and the development of BMD in children with meningomyelocele. In comparison with nonambulators, a 38% increase of BMD at the tibia and a 44% increase at the first metatarsal were reported. The use of standing and walking pro-

grams for adolescents with high-level defects (eg, thoracic lesions) is controversial, however, because, by adolescence, 70% to 90% of these individuals use wheelchairs for mobility.[63,67] Mazur and colleagues[65] compared 36 children with high-level defects who participated in a standing and walking program with 36 children for whom wheelchair use had been prescribed. The standing program guidelines were not described. The authors reported that 33% of the children in the standing and walking group were able to walk around the community, 20% walked around the home only, and 47% were nonwalkers at the completion of the study. The children who walked early had fewer fractures and were more independent in transfer skills; however, this group had also spent more days in the hospital and were not significantly different from the children who used wheelchairs with regard to skills of daily living.

Standing programs and the prolongation of walking through the use of orthoses are common for children with Duchenne's muscular dystrophy. Spencer and Vignos[68] have reported a dramatic improvement in functional capacity and increased longevity of 2 to 4 years when standing and walking is prolonged through the use of orthoses and adaptive equipment. Vignos et al[59] recommended that standing programs be incorporated into the classroom routine for the nonambulatory school-aged child for at least 3 hours daily. Contracture progression and excessive physical size are primary factors to be considered in discontinuing the standing program. Progression of contractures results in inability to wear orthoses because of skin breakdown and in inability to allow correct alignment in standing. Excessive physical size increases the risk of injury to the child or caregiver by making transfers difficult.

The use of standing programs for children with osteogenesis imperfecta is recommended by most experts; however, the recommended duration of the program has not been specified.[6–8] The use of specialized orthoses, including contoured orthoses[7] or vacuum pants,[8] is reported to provide support and reduce the risk of fracture during weight bearing.

Conclusions

Standing programs have been shown to have an effect on bone development in humans and animals. Bone mineral density has been demonstrated to increase with exercise programs that provide a physiologic stimulus for bone modeling. Intermittent loading appears to be a key stimulus during standing, as opposed to increasing the time of a static program. Therefore, active participation from the child is recommended to increase strain on the bone through muscle activity.

Reports in the literature indicate there is a decreased incidence of contractures and fractures in children with developmental disabilities who participate in standing programs.[4,6–8,65] Although suggestions related to standing have been introduced in this article, programs for contracture management and fracture prevention need to be elucidated further. No guidelines have been developed to ascertain fracture risk for children with developmental disabilities. Further study could have a significant effect on the use of standing programs as a management modality for contractures and fractures.

As loading with a constant pressure has not been found to be an effective stimulus for bone modeling in animals, an apparent controversy exists regarding the current method of using static programs in humans.[34,35] Perhaps static standing programs using orthoses or adaptive equipment are not truly static, because some motion is allowed. Anecdotal evidence for the use of standing programs for children with developmental disabilities has been demonstrated, and, until a more efficacious method of providing mechanical stimulation to the bone is identified, the use of standing programs with loading administered for at least 60 minutes, four or five times per week, is recommended

as a general guideline for bone development.[48–50,59,60,62]

References

1 Salter RB. *Textbook of Disorders and Injuries of the Musculoskeletal System.* 2nd ed. Baltimore, Md: Williams & Wilkins; 1983:5–14, 257–265.

2 Bleck EE. *Orthopaedic Management in Cerebral Palsy.* Philadelphia, Pa: MacKeith Press; 1987:142–212.

3 Tachdjian MO. *Pediatric Orthopedics.* Philadelphia, Pa: WB Saunders Co; 1990;3:1620–1622.

4 Anschuetz RH, Freehafer AA, Shaffer JW, Dixon MS. Severe fracture complications in myelodysplasia. *J Pediatr Orthop.* 1984;4:22–24.

5 Seigel IM. *Muscle and Its Diseases: An Outline Primer of Basic Science and Clinical Method.* Chicago, Ill: Year Book Medical Publishers Inc; 1986:218–245.

6 Bleck EE. Nonoperative treatment of osteogenesis imperfecta: orthotic and mobility management. *Clin Orthop.* 1981;159:111–122.

7 Binder H, Hawks L, Graybill G. Osteogenesis imperfecta: rehabilitation approach with infants and young children. *Arch Phys Med Rehabil.* 1984;65:537–541.

8 Letts M, Monson R, Weber K. The prevention of recurrent fractures of the lower extremities in severe osteogenesis imperfecta using vacuum pants: a preliminary report in four patients. *J Pediatr Orthop.* 1988;8:454–457.

9 Hassager C, Christiansen C. Usefulness of bone mass measurements by photon absorptiometry. *Public Health Rep.* 1989;104(suppl):23–33.

10 Matkovic V, Chesnut C. Genetic factors and acquisition of bone mass. *J Bone Miner Res.* 1987;1(suppl):329. Abstract.

11 Smith DM, Nance WE, Kang DW, et al. Genetic factors in determining bone mass. *J Clin Invest.* 1973;52:2800–2808.

12 Lutz J. Bone mineral, serum calcium, and dietary intakes of mother/daughter pairs. *Am J Clin Nutr.* 1986;44:99–106.

13 Santora AC. Role of nutrition and exercise in osteoporosis. *Am J Med.* 1987;82(suppl 18):73–79.

14 Martin AD, McCulloch RG. Bone dynamics: stress, strain, and fracture. *J Sports Sci.* 1987;5:155–163.

15 Lanyon LE, Rubin CT, Baust G. Modulation of bone loss during calcium insufficiency by controlled dynamic loading. *Calcif Tissue Int.* 1986;38:209–216.

16 LeVeau BF, Bernhardt DB. Developmental biomechanics: effect of forces on the growth, development, and maintenance of the human body. *Phys Ther.* 1984;64:1874–1882.

17 Issekutz B, Blizzard JJ, Birkhead NC, Rodahl K. Effect of prolonged bedrest in urinary calcium output. *J Appl Physiol.* 1966;21:1013–1020.

18 Goldsmith RS, Killian P, Inghar SH, Bass DE. Effect of phosphate supplementation during immobilization of normal men. *Metabolism.* 1969;18:349–368.

19 Donaldson CL, Hulley SB, Vogel JM, et al. Effect of prolonged bedrest. *Metabolism.* 1970;19:1071–1084.

20 Courpron P. Bone tissue mechanisms underlying osteoporosis. *Orthop Clin North Am.* 1981;12:513–545.

21 Wolff J. Die Lehre von den funktionellen Knochengestalt. *Virchows Arch [A].* 1899;155:256–262.

22 Frost HM. Mechanical determinants of bone modeling. *Metab Bone Dis Rel Res.* 1982;4:217–229.

23 Frost HM. *The Laws of Bone Structure.* Springfield, Mo: Charles C Thomas, Publisher; 1964.

24 Fukada E, Yasuda I. Piezoelectric properties of bone. *J Phys Soc Jpn.* 1957;12:1158–1163.

25 Bassett CAL, Becker RO. Generation of electric potentials by bone in response to mechanical stress. *Science.* 1962;137:1063–1064.

26 Chakkakal DA. Mechanoelectric transduction in bone. *J Mater Res.* 1989;4:1034–1046.

27 Woo S-L, Kuei S, Amiel D, et al. The effect of prolonged physical training on the properties of long bone: a study of Wolff's law. *J Bone Joint Surg [Am].* 1981;63:780–786.

28 Kisskinen A, Heikkinen E. Physical training and connective tissues in young mice: biochemistry of long bones. *J Appl Physiol.* 1978;44:50–54.

29 Bell RR, Tzeng DY, Draper HH. Long-term effects of calcium, phosphorus and forced exercise on the bones of mature mice. *J Nutr.* 1980;110:1161–1167.

30 Rubin CT, Lanyon MR. Regulation of bone formation by applied dynamic loads. *J Bone Joint Surg [Am].* 1984;66:397–402.

31 Martin RK, Albright JP, Clarke WR, et al. Load-carrying effects on the adult beagle tibia. *Med Sci Sports Exerc.* 1981;13:343–349.

32 Hert J, Liskova M, Landgrot B. Influence of the long-term continuous bending on the bone: an experimental study on the tibia of the rabbit. *Folia Morphol (Praha).* 1969;17:389–399.

33 Rubin CT, Lanyon LE. Osteoregulatory nature of mechanical stimuli: function as a determinant for adaptive remodeling in bone. *J Orthop Res.* 1987;5:300–310.

34 Carter DR, Vasu R, Spengler DM, Dueland RT. Stress fields in the unplated and plated canine femur calculated from in vivo strain measurements. *J Biomech.* 1981;14:63–70.

35 Lanyon LE, Rubin CT. Static vs dynamic loads as an influence on bone remodeling. *J Biomech.* 1984;17:897–906.

36 Rubin CT, Lanyon LE. Regulation of bone mass by mechanical loading: the effect of peak strain magnitude. *Calcif Tissue Int.* 1985;37:411–417.

37 Aisenbrey JA. Exercise in the prevention and management of osteoporosis. *Phys Ther.* 1987;67:1100–1104.

38 Goodman CE. Osteoporosis: protective measures of nutrition and exercise. *Geriatrics.* 1985;40:59–70.

39 Notelovitz M. How exercise affects bone density. *Contemp Ob/Gyn.* 1986;27:108–116.

40 Krolner B, Toft B, Porsnielsen S, Tondevold E. Physical exercise as prophylaxis against involutional vertebral bone loss: a controlled trial. *Clin Sci.* 1983;64:541–546.

41 Smith EL, Reddan W, Smith PE. Physical activity and calcium modalities for bone min-

eral increase in aged women. *Med Sci Sports Exerc.* 1981;13:60–64.

42 Ayalon F, Simkin A, Leichter I, Raifmann S. Dynamic bone loading exercises for post-menopausal women: effect on the density of the distal radius. *Arch Phys Med Rehabil.* 1987;68:280–283.

43 Dalsky GP, Stock KS, Ehsani AI, et al. Weight-bearing exercise training and lumbar bone mineral content in postmenopausal women. *Ann Intern Med.* 1988;108:824–828.

44 Nilsson BE, Westlin NE. Bone density in athletes. *Clin Orthop.* 1971;77:179–182.

45 Nilsson BE, Anderson SM, Hardrup TV, Westlin NE. Bone mineral content in ballet dancers and weight lifters. In: *Proceedings of the Fourth International Conference on Bone Measurement; University of Toronto, Toronto, Ontario, Canada.* 1978:81–86.

46 Dalen N, Olssen KE. Bone mineral content and physical activity. *Acta Orthop Scand.* 1974;45:170–174.

47 Jones H, Priest J, Hayes W, et al. Humeral hypertrophy in response to exercise. *J Bone Joint Surg [Am].* 1977;59:204–208.

48 Stuberg WA. Bone density changes in non-ambulatory children following discontinuation of passive standing programs. In: *Proceedings of the American Academy of Cerebral Palsy and Developmental Medicine Conference; Louisville, Ky; October 10, 1991.*

49 Stuberg WA. Comparison of bone density in cerebral palsy and nondisabled children. In: *Proceedings of the American Society for Bone and Mineral Research Annual Meeting; San Diego, Calif; August 29, 1991.*

50 Phelps WM. Prevention of acquired dislocation of the hip in cerebral palsy. *J Bone Joint Surg [Am].* 1959;41:440–448.

51 Beals RK. Developmental changes in the femur and acetabulum in spastic paraplegia and diplegia. *Dev Med Child Neurol.* 1969;11:303–313.

52 Harrison TJ. The influence of the femoral head on pelvic growth and acetabular form in the rat. *J Anat.* 1961;95:12–24.

53 Howard CB, McKibbon B, Williams LA. Factors affecting the incidence of hip dislocation in cerebral palsy. *J Bone Joint Surg [Br].* 1985; 67:530–532.

54 Samilson RL, Tsou P, Aamoth G, et al. Dislocation and subluxation of the hip in cerebral palsy. *J Bone Joint Surg [Am].* 1972;54:863–873.

55 Miedaner J. An evaluation of weight bearing forces at various angles for children with cerebral palsy. *Pediatric Physical Therapy.* 1990;2:215.

56 Curtis L. *The Evaluation of Weight Bearing of Children on Prone, Supine, and Upright Standers.* Chapel Hill, NC: The University of North Carolina at Chapel Hill; 1989. Thesis.

57 Birge SJ, Wheldon GD. Bone. In: McNally M, ed. *Hypodynamics and Hypogravics.* New York, NY: Academic Press Inc; 1968:213–235.

58 Overton TR, Hangartzer TN, Heath R, et al. The effect of physical activity on bone: gamma ray computed tomography. In: DeLuca HF, ed. *Osteoporosis: Recent Advances in Pathogenesis and Treatment.* Baltimore, Md: University Park Press; 1981:147–158.

59 Vignos PJ, Spencer GE, Archibald KC. Management of progressive muscular dystrophy of childhood. *JAMA.* 1963;184:89–96.

60 Tappit-Emas E. Physical therapy intervention. In: Schafer MF, Dias LS, eds. *Myelomeningocele Orthopaedic Treatment.* Baltimore, Md: Williams & Wilkins; 1983.

61 Tardieu C, Huet de la Tour E, Bret MD, et al. Muscle hypoextensibility in children with CP: parts I and II. *Arch Phys Med Rehabil.* 1982;63:97–107.

62 Smith EL. How exercise helps prevent osteoporosis. *Contemp Ob/Gyn.* 1985;25:51–60.

63 Shurtleff DB. Myelodysplasia: management and treatment. *Curr Probl Pediatr.* 1980;10: 64–71.

64 Kupka J, Geddes N, Carroll NC. Comprehensive management in the child with spina bifida. *Orthop Clin North Am.* 1978;9:97–113.

65 Mazur JM, Shurtleff DB, Menelaus MB, et al. Orthopaedic management of high-level spina bifida. *J Bone Joint Surg [Am].* 1989; 71:56–61.

66 Rosenstein BD, Greene WB, Herrington RT, et al. Bone density in myelomeningocele: the effects of ambulatory status and other factors. *Dev Med Child Neurol.* 1987;29:486–494.

67 Stillwell A, Menelaus MB. Walking ability in mature patients with spina bifida. *J Pediatr Orthop.* 1983;3:184–190.

68 Spencer GE, Vignos PJ. Bracing for ambulation in childhood progressive muscular dystrophy. *J Bone Joint Surg [Am].* 1962;44:234–242.